Government Procedures and Operations

snova
New York

Government Procedures and Operations

Sanctions in Response to the Russian Invasion of Ukraine
Eric Freitag (Editor)
2022. ISBN: 979-8-88697-154-5 (Hardcover)
2022. ISBN: 979-8-88697-189-7 (eBook)

Is the U.S. Postal Service Sustainable?
Malissa R. Rojas (Editor)
2020. ISBN: 978-1-53618-505-8 (Hardcover)
2020. ISBN: 978-1-53618-551-5 (eBook)

E-Government: Perspectives, Challenges and Opportunities
Anil Sieben (Editor)
2020. ISBN: 978-1-53617-563-9 (Softcover)
2020. ISBN: 978-1-53617-564-6 (eBook)

Public Services: Management, Opportunities and Challenges
Rosa M. Søndergaard (Editor)
2020. ISBN: 978-1-53617-477-9 (Hardcover)
2020. ISBN: 978-1-53617-478-6 (eBook)

FEMA: Emergency Management, Disaster Contracting and Grants
Naomi Stanley (Editor)
2019. ISBN: 978-1-53616-456-5 (Hardcover)
2019. ISBN: 978-1-53616-457-2 (eBook)

More information about this series can be found at https://novapublishers.com/product-category/series/government-procedures-and-operations/

Danial E. Tackett
Editor

Putting an End to Surprise Medical Billing

snova
New York

Library of Congress Cataloging-in-Publication Data

ISBN: 979-8-88697-296-2

Published by Nova Science Publishers, Inc. † New York

Contents

Preface

Surprise medical bills arise when a consumer covered by a health plan is unexpectedly treated by an out-of-network provider and is required to pay the difference between what the plan pays and the provider's charge. The issue of surprise bills, which can often expose a consumer to thousands of dollars of unforeseen medical costs, is widespread. In 2017, one in six Americans covered by an employer-sponsored plan received a surprise medical bill for out-of- network care despite having health insurance. One in ten elective hospital admissions and one in five admissions from emergency departments result in surprise bills.

Chapter 1 - This is an edited, reformatted and augmented version of Hearing before the Subcommittee on Health, of the Committee on Energy and Commerce, House of Representatives, One Hundred Sixteenth Congress, First Session, Serial No. 116–43, dated June 12, 2019.

Chapter 2 - This is an edited, reformatted and augmented version of House of Representatives; 116th Congress, 2d Session, Publication No. Rept. 116–615, Part 1, dated December 2, 2020.

Chapter 1

No More Surprises: Protecting Patients from Surprise Medical Bills*

Committee on Energy and Commerce

Wednesday, June 12, 2019
House of Representatives, Subcommittee on Health,
Committee on Energy and Commerce,
Washington, DC.

The subcommittee met, pursuant to call, at 10:02 a.m., in the John D. Dingell Room 2123 Rayburn House Office Building, Hon. Anna G. Eshoo (chairwoman of the subcommittee) presiding.

Members present: Representatives Eshoo, Butterfield, Matsui, Castor, Sarbanes, Lujan, Schrader, Kennedy, Cardenas, Welch, Ruiz, Dingell, Kuster, Kelly, Barragan, Blunt Rochester, Pallone (ex officio), Burgess (subcommittee ranking member), Upton, Shimkus, Guthrie, Griffith, Bilirakis, Long, Bucshon, Brooks, Mullin, Hudson, Carter, and Walden (ex officio).

Also present: Representative Soto.

Staff present: Waverly Gordon, Deputy Chief Counsel; Tiffany Guarascio, Deputy Staff Director; Zach Kahan, Outreach and Member Service Coordinator; Josh Krantz, Policy Analyst; Una Lee, Senior Health Counsel; Aisling McDonough; Policy Coordinator; Meghan Mullon, Staff Assistant; Kaitlyn Peel, Digital Director; Samantha Satchell, Professional Staff Member; C. J. Young, Press Secretary; Mike Bloomquist, Minority Staff Director; S. K. Bowen, Minority Press Assistant; Adam Buckalew, Minority Director of Coalitions and Deputy Chief Counsel, Health; Jordan Davis, Minority Senior Advisor; Margaret Tucker Fogarty, Minority Staff Assistant; Melissa Froelich, Minority Chief Counsel, Consumer Protection and Commerce; Peter Kielty, Minority General Counsel; Bijan Koohmaraie, Minority Counsel, Counsel, Consumer Protection and Commerce; Ryan Long, Minority Deputy Staff Director; and Brannon Rains, Minority Staff Assistant.

Ms. ESHOO. Good morning, everyone. The Subcommittee on Health will now come to order.

The Chair now recognizes herself for five minutes for an opening statement. Welcome to all of our witnesses. That's quite a table— quite a lineup, and we are eager to hear from you.

---

* This is an edited, reformatted and augmented version of Hearing before the Subcommittee on Health, of the Committee on Energy and Commerce, House of Representatives, One Hundred Sixteenth Congress, First Session, Serial No. 116–43, dated June 12, 2019.

In: Putting an End to Surprise Medical Billing
Editor: Danial E. Tackett
ISBN: 979-8-88697-296-2

Opening Statement of Hon. Anna G. Eshoo, A Representative in Congress from the State of California

Today is a bipartisan hearing about solutions to end surprise medical billing. Patients receive surprise bills when they receive care from providers who are not part of the health plan they are insured by, often referred to as out-of-network providers, and they are caught between insurers, hospitals, and doctors.

[Sounds gavel.]

Ms. ESHOO. The committee will come to order, please. There are staffers that want to have a great conversation. We have lots of side rooms for them.

These are often people who play by the rules. They bought an insurance plan, they paid their premiums, and they go to providers in their network.

Now, we all expect to receive medical bills, but the "surprise" in a surprise bill is a shock—it should be called shock billing—because it can amount to more than what most people have in a savings account, if they even have one.

In a recent Kaiser Family Foundation poll, 67 percent of the American people said they are worried about being able to afford their own or a family member's unexpected medical bills.

And it makes sense for them to be worried because receiving a surprise bill—medical bill—is incredibly common, regrettably. It has become incredibly common.

One in 5 emergency department visits result in a surprise medical bill. If you need a ground or air ambulance, you are at an especially high risk for a surprise bill.

More than half of all ambulance rides are billed out of network and the GAO found that nearly 70 percent of air ambulance trips were billed out of network.

In my region, a young woman by the name of Nina Dang broke her arm while she was riding her bike. Paramedics took her to the emergency room at Zuckerberg San Francisco General Hospital.

According to Vox reporter Sarah Kliff, who wrote a series of articles exposing surprise bills, Nina Dang left with a cast and a few months later received a bill for $20,243.

That's because Zuckerberg San Francisco General was not in her insurance network. Under current Federal law, providers are permitted to bill privately—insured patients for the balance not paid by the insurance plan.

California, New York, and several other States already have strong State protections for out-of-network emergency patients. But State law cannot regulate self-funded employer plans that cover about 100 million Americans, thus, our joint presence here today. That means that without action from Congress, millions of Americans will be left unprotected from surprise bills.

Today, we will hear testimony from those who represent each part of the system that produces surprise bills, and we welcome each one of you.

In reading the written testimonies, I found that there was a tendency to confuse the surprise billing issue with other concerns: large deductibles, narrow networks, or the pressure of high healthcare costs for both patients and what it costs our country.

I think that those are all big concerns and I want our subcommittee to tackle them. But they are not today's agenda. Our work today is not exactly simple, but I think that it is very clear. We have to protect every American from a surprise medical bill.

I am proud of the bipartisan work our subcommittee has tackled so far on this Congress. In our drug pricing hearings, we were able to put the finger pointing aside and get to the root of the issue and pass legislation to help patients, and I believe we will continue to do that.

So here is my ask of our witnesses. We need you to help us to find the best policy. We all look forward to your testimony and look forward to working—I look forward to working with my colleagues to develop a bipartisan solution to end surprise billing.

[The prepared statement of Ms. Eshoo follow:]

Prepared Statement of Hon. Anna G. Eshoo

Today is a bipartisan hearing about solutions to end surprise medical billing. Patients receive surprise bills when they receive care from providers who are not part of the health plan they're insured by—often referred to as out-of-network providers—and they're caught between insurers, hospitals, and doctors.

These are often people who play by the rules. They bought an insurance plan, they paid their premiums, and they go to providers in their network. We all expect to receive medical bills, but the "surprise" in a surprise bill is a shock that can amount to more than people have in their savings account.

In a recent Kaiser Family Foundation poll, 67% of Americans said they are worried about being able to afford their own or a family member's unexpected medical bills.

It makes sense why people are so worried. Receiving a surprise medical bill is incredibly common.

One in five emergency department visits result in a surprise medical bill. If you need a ground or air ambulance, you are at an especially high risk for a surprise bill. More than half of all ambulance rides are billed out of network, and the GAO found that nearly 70% of air ambulance trips were billed out of network.

In my region, a young woman, Nina Dang, broke her arm while riding her bike. Paramedics took her to an emergency room at Zuckerberg San Francisco General Hospital. According to Vox reporter Sarah Kliff, who wrote a series of articles exposing surprise bills, Nina Dang left with a cast and a few months later received a bill for $20,243. That's because Zuckerberg San Francisco General was not in her insurance network.

California, like New York and several other states, already has strong State protections for out-of-network emergency patients, but State law cannot regulate self-funded employer plans that cover about 100 million Americans. That means that without action from Congress, millions of Americans are unprotected from surprise bills.

Today, we'll hear testimony from the many who are part of the system that produces surprise bills. Hospitals, physicians, and health insurers know that patients can't control where they are treated in an emergency. They know that patients don't expect to receive an out-of-network bill when they go to an in-network facility. However, they still participate and contribute to a system that can bankrupt a person.

In some of our witnesses' testimony, I've seen a tendency to confuse the surprise billing issue with other concerns—large deductibles, narrow networks, or the pressure of high healthcare costs for both patients and the nation. I want our subcommittee to tackle these problems, but they are not today's agenda. Our work today is not simple, but it is clear. We must protect every Americans from a surprise medical bill.

I'm proud of the bipartisan work our Subcommittee has tackled so far this Congress. In our drug pricing hearings, we've been able to put the finger pointing aside, get to the root of the issue, and pass legislation to help patients.

I ask our witnesses to do the same. Help us find the best policy. I look forward to your testimony, and I look forward to working with my colleagues to develop a bipartisan solution to end surprise billing.

* * *

Ms. ESHOO. With that, I would like to now recognize Dr. Burgess, the ranking member of the Subcommittee on Health, for five minutes for his opening statement.

Opening Statement of Hon. Michael C. Burgess, A Representative in Congress from the State of Texas

Mr. BURGESS. Thank you, and good morning to all of our witnesses and thank you for being here today to testify on this important topic of out-of-network billing.

It is an issue that has hit home in our districts and our states and, certainly, it's a topic of conversation when I go home to Texas.

One of the most prominent out—of—network billing stories in Texas is that of Drew Calver, a 44-year-old high school teacher in Austin, Texas, who suffered a heart attack and was rushed to the emergency room at St. David's Medical Center. Good for them.

He was stented and his heart muscle was saved. And so this was an individual who was otherwise healthy. He had competed in an Ironman triathlon earlier in the year, and he was told at the outset that the hospital would accept his insurance.

He has insurance through his school district and he was billed a total of $110,000 for his 4-day hospital stay. That's more than two times his annual pay.

So problems with out-of-network billing is not an easy problem to solve but it's one where many of the stakeholders disagree on the solution.

But it is quite intentional that we have called those stakeholders who might not agree to testify at the same table today. If there is anything upon which we should all agree it is that the patient should be held harmless so that they can avoid massive bills like the one Mr. Calver received, especially in emergency situations.

And I just want to underscore what the chairwoman of the subcommittee said, and while you all are all very smart—you have differences of opinion about this—we need your help. We solicit your help.

That is why you are here today. And if you don't help us solve the problem, we will solve the problem and none of you will like it.

In addressing this issue, I hope that the stakeholders here today—physicians, insurers, hospitals, and patients—come to an agreeable conclusion, even if it is not their first choice.

My State of Texas just passed a new bill in the State legislature because the first legislative fix passed 2 years ago did not adequately address out-of-network billing.

While Texas and numerous other states have made efforts to mitigate the billing issues, states are unable to legislate what happens in cases involving multi-state employer-sponsored plans.

This is why the Energy and Commerce Committee is looking to address this issue and why the president has been so vocal in putting forth a set of guiding principles in addressing surprise medical bills.

President Trump's principles include protecting patients without increasing Federal health expenditures while maintaining choice for patients. I, largely, agree with President Trump's principles and I hope that Congress can come to a consensus upon the best way to execute a legislative effort and send something to the president's desk.

As a physician I understand the payment issues at hand when it comes to billing for healthcare services and I am really grateful that we have two physicians on our panel today.

It is important that throughout this conversation we consider the potential effect of shifting payment incentives for physicians, for insurers, for hospitals, and that we are not driving payment rates too far in one direction or another.

I do think it is critical that on such an important issue we take into account the various perspectives of the stakeholders and I am encouraged that we do have such a robust panel before us this morning.

The committee released a discussion draft a few weeks prior to this hearing and my understanding is the committee has received a lot of comments on the discussion draft.

So I am hopeful that this subcommittee will lead the charge on addressing out-of-network billing. But I think the number of proposals that members have produced shows there is serious interest to accomplish something legislatively.

Patients deserve better than to receive bills they were not expecting for the care that they needed, especially when that care is non-elective or emergent in nature.

Again, I want to thank all of our witnesses for being here today and look forward to a lively and productive discussion.

Thank you, and I will yield back.

[The prepared statement of Mr. Burgess follow:]

Prepared Statement of Hon. Michael C. Burgess

Good morning and thank you to all of our witnesses for being here today to testify on the important topic of surprise billing. This is an issue that has hit home in our districts, and it has certainly been a topic of conversation when I go home to Texas.

One of the most prominent surprise billing stories in Texas is that of Drew Calver, a 44-year-old high school teacher in Austin, who suffered a heart attack and was rushed to the emergency room at St. David's Medical Center. Mr. Calver was healthy and had completed an ironman triathlon earlier in the year. Despite being told that the hospital would accept his insurance, Mr. Calver was billed a total of nearly $110,000 for his 4-day hospital stay. This amount is more than two times his annual pay.

Surprise billing is not an easy problem to solve, and it is one where the many stakeholders disagree on the solution. It is quite intentional that we have called all those stakeholders to testify at the same table today. If there is anything upon which we should all agree, it is that the patient should be held harmless so they can avoid massive bills like the one that Mr. Calver received, especially in emergency situations.

In addressing this issue, I hope that the stakeholders—physicians, insurers, hospitals, patients, and others—are able to come to an agreeable conclusion, even if it is not their first choice. My home State of Texas just passed a new bill in the State legislature because the first legislative fix did not adequately address surprise billing. While Texas and numerous other states have made efforts to mitigate surprise billing, states are unable to legislate what happens in cases involving employer-sponsored plans. This is why the Energy and Commerce Committee is looking to address this issue, and why the President has been so vocal in putting forth a set of guiding principles in addressing surprise medical bills. The President's principles include protecting patients without increasing Federal healthcare expenditures, while maintaining choice for patients. I largely agree with these principles and hope that Congress can come to a consensus upon the best way to execute a legislative effort and send something to the President's desk.

As a physician, I understand the payment issues at hand when it comes to billing for healthcare services, and I am glad that we have two physicians on our panel today to represent the physician perspective. It is important that throughout this conversation we consider the potential effect of shifting payment incentives for physicians, and for insurers, such that we are not driving payment rates too far in one direction or the other.

I do think it is critical that on such an important issue we take into account the various perspectives that the stakeholders have. I am encouraged that we have such a robust panel before us this morning, and that the Committee has received more than 60 comments on the discussion draft.

I am hopeful that this Committee will lead the charge on addressing surprise billing, but I think the number of proposals that Members have produced shows that there is serious interest to accomplish something legislatively. Patients deserve better than to receive surprise bills for the care they needed, especially non-elective or emergency care. I would like to thank our witnesses for being here today, and I look forward to a productive discussion.

* * *

Ms. ESHOO. I thank the gentleman, and he yields back.

The Chair now recognizes Mr. Pallone, the chairman of the full committee, for five minutes for his opening statement.

Opening Statement of Hon. Frank Pallone, Jr., A Representative in Congress from the State of New Jersey

Mr. PALLONE. Thank you, Madam Chair.

I came in when Dr. Burgess was giving his opening statement and I thought, well, maybe I have to revise my remarks to be more evil. I am not usually playing good guy to his bad guy, but whatever. Maybe I didn't hear everything correctly.

[Laughter.]

Mr. PALLONE. But anyway, it's long past time for Congress to take decisive action to protect patients from the unreasonable and unacceptable practice of surprise billing.

Every day we hear new stories about American families being devastated financially and put through the tremendous emotional toll of surprise medical bills.

Stories like Stefan Kappas-Rocha of California who went to the emergency room for a kidney infection at Zuckerberg Hospital in San Francisco. She spent one night in the emergency room and was sent home a day later with Ibuprofen. Two months later, she received a bill for more than $27,000.

Then there's a story in my county of Joseph from Sea Girt who went to an in-network hospital for an emergency surgery on his leg, only to later receive a $60,000 bill from a surgeon who was out of his network.

And then there's the story of Drew Calver of Dallas, Texas, who received a $108,000 surprise medical bill from St. David's Medical Center after treatment for a heart attack.

These stories highlight a clear market failure. I know we will see a lot of finger pointing today about who's at fault for this failure, and this is the same finger pointing that has resulted in patients going into debt, ruining their credit, and questioning whether they should take their child to the hospital.

But let me be clear. I am interested in fixing this problem for consumers, not for the stakeholders who have allowed this problem to persist for decades while consumers continually paid the price. It is clear that the private sector is not going to fix this problem on its own and that Congress needs to step in and provide relief to consumers.

That being said, I want to commend the stakeholders here today for all agreeing that it's no longer acceptable to have patients in the middle of their disputes. People who need emergency care who were treated by a doctor they did not choose should be held harmless.

Now, fortunately, there's a bipartisan agreement on the committee that we must act. Ranking Member Walden and I have worked together to craft a common-sense bipartisan solution for the problem of surprise billing.

Our draft legislation would ensure that consumers with all types of private insurance are protected from surprise bills. It holds the patient harmless in surprise bill situations by ensuring that an individual's cost sharing for out-of-network care is limited to what the individual would have paid if the services were provided by an in-network provider.

This would ensure that patients are no longer penalized by the provider and the insurer's failure to contract, which is no fault of their own.

Providers would no longer be able to balance bill patients for out-of-network emergency services or for scheduled services from providers the patient was not aware would be involved in their treatment.

For the vast majority of cases, our discussion draft is simply asking providers to be more transparent about their billing practices and charges.

Insurers and hospitals also have a large role to play in making sure consumers understand their coverage. It is critical that we build some basic transparency and fairness into a system I think we all agree is incredibly difficult for consumers to navigate.

Providers, hospitals, and insurers should share this goal because the status quo is severely damaging the reputation and trustworthiness in the eyes of consumers.

Now, the discussion draft proposes resolving the payment dispute between the provider and the insurer by requiring the insuring plan to pay at a minimum the median in-network rate for that service in that geographic area.

This ensures that in the absence of balance billing every provider will be guaranteed some payment for their services and this would also create a predictable transparent means of resolving these disputes between providers and insurers who have failed to contract. It would also place little or no administrative burden on states, the Federal government, or the parties involved in the dispute.

So I look forward, Madam Chair, to hearing constructive feedback in the draft proposal. But I strongly believe that any viable solution in this space cannot result in rising healthcare costs.

This debate has shed light on the fact that some providers' charges and hospital fees are inexplicably high and I worry that if Congress chooses the wrong approach, consumers will simply end up paying those costs through higher premiums and we simply can't allow this to happen.

So I hope that today we can have a productive discussion without pointing fingers and passing the buck. We should instead focus on policy solutions that protect consumers. Ideally, such a solution will not only take the patient out of the middle and hold him financially harmless from surprise billing.

It'll also help create a lower cost, more rational healthcare system for all Americans, and I believe that the discussion draft accomplishes these goals and look forward to the feedback from our witnesses.

Obviously, Madam Chair and Dr. Burgess, you know, this discussion draft doesn't have to be the end all, and that's the reason we are having the hearing today and will continue to have discussions with people who may have alternative ideas or, you know, improving on what this discussion draft has here today.

So thank you, Madam Chair, and I—back to Dr. Burgess again, I am not used to being—he was like the bad guy today and I felt like I was——

Ms. ESHOO. No, he wasn't.

Mr. PALLONE. He wasn't?

Ms. ESHOO. No.

Mr. PALLONE. Oh, then I misunderstood then. Oh, very even tempered. OK. All right. Thank you. I yield back.

[The prepared statement of Mr. Pallone follow:]

Prepared Statement of Hon. Frank Pallone, Jr.

It is long past time for Congress to take decisive action to protect patients from the unreasonable and unacceptable practice of surprise billing. Every day, we hear new stories about American families being devastated financially and put through the tremendous emotional toll of surprise medical bills. Stories like Stefan Kappes-Rocha's of California, who went to the emergency room for a kidney infection at Zuckerberg Hospital in San Francisco. She spent one night in the emergency room and was sent home a day later with ibuprofen. Two months later, she received a bill for more than $27,000. Then there's the story of Joseph from Sea Girt, New Jersey who went to an in-network hospital for anemergency surgery on his leg only to later receive a $60,000 bill from a surgeon who was out of his network. And then there's the story of Drew Calver of Dallas, Texas, who received a $108,000 surprise medical bill from St. David's Medical Center, after treatment for a heart attack.

These stories highlight a clear market failure. I know we will see a lot of finger pointing today about who is at fault for this failure—this is the same finger pointing that has resulted in patients going into debt, ruining their credit, and questioning whether they should take their child to the hospital. But let me be clear—I'm interested in fixing this problem for consumers not for the stakeholders who've allowed this problem to persist for decades while consumers continually paid the price.

It is clear that the private sector is not going to fix this problem on its own, and that Congress needs to step in and provide relief to consumers. That being said, I want to commend the stakeholders here today for all agreeing that it's no longer acceptable to have patients in the middle of their disputes. People who need emergency care or who are treated by a doctor they did not choose should be held harmless.

Fortunately, there is bipartisan agreement on this Committee that we must act. Ranking Member Walden and I have worked together to craft a commonsense, bipartisan solution to the problem of surprise billing. Our draft legislation would ensure that consumers with all types of private insurance are protected from surprise bills. It holds the patient harmless in surprise bill situations, by ensuring that an individual's cost sharing for out-of-network care is limited to what the individual would have paid if the services were provided by an in-network provider. This would ensure that patients are no longer penalized by the provider and the insurers failure to contract, which is no fault of their own.

Providers would no longer be able to balance bill patients for out-of-network emergency services or for scheduled services from providers the patient was not aware would be involved in their treatment. For the vast majority of cases our discussion draft is simply asking providers to be more transparent about their billing practices and charges.

Insurers and hospitals also have a large role to play in making sure consumers understand their coverage. It is critical that we build some basic transparency and fairness into a system I think we all agree is incredibly difficult for consumers to navigate. Providers, hospitals, and insurers should share this goal—because the status quo is severely damaging their reputation and trustworthiness in the eyes of consumers.

The discussion draft proposes resolving the payment dispute between the provider and the insurer by requiring the insurance plan to pay, at a minimum, the median in-network rate for that service in that geographic area. This ensures that in the absence of balance billing, every provider will be guaranteed some payment for their services. This would also create a predictable, transparent means of resolving these disputes between providers and insurers who have failed to contract. It would also place little to no administrative burden on States, the Federal Government, or the parties involved in the dispute.

I look forward to hearing constructive feedback on the draft proposal, but I strongly believe that any viable solution in this space cannot result in rising healthcare costs. This debate has shed light on the fact that some provider's charges and hospital fees are inexplicably high, and I worry that if Congress chooses the wrong approach, consumers will simply end up paying those costs through higher premiums. We simply cannot allow this to happen.

I hope that today we can have a productive discussion without pointing fingers and passing the buck. We should instead focus on policy solutions that protect consumers. Ideally, such a solution will not only take the patient out of the middle and hold them financially harmless from surprise billing, but will also help create a lower-cost, more rational healthcare system for all Americans. I believe that the Pallone-Walden discussion draft accomplishes these goals, and I look forward to feedback from our witnesses.

I yield back.

* * *

Ms. ESHOO. He was in great form today, even better form. He's always in good form.

The gentleman yields back. Now I'd like to recognize my friend, the ranking member of the full committee, Mr. Walden, for five minutes for his opening statement.

Opening Statement of Hon. Greg Walden, A Representative in Congress from the State of Oregon

Mr. WALDEN. Well, thank you, Madam Chair, and thanks to Dr. Burgess and you for this hearing and to Mr. Pallone for working in the bipartisan way we are to address this surprise billing issue. The hearing really is about patients, first and foremost. We are actually going to put them first. We have all heard the stories and you heard some more today.

Patients who followed the rules, they pay their premiums, and then through no fault of their own following some sort of emergency situation or surgery, receive a 6-digit bill in the mail weeks later, which they have no way of paying.

It is not fair. It should not happen and we are going to put a stop to it one way or the other. We must protect patients from these bills and we want to get it right.

Since we released this draft last month, Chairman Pallone and I have received more than 60 comment letters on this draft from stakeholders across the healthcare industry.

That feedback is critical as we work to take the patient out of these surprise billing scenarios without raising overall healthcare costs.

I'd also like to thank all of our witnesses for being here today, many of whom have provided helpful feedback on this legislation and I'd particularly like to thank Ms. Wilkes.

Unfortunately, you have had to become an expert on this topic the hard way by living through it with your children. As a parent, I share your frustration and your desire to fix surprise billing once and for all.

Unfortunately, as you know, your experience is not unique, and I recently spoke with a doctor whose daughter's case has become pretty well known. The president had her down at the White House.

She had been in the hospital and on the way out her provider suggested she take a simple drug test. Little did she know that that test then was sent to an out-of-network lab and she soon received a bill for $17,850 in the mail. She had no reason to know or even to think to ask if the lab was in or out of network. She was just following her doctor's advice.

Situations like hers and yours, Ms. Wilkes, are why we are here today. We are going to stop this and it's why Chairman Pallone and I are moving forward with legislation to protect patients.

I am also pleased the president has taken on this issue. He was very serious about fixing surprise billing when we had a bipartisan event at the White House a couple weeks ago and I am encouraged our draft legislation lines up pretty well with the principles the president has set forth for a solution that could get his signature and into law.

So we are moving forward on this. The draft before us today, the No Surprises Act, would take a number of steps to address surprise medical bills.

First and foremost, this bill prohibits balance billing of patients and limits a patient's bill to their in-network cost-sharing amount in emergency situations.

This is common sense when a patient has little or no control over who gives them lifesaving care and can hardly be expected to make sure everyone is in network.

For scheduled care like elective surgeries, patients must receive both verbal and written notice of any out-of-network providers who will be involved in their care, and if they don't consent to that notice, they cannot be balance billed.

Under our draft bill, providers who would currently balance bill the patient will instead be paid to by the patient's insurer at the median in-network rate for the service they provided in that geographic area.

And by the way, my home State of Oregon passed legislation on surprise billing last year with a similar approach and other states have passed their own models that create an arbitration process for providers and insurers to come to an agreement on a reasonable payment, and there are combinations of the two.

Under our draft, these State laws, by the way, would remain in effect, and we know what many of the organizations represented in this room said when Oregon took up its law and what they've said since, and we know how it's playing out.

There are a number of options on how to deal with the payments to providers and I look forward to hearing from our panel on their experience with these different models.

In closing, I want to stress again this is an issue that is important to us and to our constituents and to all consumers in America. I understand there are competing interests here today. I expect we will have plenty of back and forth on the policies in this draft and that's what we are seeking.

Protecting patients, however, must be put at the forefront of this discussion and I'll continue to work with my colleagues on both sides of the aisle to do just that. We are going to resolve this once and for all.

With that, I yield back.

[The prepared statement of Mr. Walden follow:]

Prepared Statement of Hon. Greg Walden

Thank you, Madam Chair, and Dr. Burgess for holding this hearing. I'd also like to thank the Chairman of the full committee, Mr. Pallone, for working in good faith and in a bipartisan manner to release a discussion draft to address surprise billing.

This hearing is really about patients. We've all heard the stories from our constituents. Patients who follow the rules, pay their premiums, and then through no fault of their own, following an emergency situation or surgery receive a 6-digit bill in the mail weeks later, which they have no way of paying. It is not fair. It should not happen.

We must protect patients from these bills, and we want to get it right. Since we released this draft last month, Chairman Pallone and I have received over 60 comment letters on this draft from stakeholders across the healthcare industry. That feedback is critical as we work to take the patient out of these surprise billing scenarios without raising overall healthcare costs.

I'd like to thank all our witnesses for being here today, many of whom have provided that helpful feedback on this bill. I'd particularly like to thank Ms. Wilkes— unfortunately you've become an expert on this topic the hard way, by living through it with your children. As a parent I share your frustration and your desire to fix surprise billing once and for all.

Unfortunately, as you know, your experience is not unique—I recently spoke with a doctor whose daughter's case has become pretty well-known: She had been in the hospital, and on the way out her provider suggested that she take a simple drug test. Little did she know, that test was sent to an out-of-network lab and she soon received a $17,850 bill in the mail. She had no reason to know, or even think to ask, if the lab was in- or out-of-network. She was just following her doctor's advice. Situations like hers and yours, Ms. Wilkes, are why we're here today, We have to stop this. And it is why Chairman Pallone and I are moving forward with legislation to protect patients.

I'm also pleased that the President has taken on this issue. He was very serious about fixing surprise billing at a bipartisan event at the White House a few weeks ago. I am encouraged that our draft legislation lines up well with the principles the White House has set forth for a solution that could get the President's signature and become law.

The draft before us today, the No Surprises Act, would take a number of steps to address surprise medical bills. First, and most importantly, this bill prohibits balance billing of patients and limits a patient's bill to their in-network cost-sharing amount in emergency situations. This is commonsense when a patient has little to no control over who gives them life-saving care and can hardly be expected to make sure everyone is in-network. For scheduled care like elective surgeries, patients must receive both verbal and written notice of any out-of-network providers who will be involved in their care—if they don't consent to that notice, then they can't be balance billed.

Under our draft bill, providers who would currently balance bill the patient will instead be paid by the patient's insurer at the median in-network rate for the service they provided in that geographic area. My home State of Oregon passed legislation on surprise billing last year with a similar approach, and other states have passed their own models that create an arbitration process for providers and insurers to come to an agreement on a reasonable payment—and there are combinations of the two. Under our draft, these State laws would remain in place.

There are a number of options on how to deal with the payment to providers, and I look forward to hearing from our panel on their experience with these different models.

In closing, I would like to once again stress how important this issue is to our constituents. I understand there are competing interests here today and I expect plenty of back and forth on the policies in the draft. Protecting patients, however, must be put at the forefront of this discussion and I will continue to work with my colleagues on both sides of the aisle to do just that.

Thank you, Madam Chair, and I yield back.

Ms. ESHOO. The gentleman yields back. The Chair would like to remind Members that pursuant to committee rules, all Members' written statements—opening statements will be made part of the record.

I now would like to introduce all of our witnesses that are here today.

Ms. Sonji Wilkes, who is a patient advocate—thank you very much for being here; Dr. Sherif Zaafran, thank you for you being here—he is the chair for Physicians for Fair Coverage; Mr. Rick Sherlock, the president and CEO for the Association of Air Medical Services—thank you to you; Mr. James Gelfand, executive—senior vice president to health policy, the ERISA

Industry Committee; Mr. Thomas Nickels, the executive vice president of the American Hospital Association—it's nice to see you again; Ms. Jeanette Thornton, the senior vice president of product, employer, and commercial policy, America's Health Insurance Plans—welcome to you and thank you; Ms. Claire McAndrew, director of Campaigns and Partnerships at Families USA—thank you to you and the work that the organization does; Dr. Vidor—is it Vitor or Vidor?

Dr. FRIEDMAN. Madam Chairwoman, it's Vidor.

Ms. ESHOO. Vidor.

Dr. FRIEDMAN. Thank you.

Ms. ESHOO. Thank you. Vidor Friedman. Dr. Friedman, president of the American College of Emergency Physicians.

So we thank all of our witnesses for joining us today and we look forward to your testimony.

The Chair is going to begin by recognizing our first witness.

Each one of you have five minutes to give your opening statement, and you're probably all pretty familiar with what the light system.

The one you really have to pay attention to is red because it's over then, OK? So when it's yellow you have 1-minute remaining to wrap up your point.

So, Ms. Wilkes, again, thank you for being here. Tell us your story. You're recognized for five minutes.

Statement of Sonji Wilkes, Patient Advocate

Ms. WILKES. Thank you, Madam Chairwoman.

My name is Sonji Wilkes and I am a mom from Englewood, Colorado. I would like to thank the chairwoman, Congressman Burgess, and members of the subcommittee for the opportunity to discuss my family's experience with surprise billing and ask you to end this practice.

When my husband and I became first-time parents as health 20 somethings, neither of us had much experience with insurance. But we had a valuable lesson when we received a bill double what we expected.

Seems the insurance company counted me and my newborn daughter as two separate patients. Though surprised, we paid the claim and moved on.

Two years later, we decided to grow our family. A little wiser, we made sure to ask specifically if we would incur two co-pays. We double checked that our OB/Gyn and the facility that we were to deliver at were in network.

Per the documentation from our insurance provider, we were covered. My son, Thomas, was born full term. By all appearances he was a healthy boy.

Several hours after Thomas was circumcised, our pediatrician called to say that he was concerned that the circumcision site continued to bleed. The next day he called us in tears to say that Thomas had severe hemophilia A, a genetic disorder that prevents his blood from clotting.

Our doctor told us that hemophilia was a rare—excuse me, Thomas was taken to the neonatal intensive care unit so that he could be closely observed. Within the hour, a specialist from the local hemophilia treatment center was standing in our hospital room and, after asking if we had good insurance, spent the next few hours explaining hemophilia to us.

She brought a dose of clotting factor for Thomas to stop the bleeding as the hospital did not stock that medication. In the NICU, the hematologist started an IV line in my son's scalp while the NICU staff intently watched. They had never treated hemophilia.

While the hematologist was not part of the hospital or the NICU staff, we never saw a bill for the medication she administered or for her time or services.

Thomas remained in the NICU overnight for observation. Neither my husband or I left our son's side, and other than monitoring his vitals, there was no direct care give to Thomas. As a nearly 10-pound baby, he was a bit out of place in the NICU.

We were discharged within the normal post-partum period and went home to come to grips with an unexpected chronic disorder diagnosis for our baby boy.

A few weeks later, we received another shock—a $50,000 bill for Thomas' stay in the NICU. We were dumbfounded. We had been at an in-network facility. How could we possibly be responsible for that amount?

My husband and I felt we should not be held responsible. We did some research and found out that the hospital had subcontracted the NICU out to a third-party provider. This third-party provider was the one demanding payment.

We had made a good faith effort to stay in network. We refused to pay the bill and, subsequently, were sent to collections. Our credit was ruined.

Sometime later our minivan lease was expiring. As we headed to the dealership, we knew we wouldn't qualify for a new lease. I had to have a car. Thomas was being seen at the hemophilia treatment center multiple times a week. At the finance manager's desk, my husband and I explained the surprise bill. As I emptied the Kleenex box sitting on his desk, he started tapping on his computer, wiped a tear of his own, and said, we will make something happen for you. It might be at a crazy high interest rate and you'll have to keep the car until the day it dies. But I understand your situation because something similar happened to my family.

I am still driving that minivan.

When you are told your baby's body lacks the ability to stop bleeding and that he needs immediate specialized treatment, your first reaction isn't, gee, I wonder if that's in-network.

Your first reaction is, do whatever it takes to save my baby. Why would I check if the NICU, just 50 steps away from the room that I gave birth in, was in network? I think any reasonable person would assume it to be because it seems reckless and cruel that it would not be.

No family should face financial ruin because they are duped into thinking that they are at an in-network facility or because the in-network provider contracts out services like radiology, lab services, imaging, or more without the patient's knowledge.

While transparency and disclosure of any out-of-network subprovider is critical, it's not enough. Navigating health insurance is extremely difficult and especially so in crisis or for the inexperienced.

According to a recent Kaiser Family Foundation poll, four out of ten respondents said they had received an unexpected bill from a hospital, lab, or doctor in the past year.

But surprise billing is not a new issue. My personal story is from 2003. Patients need you to pass protections to stop these harmful practices.

I wish this wasn't mine or anyone else's stories to share. Please protect Americans from excessive bills and medical debt by ending this surprise billing.

My family and millions of others thank you in advance.

[The prepared statement of Ms. Wilkes follows:]

Written Testimony of Sonji Wilkes

My name is Sonji Wilkes and I am a mom and patient advocate from Englewood, Colorado. Thank you to Chairwoman Eshoo, Congressman Burgess, and Members of the subcommittee for the opportunity to discuss my family's experience with surprise billing and to ask for your help in ending surprise billing for patients.

In 2001, my husband and I become first-time parents. As healthy twenty-somethings, neither of us had much experience with medical claims and insurance, but we knew that staying in-network per our insurance policy was important. We had our first daughter at an in-network hospital, delivered by an in-network doctor. We had expected to pay $250 out-of-pocket. When the bill arrived a weeks after the delivery, it was $500. Seems that the insurance company counted myself and our newborn daughter as two separate patients. We felt a bit duped but paid the claim and moved on.

Two years later, and still with a similar insurance plan, we decided to grow our family. A little older, and a little wiser, we made sure to ask specifically if we would incur two co-pays. We doubled checked that our OB/GYN and the facility we were to deliver at were still in-network. Per the documentation we had from our insurance provider, we were following the rules.

My son, Thomas, was born full-term and came into the world just under 10 pounds. By all appearances, he was a healthy boy. Within a few hours of birth, Thomas was circumcised. But several hours later, our pediatrician called to say he was concerned that the circumcision site was continuing to bleed and that he wanted to run a few tests. By the next day, our pediatrician called us back, in tears, to break the news that Thomas had severe hemophilia A, a genetic disorder that prevents his blood from clotting. The pediatrician told us that hemophilia was a rare, lifelong disorder and that he didn't know much about it, but he had a hematologist waiting on the other line to talk to us. They decided to take Thomas to the Neonatal Intensive Care Unit so he could be closely observed. Within the hour, the hematologist for the local Hemophilia Treatment Center was standing in our hospital room, and after opening the conversation by asking if we had good health insurance, spent the next few hours explaining hemophilia to us. She had brought a dose of anti-hemophiliac clotting factor to administer to Thomas to stop the bleeding, as the hospital facility we were at did not stock the medication in the pharmacy. In the NICU, the hematologist prepared the IV, and started an intravenous line in my newborn's scalp while the NICU staff intently watched, as they were unfamiliar with hemophilia and did not know how to treat it. The hematologist was not part of the hospital or NICU staff; she was simply there as a caring, knowledgeable provider. We never saw a bill for the medication she administered or for the hematologist's time and services.

Thomas remained in the NICU overnight for observation. As a nearly 10-pound baby in the NICU, he was a bit out of place. Neither my husband or I left Thomas's side and other than monitoring his vital signs, there was no other direct care given to Thomas. We were discharged within the normal post-partum period and went home to come to grips with the unexpected diagnosis of a chronic disorder for our baby boy.

A few weeks later, we received another shock. Opening the mail, we found a bill for $50,000 for Thomas's stay in the NICU. My husband and I were dumbfounded. We had been in an in-network facility. How could we possibly be responsible for that amount?

The insurance company was adamant. According to them, we had a $50,000 debt that needed to be paid. My husband and I were equally adamant – we should not be held responsible. We did some research and found out that the hospital had subcontracted the NICU out to a third-party provider. This third-party provider was not part of any insurance company's network.

We felt we had made a good faith effort to stay in-network based on the information that was provided to us. We refused to pay the bill and were subsequently sent to collections. Our credit was ruined, but our resolve was not. Several years later, the debt was dismissed as part of a class action lawsuit, but nevertheless, we struggled with the effects of a bad credit rating.

Before the bill was resolved, but after our credit was trashed, our mini-van lease was expiring. We had to either turn it in or buy it, and neither option was going to be easy. We knew we wouldn't qualify for a new lease and we had very real concern that the dealership wouldn't enter a contract with us to buy out the existing lease. We went into the dealership to talk with them and it was not looking good with the first guy we talked to. We asked to talk to the finance manager and I completely broke down in front of him when he said he didn't think he would be able to help us. I had to have a car: Thomas was being seen at the Hemophilia Treatment Center multiple times a week and getting there without a car was nearly impossible. My husband and I explained how the surprise health care bill had led to our credit rating as I emptied the Kleenex box sitting on the finance manager's desk. He started tapping on his computer keyboard, wiped a tear of his own, and said, "We'll make something happen for you. It might be at a crazy high interest rate and you'll have to keep that car until the day it dies, but I understand your situation. My family also got hit with an expensive medical bill we weren't expecting." Twelve years later, I'm still driving that mini-van.

When you are told that your baby is bleeding and his body lacks the ability to stop and that he needs immediate specialized treatment, your first reaction isn't, "Gee, I wonder if that's in-network;" your first reaction is, "By all means, do whatever it takes to help my baby." I would have never thought to check if the NICU, just 50 or so steps from the room I gave birth in, was in-network. I think any reasonable person would assume it to be because it seems reckless and cruel to me that it would not be. After all, when newborns end up in the NICU, it is an occasion of maximum family vulnerability, and it will inevitably entail high-cost care.

Consumers should be protected from expensive surprise medical bills in emergency situations or when they believe that they are appropriately seeking care from in-network providers. No family should face financial ruin because they are duped into thinking they are at an in-network facility or because their in-network provider contracts out services like radiology, lab services, imaging, or more without the patient's knowledge. While transparency and disclosure of any out-of-network sub-providers is critical, it's still not enough. My husband and I consider ourselves to be health literate, but navigating the nomenclature of health insurance policy is extremely difficult, and especially so for people who are dealing with the stress of a medical crisis, or for people who have not had many experiences in a health care setting. These families aren't often equipped to know how to appeal the bill, and even if they do begin that process, the collections agency can start calling.

According to a recent Kaiser Family Foundation poll, four out of 10 respondents said they had received an unexpected bill from a hospital, lab or doctor in the past year. But surprise billing is not a new issue: the personal story I just shared with you is from 2003. Patients need Congress to pass protections to stop these harmful practices.

While serious policy disagreements need to be worked out, you cannot let this effort grind to a halt. My family incurred a devastating surprise bill 15 years ago. Every year, millions of other families get similar bills. The time has come for this egregious practice to stop. Failing to pass meaningful legislation means you are letting millions more families experience the fear and pain my family faced. Please get this done.

Thank you for listening to my family's experience with surprise billing. Please protect patients from excessive bills and medical debt by ending surprise billing. My family and millions of others thank you in advance.

* * *

Ms. ESHOO. Thank you, Ms. Wilkes. How is your son today?

Ms. WILKES. He's very good. Ms. ESHOO. Good. That's great.

Ms. WILKES. Fifteen years old and learning how to drive in that minivan.

Ms. ESHOO. Isn't that wonderful? Isn't that great? Isn't that great? I just want to make a suggestion. I think that the witnesses all need to direct their comments attached to Ms. Wilkes' story. I mean, this is—I don't know—I don't think there's anyone here that can defend it. But it's just a suggestion.

I am now pleased to recognize Dr. Zaafran for five minutes for his testimony. Thank you and welcome.

Statement of Sherif Zaafran, M.D., FASA, Chair, Physicians for Fair Coverage

Dr. ZAAFRAN. Thank you. Good morning, Chairman Eshoo, Ranking Member Burgess, and distinguished members of the committee.

Thank you for inviting me to testify today on behalf of Physicians for Fair Coverage. My name is Sherif Zaafran and I serve as chair of the board of PFC and I am a practicing anesthesiologist.

PFC is a non-profit nonpartisan multi-specialty association of tens of thousands of physicians partnered with patient advocates to end surprise medical billing.

We are committed to finding a solution that creates strong patient protections, ensures access to care, and improves transparency.

To be clear, PFC-affiliated physicians prefer to be in-network and are actually in-network with the vast majority of the patients we see. These numbers are actually representative of the larger market for emergency medicine, anaesthesiology, radiology, and other hospital-based physicians.

On behalf of PFC, I want to commend all of you for working to address out-of-network surprise billing for our patients. As a physician, I live and work by the creed do no harm and believe that any solution to surprise billing should meet this test as well.

In this spirit, PFC believes that protecting patients from potential financial stress by eliminating balance billing for unanticipated out-of-network care and ensuring patients pay no more than their in-network cost sharing is the right thing to do.

It is important, however, to understand what causes surprise billing before we talk about the solution. There are two key factors: an increasing proliferation of high deductible plans, many of which can be $5,000 or more, which has resulted in a significant financial burden on patients that is unanticipated; and two, complicated plan designs with tiered and narrowing networks which force doctors to be out of network and in many instances not by their choice.

Understandably, a Federal solution is key to solving the problem of unanticipated out-of-network costs. We want to recognize the leadership of Congressmen Ruiz and Bucshon for putting for a very thoughtful proposal, and we appreciate the proposal offered by full committee Chairman Pallone and Ranking Member Walden.

PFC does have concerns, however, that the median in-network benchmark currently in the full committee's discussion draft could have the unintended consequences of potentially driving more patients and their physicians out of network.

Our recommendation is to turn the benchmark payment concept into an interim payment with the ability of either side to go to a baseball-style independent dispute resolution process if there is a disagreement.

The care provided by different physicians is not always uniform. There can be variability in quality and the cost of providing high-value care, especially when providing certain types of care in different geographical areas.

While there may be a desire by some to reduce spending in critical pinnacle areas for patients in order to increase their own profitability, physicians would prefer to decrease overall healthcare costs by investing in resources that allow for better patient outcomes.

To be sure, the best arbitration process is one that does not need to be utilized. We believe an appropriate interim payment will resolve most disputes. For those that it does not, IDR provides the opportunity to appeal the payment in a fair and expedited way.

And this cut both ways. Plans and providers alike will have the opportunity to appeal. PFC has been very involved in the debate on this issue in the states and we note that solutions incorporating IDR such as New York and, most recently, in Texas, have proven successful.

Indeed, in New York, such a process resulted in out-of-network rate dropping from 20.1 percent to 6.4 percent after IDR solution was put in place. According to a recent study by the Georgetown University Center on Health Insurance Reforms, the independent dispute resolution process has resulted in a decrease in out-of-network claims, a dramatic decline in consumer complaints about surprise bills, and no indication of an inflationary effect on insurers' annual premium rate filings.

The law has also led to stronger protections for patients and more patient-centric health plans, enhanced transparency from health insurers, and increased network participation and fewer out-of-network claims.

We believe a Federal solution should build on this proven success and we encourage the committee to include the IDR process in future iterations of the legislation.

Doing so will preserve existing in-network arrangements, ensure both providers and payers have the ability to achieve a fair rate, take the patient out of the middle, and avoid significant disruption that would result from moving the market to a set benchmark rate.

On the other hand, a poorly constructed untested solution could threaten patients' access to quality care and the provider's ability to serve their communities.

For example, the experience in California shows that a benchmark approach does not work. The law has had unintended consequences, resulting in insurers refusing to renew longstanding contracts or offering significantly reduced rates that undermine good faith contracts.

Insurers in the State now have little incentive to contract with physicians.

Finally, we urge you to reject the false narrative advanced by some that arbitration necessarily involves a choice between so-called reasonable rate and providers' full billed charges.

Arbitration guardrails can and should be designed to guide the parties to market-based rates while preserving appropriate variation based on performance and local conditions which economic studies have shown is the outcome produced with baseball-style former in particular.

In conclusion, PFC advocates for and supports a ban on balance billing for unanticipated out-of-network care with strong patients' protections, fair reimbursement backed by an IDR process to ensure access to care, greater network adequacy standards, and improved transparency for all patients.

Madam Chair, members of the committee, we appreciate your leadership on this important issue and thank you for the opportunity to testify.

PFC stands ready to work with you in the best interests of our patients and physicians who care for them, and I am happy to answer any questions you may have.

[The Prepared Statement of Dr. Zaafran follows:]

Written Testimony of Sherif Zaafran, M.D.

Chairwoman Eshoo, Ranking Member Burgess, and distinguished Members of the Committee, thank you for inviting me to testify on behalf of Physicians for Fair Coverage (PFC). I serve as Chairman of the Board of PFC. I also serve as the President of the Texas Medical Board, and the National Legislative Liaison for US Anesthesia Partners (USAP) and continue to treat patients as a practicing anesthesiologist. While I wear many hats, today I am providing testimony through my role as Chairman of PFC.

PFC is a non-profit, non-partisan, multi-specialty association of tens of thousands of physicians partnered with patient advocacy groups. PFC members care for more than 50 million patients each year in more than 3,000 facilities nationwide. We are committed to finding a solution to surprise medical bills that creates strong patient protections, ensures access to care, and improves transparency. PFC-affiliated physicians prefer to be in-network and are actually in-network with 95 to 99 percent of the patients they see. The data indicates that these numbers are representative of the larger market for emergency medicine, anesthesiology, and radiology and that the vast majority of these doctors are in-network.[1] We would also remind the Committee that hospital-based physicians treat a significantly higher portion of uninsured, Medicaid, and Medicare patients than most other practices. We treat all patients who need care at our facilities, without regard to their insurance status or their ability to pay.

On behalf of PFC, I want to commend all of you, as well as the Chairman and Ranking Member of the full Energy and Commerce Committee, for working to address out-of-network

[1] https://www.cdc.gov/nchs/data/nhamcs/web_tables/2015_ed_web_tables.pdf; https://hcupnet.ahrq.gov/#setup; https://www.brookings.edu/research/state-approaches-to-mitigating-surprise-out-of-network-billing; https://www.ama-assn.org/sites/amaassn.org/files/corp/media-browser/public/health-policy/PRP-2017-physician-benchmark-survey-patient-mix.pdf.

surprise billing for our patients. As a physician, I live and work by the creed "do no harm." I believe that any solution to surprise billing should meet this test as well. PFC supports the intent of the Committee's draft legislation, as we strongly believe patients should be protected from the potential financial stress associated with unanticipated out-of-network care.

We believe protecting patients by eliminating balance billing and ensuring patients pay no more than their in-network cost-sharing is the right thing to do. We also support many of the transparency requirements that work towards ensuring no patient is surprised with an out-of-network provider as part of scheduled care.

However, federal intervention to protect patients also requires careful federal intervention to deal with the dispute that arises between the plan and physician over reimbursement as a result of eliminating the ability of the physicians to bill for their services.

PFC believes the federal intervention to resolve this dispute should comport with the following principles: 1) ensure fair reimbursement for specific physicians case-by-case, who end up providing services to patients who are out-of-network; 2) protect the vast majority of the in-network contracted marketplace so that the solution doesn't incentivize and generate a greater volume of out-of-network claims; and 3) create an incentive for currently out-of-network plans and physicians to go in-network. PFC is concerned that the "median in-network" benchmark currently in the Energy and Commerce discussion draft falls short of these principles and could potentially drive more patients out-of-network.

The median in-network benchmark will not represent fair reimbursement for specific physicians case-by-case who end up providing services to patients who are out-of-network. There are significant differences from one patient encounter to another such as training and experience of the physician, circumstances and complexity of the episode, the cost intensity of the location, and the quality of the care provided. The median in-network rate doesn't recognize any of these differences and would reimburse based on an artificial formula set in statute that simply can't reflect the tremendous diversity of reimbursement rates needed to sustain a complex, dynamic market.

However, perhaps the greatest concern is the negative effect that a benchmark approach for out-of-network care would have on the contracted marketplace throughout the country (which represents the vast majority of patient volume). Under this formula, half the in-network rates in a given area would be above this number and half would be below by definition. Health plans would be greatly incentivized to NOT renew contracts with practices with existing contracts above the median in-network rate. Doing so would immediately reduce their expenditures and would also drive down the median in-network rate over time, leading to a vicious cycle of jamming down physician reimbursement to unsustainable levels. Ultimately, this would harm patients by creating an unsustainable economic environment, especially for physician practices that treat over 200 million patients a year. The public health risks are substantial and foreseeable if a policy is implemented that would erode access to and quality of care for patients.

Our recommendation for revising the draft to meet the principles laid out above is to turn the benchmark payment concept into an interim payment with the ability of either side to go to a baseball-style Independent Dispute Resolution (IDR) process for recourse if the payment is inappropriate.

The interim payment should be higher than the median in-network rate in order to mitigate the volume of disputes going to IDR and should be set in a way that doesn't allow health plans to manipulate it by canceling contracts with the highest reimbursement. We believe that the interim payment will resolve most disputes; for those that it does not, IDR provides the opportunity to appeal the payment in a fair way. And this cuts both ways – plans and providers alike will have the opportunity to appeal.

PFC has been very involved in the debates on this issue in the states and we note that solutions incorporating IDR have proven successful. Twelve states have now adopted a solution incorporating baseball-style IDR including Washington state, Nevada, and Colorado this year and most recently my home state of Texas.[2]

Each state sets their model up a bit differently, but they all have the same basic framework in common—the patient is protected; both parties have recourse to a neutral third-party in the out-of-network payment dispute if they believe the other party is unreasonable; each party is incentivized to provide their most reasonable offer; and the parties are incentivized to remain or go in-network and avoid the dispute resolution process.

Perhaps what is most telling about these four state efforts this year is that the key stakeholders— providers, insurers, and patient groups—all supported that framework which then passed with bipartisan support in their state legislatures. We believe a federal solution should build on this success by incorporating these key features for resolving payment issues between providers and payers. We encourage the Committee to include this IDR process in future iterations of the legislation.

The inclusion of an IDR process is a critical aspect of a solution that will preserve existing in-network arrangements, ensure both providers and payers have the ability to achieve a fair rate, take the patient out of the middle, and avoid significant disruption that would result from moving the market to a set benchmark rate. A poorly constructed solution could threaten patients' access to care and providers' ability to serve their communities.

Economic Realities Hospital-Based Physicians Face

The overwhelming majority of PFC-affiliated physicians are hospital-based physicians that provide around-the-clock care every day of the year, regardless of a patient's coverage status. The provision of these services ensures that patients with a middle-of-the-night heart attack or emergency C-section can seek and receive immediate care from qualified professionals.

Hospital-based physicians face a fundamentally different set of economic realities than other specialties who provide primarily scheduled care. Unlike physicians who have the ability to select whether they will see a patient based on their health insurance coverage, hospital-based physicians have no control over payer mix or plan type. This is because efficient, consistent care typically requires an emergency medicine, radiology, anesthesiology, or pathology group to cover all the patients at a given facility. Further constraints are already embedded in federal law, as the Emergency Medical Treatment and Labor Act (EMTALA) requires physicians to provide emergency care regardless of a patient's ability to pay.

The payer with the highest percentage of patients with an emergency department visit is Medicaid (32 percent), followed by private insurance (31 percent), Medicare (23 percent), and the uninsured (14 percent).[3] Thus, 46 percent of the patients seen by emergency medicine

[2] Reflects data reported by the Commonwealth Fund and recently enacted bills in Colorado, Nevada, and Washington. https://www.commonwealthfund.org/blog/2019/state-efforts-protect-consumers-balance-billing.

[3] *Ibid.*

physicians are uninsured or Medicaid patients. Compare this to orthopedic surgery which has just 6 percent of uninsured and Medicaid patients.[4] Moreover, commercial rates cannot be discussed in a vacuum. They must be viewed in the context of the overall economic reality of the practice. After taking all these types of payers into account, the weighted average reimbursement per patient is about $155 per visit, or just 107 percent of Medicare.[5]

If new policies go into effect that jam down commercial rates for emergency medicine, the economics of the practice will become untenable with virtually half their patients paying nothing or significantly underpaying relative to the cost of care. EMTALA rightfully eliminates the ability of hospital-based physicians (which includes not just emergency physicians, but also radiologists, surgeons, and anesthesiologists) to turn away patients, but this inherently means physicians have no ability to adjust their patient-payer mix, and with Medicaid and Medicare only reimbursing through artificially low set rates, providers cannot negotiate higher rates there to make up the difference.

It is also worth considering hospital-based physician fees in the overall context of health care costs. Despite statements to the contrary, hospital-based physician professional fees are not large enough to drive overall health care cost inflation. Combined emergency department, anesthesiology, and radiology professional fees are 2.3 percent of the total private insurance spending per beneficiary.[6] So if the policy goal is to drive down health care costs, driving down physician fees will have very little impact—particularly when you consider that such an impact would destabilize the EMTALA-based emergency care safety net in this country. Frankly, my emergency medicine colleagues should be celebrated for providing high quality care under inherently unpredictable circumstances to 140 million patients a year for only $155 a visit, not vilified based on highly selective, misleading data as we've recently seen published as part of this policy debate.

Concerns with Median In-Network Rate as Benchmark

PFC believes it is equally important to not only protect patients from unexpected out-of-pocket costs, but also to ensure they have access to care where and when they need it. As highlighted above, we have serious concerns that setting payment at the median contracted rate for services in the same geographic area will threaten access to care. Basing the reimbursement mechanism on the median contracted rate is challenging and subject to insurer manipulation. This lacks transparency and visibility in what is regarded by insurers as highly-protected, confidential,

---

[4] https://hcupnet.ahrq.gov/#setup; https://www.beckersasc.com/asc-turnarounds-ideas-to-improve-performance/payer-mix-at-orthopedics-driven-ascs-6-statistics.html; https://www.ama-assn.org/sites/ama-assn.org/files/corp/mediabrowser/public/health-policy/PRP-2017-physician-benchmark-survey-patient-mix.pdf.

[5] https://hcupnet.ahrq.gov/#setup; www.cms.gov/apps/physician-fee-schedule/search;Truven Payer Claims Database; https://www.aap.org/en-us/professionalresources/Research/Medicaid%20Reimbursement%20. Reports/medicaid_reports_ national_all.pdf; Medicare PUF file.

[6] Determined using data from: https://www.cbo.gov/sites/default/files/recurringdata/51298-2017-09healthinsurance.pdf; https://www.healthcostinstitute.org/research/annual-reports/entry/2017-health-care-cost-and-utilization-report; Truven payer claims database; https://www.prweb.com/releases/2011/2/prweb8127064.htm; Truven payer claims database; https://hcupnet.ahrq.gov/#setup; https://www.cdc.gov/nchs/data/nhamcs/web_tables/2015_ed_web_tables.pdf http://monitor.pubs.asahq.org/article.aspx?articleid=2705479; https://www.hcup-us.ahrq.gov/reports/statbriefs/sb223-Ambulatory-Inpatient-Surgeries-2014.jsp; https://www.ama-assn.org/sites/ama-assn.org/files/corp/mediabrowser/public/health-policy/PRP-2017-physician-benchmark-survey-patient-mix.pdf.

and guarded information. The median contracted rate is not a viable standard that ensures transparency and market standards.

Additionally, a single payment standard doesn't allow for differentiation in the marketplace based on value, quality or complexity and cost intensity of the practice location. In particular, the inability to be compensated for the types of quality metrics that ultimately decrease the overall cost of care will inhibit providers who invest to create this value and drive everyone to an inefficient "one-size-fits-all" reimbursement standard.

To be clear, PFC physicians prefer to be in network because it means higher patient volume, greater referrals, lower administrative costs, fewer denials, and guaranteed payment including assurances of direct pay through assignment of benefits. To secure optimal, market-based, in-network rates requires physicians and insurers to negotiate reimbursement on equal footing and under arms-length transactional settings; optimal negotiations implies concessions will generally be made on both sides. The contracted in-network rate is a heavily discounted one that physicians accept in return for these considerations which are not available to out-of-network physicians.

The current benchmark in the draft bill will remove incentives for insurers to negotiate in good faith during contract negotiations. By using the median contracted rate as a payment standard, we contend that health plans may simply cancel contracts, refuse to negotiate rates that are above the median, or drive rates down over time to lower the median. Insurers will have an incentive to lower contracted rates because all care will be subject to the payment standard and there will be no ability for non-contracted providers to charge more than contracted rates.

Physicians have already experienced this type of behavior by health plans in states such as California which took a similar approach to the committee's discussion draft. California's 2016 surprise billing law uses the weighted average of in-network rates. *The experience in California shows that this benchmark approach does not work.* The law has resulted in insurers refusing to renew long-standing contracts or offering significantly reduced rates that undermine good faith contracts. Insurers in the state have little incentive to contract with physicians. Some physician groups are reporting that their insurers are seeking unreasonable and unjustified payment reductions of 21-40 percent.

In fact, since insurers often pay a smaller percentage of the allowed amount for out-of-network services, the insurance companies are further incentivized to cease contracting efforts or refrain from negotiating or renegotiating contracts where network adequacy standards are lacking. At a time when there are already physician shortages in many rural and economically disadvantaged communities, setting payments at unsustainable levels will ultimately exacerbate the current predicament and harm access to care.

Recommended Framework: Interim Payment With IDR

PFC supports proposals that would establish a process that both protects patients and preserves the broader market which is largely functioning. As discussed, we believe the correct framework to accomplish this goal is one that 1) eliminates balance billing; 2) sets a reasonable interim payment for out-of-network payments; and 3) provides recourse to either party through an IDR process if they believe the other party is not being reasonable.

PFC supports the concept of an appropriate benchmark as part of an Interim Direct Reimbursement payment as long as it is reasonable and coupled with a process for physicians to appeal that rate. An additional dispute resolution process would ensure a level playing field and that neither side would gain an unfair edge during contract negotiations. Additionally, setting an appropriate interim payment would also reduce the number of claims that go to the dispute resolution process. Such a process would ensure that incidental claims are paid with minimal increased cost to the system and the parties involved.

PFC recommends the process include several guardrails around the dispute resolution process that would ensure the arbiter has a clear picture of the factors involved in determining a fair and appropriate payment. These factors should include:

- The previously contracted rate and contracting history between the plan and provider under dispute. This provision is particularly important to maintaining a balanced environment and ensuring that the contracted market remains stable, which benefits everyone: patients, insurers, self-insured employers, physicians and hospitals;
- The physician's level of training, education, experience, specialization, the acuity level of the patients, and physician quality and outcome metrics;
- Past compliance with contract terms;
- The circumstances and complexity of the case; and
- Other relevant economic aspects of physician payment for that specialty in the same geographic area.

PFC believes these parameters would ensure the process has a stabilizing effect on insurance networks.

It is important to emphasize that we expect such an IDR model to be used relatively rarely. The purpose of the IDR is to provide fair recourse to either the plan or provider if the other party is being unreasonable. Thus, it is important as a backstop, but in practice it will be rarely used because each party will now be incentivized to be reasonable in their private negotiating. They will know that they will lose if they are unreasonable and the other party initiates the dispute resolution process.

Indeed, as we saw in New York, the out-of-network rate dropped 68 percent from 20.1 percent to 6.4 percent after their IDR solution was put in place. This suggests that the plans and providers in that state found it more beneficial to negotiate an in-network contract than to fight out-of-network reimbursement through arbitration.

State Experience

PFC's support for an independent dispute resolution process is largely based on our work in the states. We looked to the success of the bipartisan model used in New York State. That model is both effective and has the support of consumer and patient groups.[7]

[7] https://advocacy.consumerreports.org/wp-content/uploads/2014/07/NY.OON_.Case_.Study_.pdf.

According to a recent case study by researchers at the Georgetown University Center on Health Insurance Reforms,[8] *the independent dispute resolution process has resulted in a decrease in out-of-network claims, a "dramatic" decline in consumer complaints about surprise bills, and no "indication of an inflationary effect in insurers' annual premium rate filings." The law has also led to stronger protections for patients and more patient-centric health plans; enhanced transparency from health insurers; increased network participation; and fewer out-of-network claims.*

Other states—from Colorado and Nevada to Texas and Washington—have recently passed legislation based on a dispute resolution process. For example, Washington Governor Jay Inslee recently signed legislation into law that would protect patients by paying out-of-network providers a "commercially reasonable" amount based on payments for the same or similar service in the same geographic area. There is then a binding arbitration process for when an insurer and provider cannot agree on a price for the covered service.[9]

Also, the Texas Legislature has approved legislation (SB 1264) that prohibits surprise billing; establishes an initial payment of the usual and customary rate, the agreed amount, or the amount from the appeals process; and sets up an arbitration process to resolve payment disputes. These two examples are from states that have been examining and working toward addressing the issue of out-of-network billing for years.

The trend of states legislating an interim payment coupled with a dispute resolution process is not something that Congress should overlook. The fact that key stakeholders in those states—patient groups, providers, insurers—all agreed on this framework is critical to ensuring a bill can ultimately be passed. In total 12 states have a dispute resolution process that has been approved by their legislature or has been implemented.

While we support these state efforts, PFC believes that state protections should not apply unless they meet the minimum federal standard. Federal patient protections and independent dispute resolution standards for physicians must set a floor in order to protect access to the safety net in all 50 states. State approaches should only apply if they provide even greater patient and physician protections. Moreover, physicians should have sufficient and adequate access to the IDR process under applicable state provisions and, if they do not, they should have access via the federal IDR process.

All Payer Claims Databases

PFC believes it is imperative that a verified, statistically representative benchmarking database independent from both providers and payers be utilized when determining rates. The PFC proposal specifies that the Interim Direct Reimbursement be determined using a benchmarking database maintained by a nonprofit organization that is not affiliated with or receives funding from a health insurance company.

While the draft bill leaves the methodology to the rulemaking process, it does include grant money for states to establish or maintain All Payer Claims Databases (APCD). We have concerns about relying on individual state APCDs to determine rates. There will be a significant

[8] Georgetown University Health Policy Institute Centers on Health Insurance Reforms, *New York's 2014 Law to Protect Consumers from Surprise Out-of-Network Bills Mostly Working as Intended: Results of a Case Study*, May 2019; https://georgetown.app.box.com/s/6onkj1jaiy3f1618iy7j0gpzdoew2zu9.

[9] Washington HB 1065. https://app.leg.wa.gov/billsummary?BillNumber=1065&Year=2019&Initiative=false.

lag time for states to pass legislation authorizing the collection of claims, apply for federal grant money, and build the infrastructure. It is also very expensive to establish and maintain.

PFC would ask you to use FAIR Health, which is a non-profit, independent, national data repository established to bring clarity to health care costs and health insurance information. The database includes more than 28 billion privately billed medical and dental procedures covering more than 150 million privately and publicly insured individuals, is used widely (including by state and federal governments), is one of only four qualified entities to utilize Medicare and Medicaid data, and provides the greatest transparency of pricing and costs in the health care market of any national database.

Creating Greater Transparency

In addition to rising out-of-pocket costs, patients often face frustration with a lack of transparency in the health care system, especially when it comes to understanding which physicians are currently in the network of their health insurance plan. Unfortunately, the accuracy of such information is highly inconsistent among insurers and even within the various plans of the same insurer.

PFC recommends requiring all insurers to update their provider network directories online at least monthly with easy access for all plan beneficiaries, and to perform an audit annually to ensure accuracy. Furthermore, health plans should be required to disclose a detailed description of the enrollee's health plan on their health insurance card to reduce errors and help providers properly adjudicate claims.

This includes the requirement that insurers disclose on the members' plan information and identification card, the state by which the plan is regulated, and the state laws it operates under, or if federally regulated, a requirement that it disclose that it is governed as a group benefit plan under federal law such as the Employee Retirement Income Security Act (ERISA).

Finally, we know that when patients are empowered to make their own decisions in the medical marketplace, quality can go up and costs can go down. This can better be achieved with greater price transparency, with one key to this being to require providers to share cost estimates of their health care services to patients.

In Conclusion

PFC advocates for and supports a ban on balance billing for unanticipated out-of-network care with strong patient protections, fair reimbursement backed by an Independent Dispute Resolution process to ensure access to care, greater network adequacy standards, and improved transparency for all patients.

We appreciate your leadership on this important issue and thank you for the opportunity to testify. PFC stands ready to work with you in the best interest of our patients and the physicians who care for them.

* * *

Ms. ESHOO. Thank you, Doctor.

The Chair now is pleased to recognized Mr. Sherlock for five minutes for your oral testimony, and thank you for being here again.

Statement of Rick Sherlock, President & CEO, Association of Air Medical Services (AAMS)

Mr. SHERLOCK. Thank you. Good morning, Chairwoman Eshoo, Ranking Member Burgess, and distinguished members of the subcommittee.

On behalf of the association of Air Medical Services, we look forward to working with you to ensure everyone in America has access to lifesaving emergency air medical services when they need it most.

Emergency air medical services are highly effective medical interventions appropriate in cases where getting a patient directly to the closest most appropriate medical facility can make a significant difference in their survival and recovery.

Today, because of air medical services, 90 percent of Americans can reach a level one or level two trauma center within an hour. However, since 2010, 90 hospitals have closed in rural areas and an estimated 20 percent more are at risk of closing.

Our members fill the gap created by closures, but this lifeline is fraying as 31 air medical bases have also closed in 2019. Emergency air medical providers never make the decision on who to transport. That decision is always made by a requesting physician or medically trained first responder.

Air medical crews then respond within minutes, 24 hours a day, 7 days a week without any knowledge of a patient's ability to pay for their services.

Our members are unique in the healthcare system. The service is heavily regulated by the states for the purposes of healthcare as ambulances and the Federal government for aviation safety and services as air carriers. It is their status as air carriers that allow rapid transport of patients over significant distances.

Over 33 percent of our flights cross State lines every day. For that reason, the Airline Deregulation Act's uniform authority over the national airspace is essential to the provision of this lifesaving service.

Exemption air medical services from the ADA would allow states to regulate aviation services including where and when they are able to fly, limiting access to healthcare for patients in crisis.

Congress took significant action on emergency air medical billing in 2018. In the FAA reauthorization act, Congress established the Advisory Committee on Air Ambulance and Patient Billing.

Congress would benefit from reviewing the work of the Advisory Committee, which was tasked to recommend actions to provide relief for patients while taking into account the unique operational, regulatory, and financial aspects of emergency air medical services.

To prevent balance billing, our members are actively negotiating with insurance companies to secure in-network agreements. One member alone has increased their participation from five percent to almost 43 percent in the last three years.

Despite that, some insurers have refused to discuss in-network agreements. That hurts both patients and caregivers. Air medical services are not a cost driver for insurance. According to testimony before the Montana legislature Joint Economic Affairs Subcommittee in 2016, supported by national health insurance data, covering air medical services in full represents about a $1.70 of the average monthly premium. More than 70 percent of the 360,000 patients transported by helicopter air ambulances each year are covered by Medicare, Medicaid, or are uninsured. According to a study conducted by Xcenda in 2017, $10,199 was the median cost of providing a helicopter transport, while Medicare paid $5,998, Medicaid paid $3,463 and the uninsured paid $354.

This results in an ongoing imbalance between actual costs and government reimbursement and is the single biggest factor in increasing costs.

AAMS strongly supports legislation that would increase transparency regarding air medical services and reform the Medicare reimbursement system for those services, which is a primary driver of balance billing.

Legislation introduced in the 115th Congress supported on this committee by Congressman Ruiz and Johnson and co-sponsored by Chairwoman Eshoo, the Ensuring Access to Air Ambulance Services Act, would mandate 100 percent industry reporting of comprehensive cost data to the Centers for Medicare and Medicaid and then rebase Medicare fees for emergency air medical transport using that data, which would address the gap between reimbursements and costs.

Additionally, there are reported incidents where individuals receive high bills for cases of prescheduled nonemergent private airplane transports. AAMS refers all such inquiries and reports to the Department of Transportation consumer protection division in the hopes that the agency exercises its already existing authority to protect consumers.

Finally, AAMS would ask the committee to recognize the tremendous commitment our industry members and caregivers make who have dedicated their life's work to serving others and to ensure critical emergency medical response is always available to the communities they serve.

AAMS believes in protecting patients. Our members protect them every day. AAMS thanks the committee for the opportunity to offer this testimony and asks the committee to recognize the unique aspects of this essential service and not to curtail access to healthcare for patients in crisis.

[The Prepared Statement of Mr. Sherlock follows:]

Written Testimony of Rick Sherlock

The Association of Air Medical Services (AAMS) is the leading international organization representing the air medical industry and over 250 air ambulance services across the United States, offering emergency helicopter and fixed wing air medical services. Our vision is to assure that every person has access to high-quality air medical and critical care transport in their time of crisis. Our members are actively working to address balance billing issues related to their services through patient advocacy programs and dramatic increases in their in-network agreements, which take patients out of the middle and hold them harmless. AAMS supports solutions that take patients out of the middle while preserving access to our critical life-saving services. During the last Congress, AAMS supported the bipartisan, bicameral language in the FAA Reauthorization Act that mandated the Air Ambulance Patient Billing Advisory Committee determine appropriate solutions to address billing and cost issues and recommend best practices and steps that can be taken to protect consumers. We request that Congress do no harm and protect access to the critical, life-saving medical interventions and the access to critical care levels of health care that our services provide. In time-sensitive, life-threatening illnesses and injuries, when seconds matter, we want to continue to keep these patients alive.

In summary, AAMS recommends that Congress take the following steps:

- Support and encourage immediate implementation of the Department Of Transportation's Advisory Committee On Air Ambulance And Patient Billing (AAPB) which is to identify actions to "protect consumers from balance billing" as directed by Congress in the 2018 FAA Reauthorization Act.
- Enact legislation that would require all air medical providers to submit cost and quality data to the Centers for Medicare and Medicaid Services (CMS) and give CMS the authority to update the reimbursement fee schedule. This allows the Federal government, in addition to other stakeholders and the public, to better understand the true costs of emergency air medical services and how the industry operates to provide these services. Moreover, this will enable CMS to update the outdated Medicare reimbursement rate to accurately reflect true industry costs. Requiring all air medical providers to report this data and CMS to reimburse emergency air medical services based on the actual costs of transport will help reduce cost shifting to the private market and increase the number of in-network agreements, which would eliminate the balance billing issue.
- Encourage the Department of Transportation to use its existing authority to investigate charges of certain non-emergency, on-demand private airplane transports that may exceed standard industry charges for similar services, including investigating how such services are arranged.

AAMS offers the following written testimony in support of these recommendations.

Background on Emergency Air Medical Services

AAMS represents both helicopter and fixed-wing air medical providers and operators who deliver life-saving emergency transports every day. AAMS members transport approximately 360,000 critically ill and injured patients per year via emergency helicopter transport and an additional 100,000 per year via fixed-wing airplanes, some of which are also emergency transports. Emergency air medical services (EAMS) go beyond typical ambulance services, as they are essentially flying emergency rooms and critical care units, capable of a level of care beyond most ground ambulance services. They are highly-effective medical interventions, but they are an expensive service that should only be used according to pre-existing protocols developed by local medical and emergency response authorities.

It's important to note that emergency air medical services do not decide which patients are transported by air medical or ground ambulance services. They never self-dispatch; they only respond to requests from medically-trained first-responders or physicians. Medically-trained first responders or physicians determine whether patients need emergency air medical services based on a variety of factors, including but not limited to, the higher level of care offered by an air medical crew (e.g., airway stabilization, blood transfusions, etc.); the need for more rapid transport than a ground transport would allow based on the patient's condition; or the geography in remote or rural areas and the distance to travel to tertiary care. Emergency air medical providers are called to respond to both on-scene requests from first responders and emergency inter-facility requests from physicians.

Emergency air medical crews respond to those requests within minutes, day or night; they are ready to respond to the most seriously ill or injured patients on a 24 hours-per-day 7 days-per-week basis. Air medical crews are dedicated critical care providers, with higher levels of training, equipment, and experience than most ground ambulance providers. Air medical pilots are some of the most experienced in aviation. Through both voluntary industry commitments and industry-supported regulations, air medical helicopters operate at a higher level of aviation safety than the rest of the on-demand aviation segments, with several regulations designed solely to address the unique risks associated with the emergency air medical environment. *AAMS would ask the Committee to recognize the tremendous commitment that these individuals make to ensure critical emergency medical response is always available to the communities they serve.*

Approximately 90% of the patients transported by emergency air medical helicopters are for stroke, cardiac, and trauma conditions; the remaining 10% encompass specialty pediatric care, burns, neonatal, high-risk obstetrics, neurological, and other conditions. Because these age-related conditions are more prevalent in Medicare and Medicaid populations, our members' transport volume directly impacts that patient mix.[10]

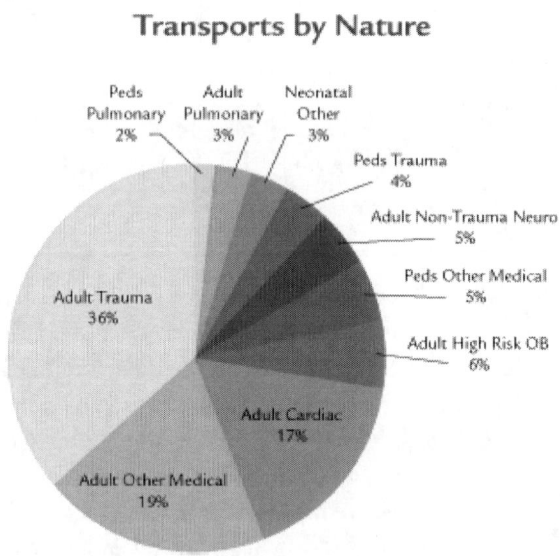

The Increasing Need for Emergency Air Medical Services

EAMS is a critical component of the health care delivery system in the United States, ensuring that critically injured patients are able to quickly and safely access trauma care and other critical

[10] https://www.healthsystemtracker.org/chart-collection/know-cardiovascular-disease-spending-outcomes-united-states/#item-mortality-rates-within-30-days-hospital-admission-heart-attack-stroke-decreased-version-2.

tertiary care. Nearly 85 million Americans can only access a Level I or Level II trauma center within 60 minutes via helicopter. Another 30 million Americans do not have access to these centers within this time sensitive window - sometimes called the "golden hour - even by air. Nonetheless, EAMS serves as a critical lifeline to these individuals who often live in rural areas.

On March 20, 2019, the Government Accountability Office (GAO) published its report, "Air Ambulance: Available Data Show Privately-Insured Patients Are at Financial Risk." Congress required the GAO to produce the report in the "Explanatory Statement" for Division H of the "Consolidated Appropriations Act, 2017" (H.R. 244). That language directed the GAO "to submit a report to the Committees on Appropriations of the House of Representatives and the Senate on fixed-wing and helicopter air ambulance services, operational costs, and, as available, payment structures no later than 18 months after the enactment of this Act." GAO reported that "there were 752 bases in the 2012 data and 868 bases in the 2017 data." The report also notes that the added bases:

- "increased the total area served by helicopter bases by 23 percent." "About 60 percent of the new helicopter bases and about half of the new fixed-wing bases…were in rural areas."
- "For just under half of the new helicopter bases…the area served overlapped with existing air ambulance coverage by more than 50 percent." Added bases "increased the total area served by helicopter bases by 23 percent."

EAMS expansion in rural areas helped fill the gap in rural health care created by closing rural hospitals. As recent media reports from Fort Scott, KS[11]; Fairfax, OK[12]; and Port Arthur, TX[13] show, rural communities are devastated by the loss of their hospital facilities and the anxiety over who will provide access for emergency health care needs. Those closures follow the closing of 64 rural hospitals in 2013-2017, according to the GAO. Most closures were in southern states, with Texas experiencing 14 closures, but the Midwest, West and Northeast regions also lost hospitals. Furthermore, Navigant recently published an analysis that indicates as many as 21 percent of rural hospitals could be at risk for closing due to changes in payer reimbursements[14].

The ability of EAMS to fill the gap in access to health care in rural America, is diminishing. Due to mounting financial pressure, since January 1, 2019, 31 helicopter air ambulance bases have closed and the third largest helicopter air ambulance provider in the United States is only now on the path for emergence from voluntary bankruptcy protection filing in March, 2019. Many of the closed bases were located in rural areas where they did not suffer from lack of transport demand but suffered economically due to a larger portion of Medicare, Medicaid, and uninsured patients.

The combination of fewer air medical bases and fewer rural hospitals should be of great concern to Congress. At a time when rural hospitals are closing, it is critical to maintain, or

[11] https://www.npr.org/sections/health-shots/2019/05/14/722199393/no-mercy-how-a-kansas-town-is-grappling-with-its-hospitals-closure.

[12] https://www.washingtonpost.com/news/national/wp/2019/05/11/feature/whos-going-to-take-care-of-these-people/?noredirect=on&utm_term=.504dc41b782d).

[13] https://www.beaumontenterprise.com/opinions/editorials/article/ENTERPRISE-EDITORIAL-St-Mary-closing-is-part-of-13937084.php.

[14] https://www.modernhealthcare.com/article/20190220/NEWS/190229999/nearly-a-quarter-of-rural-hospitals-are-on-the-brink-of-closure.

even to increase access to emergency transportation for rural and underserved Americans. An increase in the time required to transport a critically ill or injured patient from an incident scene to the appropriate facility brings with it the risks of life-altering complications or even death. Unfortunately, with the closure of air medical bases and the continued closure of rural hospitals, it seems inevitable that transportation times will increase.

AAMS' members also serve a vital role in our homeland security infrastructure. Notably, our members respond to disasters working in partnership with FEMA and other Federal and State agencies. If federal policy to remedy economic issues effecting emergency air medical services are not implemented, the current capacity of EAMS to surge to support robust participation in disaster response may also be at risk.

The Economics of Air Medical Transport

As of 2017, over 70% of air medical flights are under-reimbursed as they transport Medicare, Medicaid or uninsured patients. EAMS are rarely publicly funded; less than 10% of EAMS nationwide are through a publicly funded agency. This results in an ongoing imbalance between actual costs and government reimbursement and is a significant change from just 10 years ago, when the Medicare and Medicaid populations were significantly smaller. As those populations increased as a percentage of the overall number of transports conducted, the uncompensated cost of those transports multiplied, increasing the cost for all transports. Today, the single biggest factor increasing cost is the Medicare reimbursement gap. According to a study conducted by Xcenda in 2017[15]:

- $10,199.00: Median cost of providing one helicopter transport
  - $5,998.00: Median Medicare reimbursement (base rate plus mileage) per transport
  - $3,463.00: Median Medicaid reimbursement per transport
  - $354.00 Median self-pay (uninsured) reimbursement

Seven out of ten of patients transported by EAMS are either Medicare, Medicaid, or uninsured; the remaining three out of ten patients must subsidize the remaining cost. This is unsustainable, and drives a significant cost-shift to private insurance-compensated transports.

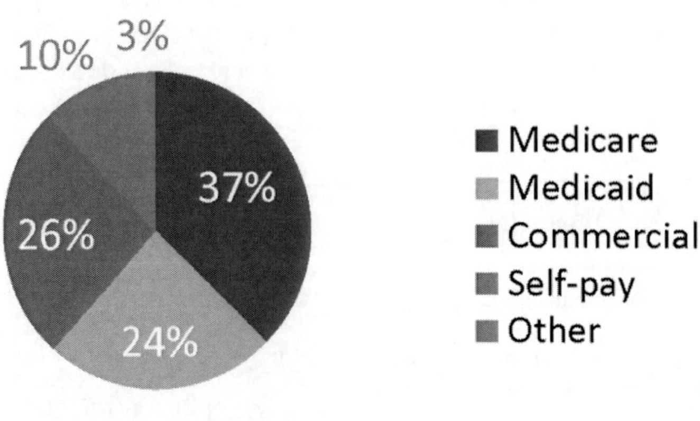

[15] https://aams.org/aams-publishes-findings-air-medical-cost-study/.

Of the approximately 360,000 patients transported by EAMS per year:

- ~133,200 are Medicare patients (37%);
- ~86,400 are Medicaid patients (24%);
- ~36,000 are uninsured patients (10%);
- ~93,600 are commercially insured (26%) (approximately 40% of those patients would be in-network);
- ~10,800 are covered by "other" insurance (3%).

The study further found that uncompensated care incurred by serving Medicare, Medicaid, and uninsured patients creates cost deficits that require private payers to cover more than $26,000 per transport to allow providers to just break even. Resolving the Medicare cost gap would reduce the pressures that drive higher pricing, as well as to limit a patient's potential exposure to a balance bill.

These numbers-both the high fixed cost of providing the service and the mix of patients transported-become significantly worse in rural areas. Rural areas carry the highest demand (mostly due to hospital closures), as well as a significantly higher ratio of Medicare, Medicaid, and uninsured patients. As the recent EAMS base closures show, we are less likely to have the ability to serve the areas where emergency air ambulance transports are needed most.

AAMS strongly supports legislation that would reform the broken Medicare reimbursement system for EAMS, which is a primary driver of balance billing. Legislation introduced in the 115th Congress, the "Ensuring Access to Air Ambulance Services Act" (H.R. 3378), would rebase the Medicare fees for emergency air medical transports utilizing comprehensive cost data collected from providers. This rebasing would address the growing gap between Medicare reimbursements and the actual costs of providing the service.

Air Medical Services and the Airline Deregulation Act

EAMS are unique in the health care system. Air ambulance medical services provided in flight are done so in a unique environment and with concerns for aviation and patient safety that only exist in the air. The service is heavily regulated by the states for the purposes of health care (as ambulances) and the federal government for aviation safety and services (as air carriers). Emergency air medical services are ambulances in that they transport critically ill and injured patients, but it is their status as air carriers that allows rapid transport of those patients over longer distances; over 33% of EAMS flights cross state lines every day and nearly all of them will cross a county or municipal boundary.

The Airline Deregulation Act's (ADA) uniform authority over the national airspace is essential to the provision of this life-saving service. Air medical services were always meant to be included as air carriers under the ADA; a Senate floor colloquy directly discussed "the need for air ambulance services" during debate on the ADA on April 19, 1978.[16]

Exempting air medical services from the ADA would allow states to regulate a wide range of issues in relationship to the aviation aspects of a licensed air-carrier, including where and when they are able to fly, creating borders in the sky and limiting access to critical care. Rate

[16] https://aams.org/wp-content/uploads/2018/06/ADA-Leg-Hx-involving-Air-Ambulances-1978.pdf.

regulation is only the latest argument in a long history of attempts by some states to regulate the following issues:

- Competition in air medical transport;
- Aviation safety regulations;
- The size of the aircraft;
- The areas in which the aircraft can operate;
- The distances an aircraft can travel; and
- The relationship to hospitals or existing medical services.

Emergency air medical services are already heavily regulated by states; they are licensed ambulance providers overseen by state-licensed medical directors. States have full and unfettered authority to regulate every aspect of the provision of medical care within the aircraft. Further, states and local communities often regulate the triage protocols for requesting an emergency air medical service, and whether that patient should be taken by air or ground.

Should there be a change to the 40-year-old federal primacy over aviation and air carrier regulation, there would be enormous consequences for air medical operations, including:

- Negative Impact on Safety: Allowing states to regulate prices or billing would reduce financial compensation needed to invest in both required and voluntary safety enhancements. EAMS operators support enhanced safety regulation and stand fully committed to additional safety enhancements beyond regulation (night vision goggles, Crash Resistance Fuel Systems, and robust flight operational quality assurance systems). All of those safety enhancements would be severely hampered by state rate regulation that reduces the ability to make these investments.
- Borders in the Sky: The ADA protects airlines from state regulation on air carrier routes. By exempting EAMS from the ADA, state authorities would be allowed to regulate where air medical services fly, usually in attempts to restrict competition. For example, an aircraft in South Carolina transported a critically injured child to a North Carolina hospital. The hospital, acting under the state's then-existing Certificate of Need (CON) law, attempted to bar the aircraft from the helipad, going so far as to threaten the impoundment of the aircraft and the arrest of its crew. A federal court affirmed the ADA's protection of that aircraft's ability to cross borders and ensure that the closest appropriate aircraft can transport a patient to the closest appropriate hospital or trauma facility for their time-sensitive medical condition.
- Decrease in Access to Critical Air Medical Transport, especially in Rural Areas: Limiting the number of air medical services in an area (including through CON laws) will cause a significant decrease in access, especially in rural areas, in cases where state-regulated systems arbitrarily determine a lack of sufficient "need."
- Limit Patient Care Decisions by Referring Physicians: In the case of inter-facility transports, physicians are currently able to make a transport determination based on their expertise and the condition of the patient. Altering the ADA would limit that decision-making ability.
- Restrict access to choose: A state could restrict the ability of a health care entity to choose to possess their own Part 135 certificate, or to freely choose the Part 135

operator that meets their needs. Restrictions on the ability of an air carrier to operate where needed means that a state could choose to not allow an operator to provide services within its boundaries.

Current Efforts to Address Balance Bills: Patient Advocacy and Network Participation

AAMS' members are addressing balance billing in a number of ways, including through patient advocacy programs and increased insurance network participation. AAMS is concerned that recent insurance industry behavior toward emergency air medical transport has only worsened problems of balance billing and air medical program stability, especially in the rural environment.

States possess the ability to regulate insurance plans offered within their borders, with the exception of federally-regulated Employee Retirement Income Security Act (ERISA) plans. Together, either the state or the federal government has the authority to compel insurers to offer insurance products that provide fair compensation for emergency air medical services. Yet, private insurance has responded by increasingly setting rates arbitrarily or denying payments through medical necessity denials, underpayments, and other tactics. For example, nearly half of all claims are initially denied reimbursement by the health plan. Almost 40% of these denials are for medical necessity – a decision made by the attending physician or first responder based on medical protocols and state EMS protocols, not the air medical program. If insurance companies are allowed to disregard decisions made in emergency situations, by a medical professional that are in the best interest of the insured patient, then what is the purpose of health insurance? Health care providers, especially in emergency situations, cannot be concerned with their decisions being second-guessed after-the-fact by insurers, whose intent may be more focused on financial concerns than patient needs.

Our members are actively negotiating with insurance companies to secure in-network contracts where such negotiations are available. Despite that willingness to negotiate in-network rates, some insurers, citing low volumes and infrequent need for transports, have outright refused to even discuss an in-network agreement with emergency air medical providers. AAMS finds that refusal simply unconscionable; while it may make sense to the insurer, it hurts both the patients they are insuring and the health care providers. Despite this, our members have managed to increase network participation significantly; one member alone has increased their overall network participation from 2% to almost 30% in the last three years. Insurance companies must recognize the need for this service and limit questions of medical necessity, enter into network negotiations with emergency air medical providers, and stop the practice of slow payments or payments directly to the patient (which only places patients in the middle).

It is important to note that emergency air medical transports are not a cost driver for health insurance companies – in fact, this life-saving service is less than one percent of all health care costs. According to testimony before the Montana Legislature Joint Economic Affairs Subcommittee in 2016, and supported by national health insurance data, covering air medical services in full represents about $1.70 of the average monthly premium. While these services are expensive to operate and expensive per transport due to the nature of the service, the math shows that they can be covered easily by health insurers for a tiny fraction of a monthly insurance premium. Emergency air ambulance transport is an extremely rare service and a very small part of the entire health care delivery system. According to the 2018 Milliman Medical Index Study on health care costs, emergency air ambulance services represent a tiny fraction of the "other" 4% of premium costs ("other" costs also includes ground ambulance, durable medical equipment (DME), home health, and all medical supplies)[17]. To break it down even further, air ambulance transports account for less than 1% of all ambulance transports.

Many of AAMS' members have patient advocacy programs that allow dedicated patient advocates to work side-by-side with patients to help them and their families navigate the complex world of insurance claims. If, and when, the insurance company underpays or rejects a first responder or physician's decision, our members' patient advocacy programs intervene by advocating on the patients' behalf to appeal these decisions and ensure they are covered fairly by the health plan for which they pay their premiums. Our members are committed to helping our patients from the start of their medical emergency until their claim is resolved. For one of our largest members, *through their growing in network relationships, patient advocacy and robust financial assistance program, the average out of pocket for their patients including copays and deductibles is less than $400.*

Emergency Air Medical Services vs. Non-Emergent Medical Transport

EAMS provide emergency medical response 24 hours-per-day, seven days-per-week to ensure that patients have access to, and receive, the best care and transport possible, regardless of when or where an emergency happens. Providers transport a patient only when a physician or medically-trained first responder has deemed air medical transport medically necessary. Whether these transports are from the actual scene of an accident or injury (such as the side of the road or a football field) or inter-facility (from a smaller less-equipped hospital to more advanced care at a tertiary health care center), they are all deemed emergency situations by the requesting physician or first responder. After determining whether the flight conditions allow for a safe flight, EAMS respond to every request within minutes and without knowledge or regard for a patient's ability to pay.

Emergency air medical services include all helicopter transports. In some cases of extreme distances fixed-wing airplanes are used in emergency patient response; while these flights are less frequent, they are by no means less critical.

There are also services that offer non-emergency private fixed-wing airplane medical transport by air. Those services are not always requested by physicians; they can be requested by anyone with an ability to pay, and are most often arranged through hospital case managers or by patients' families using internet directories. Traditionally, and like any pre-arranged private air-taxi service, the fees for private airplane medical transportation would be paid up-front by the person arranging the flight; these flights would rarely be covered by Medicare, Medicaid, or private insurance.

AAMS is aware of several companies currently offering different options to arrange and finance these types of flights; AAMS has also received questions regarding these types of privately arranged airplane transports. It should be noted that these flights are no different in their arrangement than any other on-demand private aircraft transport. These flights should also

[17] http://www.milliman.com/uploadedFiles/insight/Periodicals/mmi/2018-milliman-medical-index.pdf.

never be confused with emergency air medical services or the economic issues faced by emergency air medical services or providers.

AAMS refers all questions and concerns regarding billing to the Department of Transportation's Consumer Protection Division (DOT CPD). DOT CPD has full authority to regulate the economic aspect of these services and AAMS strongly recommends that DOT exercise this authority wherever necessary to ensure that patients and their insurers are informed of the full cost estimate of the services before the non-emergent flight and are not excessively charged following the flight.

Legislative Actions Already Taken to Address Air Medical Balance Billing

In order to address possible billing concerns, and because EAMS is both ambulance and air-carrier, Congress took significant action on emergency air medical balance billing in 2018. In the "FAA Reauthorization Act of 2018" (H.R. 302):

- Congress established the "Advisory Committee on Air Ambulance and Patient Billing," which is composed of all stakeholders in air medical services and is directed to identify actions to "protect consumers from balance billing." The Committee includes the Secretary of Health and Human Services and is further required to make recommendations for "consumer protection...and the prevention of balance billing," including "options, best practices, and identified standards to prevent instances of balance billing." The provision requires the Committee to deliver its final report to Congress, and further directs the Secretary of Transportation to issue any necessary regulations or guidance to enhance the transparency and data reporting of emergency air medical providers and establish "consumer protections for customers of air ambulance providers."
- Another provision of the FAA Reauthorization Act requires the Secretary of Transportation to provide a separate report to Congress on plans for additional "oversight of air ambulance providers."
- A third section of the legislation establishes additional requirements for emergency air medical services, including providing contact information for the Department of Transportation's Aviation Consumer Advocate.

We would urge both the Committee and Congress to allow the Advisory Committee to carry out its mandate, which is specifically required to identify solutions to EAMS balance billing issues. Congress structured the Advisory Committee to bring together insurers, insurance regulators, consumer groups, physicians, and air medical providers to perform a comprehensive review and to recommend actions to provide relief for patients while taking into account the unique operational, regulatory, and financial aspects of emergency air medical services.

Even before enactment of the FAA Reauthorization Act, the Department of Transportation took action, using its existing authority, as described in the 2017 Government Accountability Office (GAO) report on air medical billing and cost issues. The Department's Aviation Consumer Protection Division established a portal for addressing air ambulance consumer complaints, and is responding to those complaints. In 2018, of over 350,000 air medical transports, DOT has received 24 complaints, which represents approximately .007% of all patient transports. To date in 2019, 6 complaints have been reported to DOT.

In Conclusion: Increase Transparency, Preserve the Service, and Do No Harm

AAMS also supports efforts to increase transparency regarding emergency air medical services, costs, and prices. The FAA Reauthorization Act tasks the Advisory Committee with developing recommendations for the federal collection of additional data on costs, charges and payments, operations, and competition.

The "Ensuring Access to Air Ambulance Services Act" would also enhance transparency, not only by collecting comprehensive cost data, but also by directing the GAO to compile this data into a report to Congress. The legislation would also establish a data collection program for reporting of quality metrics for health care provided by emergency air medical services.

As rural hospitals continue to close, air medical transports provide an essential, life-saving service for rural patients. The ongoing and growing shortfall in Medicare and government payments for the service is undermining the ability of providers to continue to serve patients-in-need. It is therefore vital for Congress to both reform Medicare reimbursements and avoid taking any action that would accelerate the closure of bases and further limit access to critical levels of health care for millions of Americans.

We believe that some current ideas to solve for balance billing for patients are misguided, such as a proposal to require air medical providers to separate "aviation" costs from "health care" costs in bills. Emergency medical care provided in flight is done so in a unique environment and with concerns for aviation and patient safety that only exist in the air. Health care and aviation services are inextricably linked and impossible to separate in any meaningful way. For example, many aircraft are fitted with external oxygen tanks to decrease the risk of cabin fire, thus changing the nature of delivering oxygen to patients. The costs for that service are increased by its use in an airborne environment, and should not be compared to similar services on the ground. Most importantly, the separation of bills in this manner would provide no discernable benefit for patients, and does nothing to reduce the costs of emergency air medical services or protect patients from receiving balance bills caused by extraordinarily low payments made by insurers or insurer's refusal to discuss in-network agreements with air medical providers.

Additionally, proposals to limit air ambulance charges by using Medicare as a metric would be devasting to EAMS. As we have shown, and as independent studies have clearly indicated, the current Medicare fee schedule was developed without a study of costs and since its implementation CMS has never collected a single cost data point nor undertaken an analysis of the cost of providing the services. By capping rates at 125% of Medicare as some propose, EAMS would essentially collect the following:

- $10,199.00: Median cost of providing one helicopter transport
  - $7,497.50 Proposed Median Commercial Insurance reimbursement per transport
  - $5,998.00: Median Medicare reimbursement (base rate plus mileage) per transport
  - $3,463.00: Median Medicaid reimbursement per transport
  - $354.00 Median Self-Pay Reimbursement

This proposal would end emergency air medical transport in the United States, limiting services only to those communities who choose to provide them as a public service or hospitals willing to subsidize the bulk of the cost.

Finally, we believe that the entire discussion of balance and surprise billing, at least as it has applied to emergency air medical services, seems to ignore a simple but important principle: "do no harm." Do no harm to patients who may receive these bills, but also do no harm to the caregivers who have dedicated their life's work to serving others, either in the back of helicopter, a ground ambulance, an emergency room, or at a patient's bedside. AAMS believes in protecting patients; our members protect them every day. AAMS believes in protecting them from the devastating disability of strokes and heart attacks, protecting their lives from horrible injuries caused by accidents, and protecting them from worsening injuries sustained during floods, storms, mass shootings, and other natural disasters.

AAMS thanks the Committee for the opportunity to offer this testimony and welcomes continued dialogue on this important topic. Again, we ask the Committee to recognize the unique and distinct regulatory, economic and operational aspects of this essential service and to take care that any legislation does not inadvertently curtail access to EAMS for patients-in-need.

* * *

Ms. ESHOO. Thank you, Mr. Sherlock.

Now I would like to recognize Mr. Gelfand for five minutes for your testimony.

Statement of James Gelfand, Senior Vice President, Health Policy, The ERISA Industry Committee

Mr. GELFAND. Chairwoman Eshoo, Ranking Member Burgess, and members of the subcommittee, thank you for this opportunity to testify.

I am James Gelfand, senior vice president for health policy at the ERISA Industry Committee, a trade association representing large employer plan sponsors.

Our member companies offer comprehensive health benefits and as self-insured plans pay around 85 percent of healthcare costs for our beneficiaries. About 181 million Americans get insurance through a job and surprise billing fundamentally frustrates the goal of providing quality affordable employer-sponsored coverage.

The vast majority of our employees are not doctors, HR executives, or medical billing experts, nor should they have to be. But patients are falling victim to impossible complexities. Employers are ready to work with Congress to right the ship. We are focused on three scenarios in which patients end up with big bills they couldn't see coming or avoid.

Number 1, a patient receives care at an in-network facility but is treated by an out-of-network provider. Number 2, a patient requires emergency care, but the provider's facility or transportation are out of network. And number 3, a patient is transferred or handed off without sufficient information or alternatives. It is usually not the providers you're planning to see.

It is the anesthesiologists, radiologists, pathologists, or emergency providers or transport for an unexpected trip to the NICU.

Many work for outsourced medical staffing firms that have adopted a scam strategy of staying out of networks, practicing at in-network facilities, and surprise billing patients. It is deeply concerning but the problem is narrowly defined and therefore we can fix it.

ERIC applauds the committee for taking the lead on solving this. The No Surprises Act nails it. It takes patients out of the middle and creates a market-based benchmark rate to pay providers fairly.

The benchmark is not developed by government and it is not price setting. The committee might also consider network matching. It is simple.

If a provider practices at an in-network facility, they take the in-network rate, or they go work somewhere else. Or base the benchmark on Medicare. You could set the rate higher, say, 125 percent of Medicare, and still make the system more affordable, sustainable, and simpler.

These approaches will eliminate the surprise bills. That's a huge win for patients and improves the system by creating certainty for payers and fair pay for providers.

But not everyone wants to stop surprise bills. Some provider specialties are saying, let us keep doing what we are doing—just use binding arbitration to make someone else pay these bills. They're asking for a nontransparent process that could force plans and employers to pay massive and fake medical list prices.

It is essentially setting money on fire. Funds that would have been used to pay for healthcare will instead be spent on administrative costs such as lawyers, arbitrators, facility fees, and on unreasonable settlement amounts. Make no mistake, patients will pay these costs.

The ground and air ambulance companies are asking Congress to let them keep surprise billing, too. Do nothing, wait for another study, another report, and there have already been four.

They know patients cannot shop for them and many participate in no networks. State insurance commissioners are begging for help with air ambulances. But Congress has tied their hands.

Employers think Congress should end this. Treat medical transport the same as emergency care. We should end surprise billing in the ER and on the way there.

Other providers figure they're willing to stop surprise billing but only if they can increase in-network rates. They're calling for network adequacy rules to force insurers and employers to add more providers to their networks, even if those providers demand astronomical payments.

Does anyone here actually believe that these hospital-based doctors whose services cannot be shopped for, who are guaranteed to see our patients, are begging to be included in our networks but nobody will return their calls? That they have no choice but to go and join these out-of-network Wall Street-owned firms?

It doesn't make sense. Employers design health benefits to help our beneficiaries. We don't sell insurance. We want networks that meet our patients' needs. Why would we want to cover an operation but leave out the anaesthesia?

We want our employees to be able to afford their health insurance, too, and that means we must be able to say no when providers are gaming the system. We are here to solve a specific problem, not to create new ones. Network adequacy is a distraction. Let's focus on protecting patients from surprise medical bills.

In conclusion, thank you for this opportunity to share our views. The ERISA Industry Committee is eager to work with Congress towards a bipartisan comprehensive solution that protects access to care and ends the surprise billing crisis without driving up health insurance costs.

And I am happy to answer any questions.

[The prepared statement of Mr. Gelfand follows:]

Written Testimony of James Gelfand

Intro and About ERIC

Chairwoman Eshoo, Ranking Member Burgess, and members of the Subcommittee, thank you for this opportunity to testify on the surprise medical billing crisis. I'm James Gelfand, Senior Vice President for Health Policy at The ERISA Industry Committee – ERIC for short – the only national association that advocates exclusively for large employers on health, retirement, and compensation public policies at the federal, state, and local levels. ERIC member companies are leaders in every sector of the economy, with employees in every state, and we represent them in their capacity as sponsors of employee benefit plans for their own workforce.

Each of you and your constituents likely engage with an ERIC member company when you drive a car or fill it with gas, use a cell phone or a computer, visit a bank or hotel, fly on an airplane, watch TV, benefit from our national defense, go shopping, receive or send a package, wear makeup, or enjoy a soft drink.

Our member companies offer comprehensive health benefits to employees, their families, and often retirees, too. On average, large employers pay around 85 percent of health care costs on behalf of our beneficiaries – that would be a gold or platinum plan if bought on an Exchange. But we don't generally buy or sell health insurance; these plans are self-insured. In other words, ultimately it is the company that is on the hook for the vast majority of the costs of our patients' care. There are about 181 million Americans who get health care through their job, and over 100 million of them are in self-insured plans like ours.

We offer these great health benefits to attract and retain employees, to be competitive for human capital, and to improve health and provide peace of mind. Large employers, like ERIC member companies, roll up their sleeves to improve how health care is delivered in communities across the country. They do this by developing value-driven and coordinated care programs, implementing employee wellness programs, providing transparency tools, and a myriad of other innovations that improve quality and value to drive down costs. These efforts often use networks to guide our employees and their family members to providers of higher quality and lower cost. Surprise billing undermines all of this and fundamentally frustrates the goals of providing quality, affordable employer-sponsored health benefits.

ERIC is the only national association that advocates exclusively for large employers on health, retirement, and compensation public policies at the federal, state, and local levels.

No doubt you have heard from your constituents about this. ERIC has also heard from our member companies about beneficiaries who have fallen victim to devastating surprise bills. We can provide examples upon request. Again, these are beneficiaries with some of the most robust insurance coverage available, and still they are experiencing immense, and in our view, unnecessary hardship.

Often these employees do everything right. They look up in-network providers. They call ahead. They ask questions at the hospital. But still, they later receive enormous, unexpected bills. These horror stories of surprise bills have our beneficiaries afraid to go to the hospital at all – even with a platinum plan! They're skipping care, they're worried while at work, and we have no choice but to call for bold action from Congress to address what has become a surprise billing *crisis.*

This crisis is narrowly confined and straightforward to resolve. There is a bipartisan path forward. We commend Congress for rolling up its sleeves to look into why surprise bills are generated, and how you can stop them. For large employers, this is not a question of who should pay, but rather how to stop these bills from ever being generated, because these surprise bills are unfair and should never happen.

About Surprise Medical Bills

The vast majority of health care providers rarely or never generate surprise bills. It's almost exclusively confined to specific and small subsets of the health system that the patient does not have the ability to choose or shop for. Primarily, these are ancillary providers working in a hospital (such as pathologists, radiologists, anesthesiologists, assistant surgeons), emergency care providers such as ER doctors, neonatologists, ambulances and air ambulances whose service the patient cannot refuse or negotiate, or surprise fees from the hospital itself.

Patients are experiencing three scenarios that consistently give rise to a surprise medical bill:

- A patient receives care at an in-network facility, and at some point, during the course of care, (without the patient's advance knowledge or consent, or without presenting the patient with a meaningful alternative), the patient is treated by an out-of-network provider;
- A patient requires emergency care, and the providers, facility, or medical transportation are outside of the patient's insurance network; and
- A patient is transferred or handed off to care, but not properly informed that this care is out-of-network, and not offered sufficient alternatives.

It is true that there are other situations that can potentially lead to bills for the patient, but most of these are not what the public is talking about in the national conversation regarding surprise medical bills. For example, some have suggested that a surprise medical bill is when an individual receives care and doesn't realize they have not yet reached their insurance deductible. Others have cited instances where an individual violates the terms of their plan and goes to the emergency room for non-emergency care. Some provider groups are seizing on the opportunity to try and dismantle existing standards related to step-therapy and prior authorization, mental health parity rules, and formulary management, too. We urge Congress not to deviate from the core three scenarios above.

There are those who are trying to use this debate about surprise billing to unravel the system of networks that has developed, but employers and insurers need networks in order to ensure beneficiaries obtain the highest quality care, to control costs, and to ensure access for our patients. We believe the best course of action is to work to directly address the crisis at hand, and avoid relitigating "network adequacy" or the rules established in the Affordable Care Act.

ERIC's Solutions to Surprise Medical Bills

ERIC, along with many other groups representing employers, believes that Congress can, and should solve this problem – and that the best solutions will be simple, straightforward, and transparent. We propose three core policy changes to decisively end the surprise billing crisis. Here's how to do it:

1. "*In-network matching rate guarantee.*" This is a simple concept – if a patient goes to an in-network facility, every provider they see should be required to accept in-network rates as payment in full. This one change would eliminate any instance of surprise medical billing for a patient going to an in-network facility.
2. "*An emergency, last-resort, benchmark backstop.*" In most instances when a patient needs emergency care, and that care is out-of-network, the insurer or plan sponsor comes to an agreement on payment with the provider. When they cannot, a benchmark is needed to determine an appropriate payment amount. The most straightforward solution would be to designate a percentage of Medicare – we suggest 125 percent of what Medicare would pay that provider, in that market, for that service.
   If Congress prefers to set a benchmark based on private markets, rather than Medicare, another option would be to look at the average contracted rate in a given market – rates mutually agreed to between insurers and doctors, without government involvement. But if the benchmark rate is equal to or higher than the average… then the average provider will make more money out-of-network. We suggest something like 80 percent of the average. That would ensure fair payment to providers, while encouraging network participation.
3. "*Require informed consent.*" When a transfer or handoff takes place, Congress can require the provider to tell the patient if the care will be out-of-network. If so, they should offer the patient an in-network alternative whenever possible.

Enacting a variation of these three policies would wipe out the vast majority of surprise medical bills, while ensuring patients' access to care, and guaranteeing fair reimbursement to providers. There is still more Congress could do, including cracking down on abusive behavior by outsourced, medical staffing firms, banning certain kickback agreements, and the like. But just the three policies described above would be an incredibly effective start.

About the "No Surprises Act"

ERIC applauds the Energy and Commerce Committee for being early out of the gate with a thoughtful and effective legislative draft to address the surprise billing crisis. The *"No Surprises Act"* creates a reasonable, market-based benchmark in surprise billing situations, taking the patient out of the middle, and providing certainty to plans, plan sponsors, patients, and providers. This is a fair solution, that does not inappropriately "tip the scales" in favor of one sector over another – even so, it addresses some of the deep iniquities currently present in the health care system. Those iniquities have resulted in a system in which, right now, there are winners and losers – and the losers are patients (along with the plans and plan sponsors working and paying on their behalf). The "*No Surprises Act*" brings needed fairness and clarity where currently both are lacking.

Paying Providers Fairly

The legislation creates a benchmark payment rate based on median prices that have been agreed to under contract by providers and insurers in a given geographic region. This proposal leverages market forces to enhance and improve networks for patients, without harming providers' bottom lines. Because the benchmark is based on rates agreed to by both sides of the interaction, without government involvement, any suggestion that this constitutes "price-setting" is simply untrue.

While the Committee deliberates on a benchmark payment rate, we ask that you consider ways to simplify and enhance this approach.

First, in cases of a provider practicing at an in-network facility, we urge the Committee to bypass any need for a benchmark, by simply enacting a "network matching" guarantee. This would completely remove the government from influencing prices in these scenarios, simultaneously protecting patients from most surprise bills, and complementing the Committee's approach thus far. There is bipartisan interest in such an approach: it has been praised by the Brookings Institution and the American Enterprise Institute, the Manhattan Institute, and many others, including more than 40 business groups who are united in supporting network matching.

Network matching preserves complete freedom of choice for providers who don't like the rates in a given facility – they can simply work somewhere else. If sufficient volume and quality of providers cannot be obtained for a facility, then the network rate will necessarily increase. Employers offering health plans for their workforce want high quality providers to be available to care for employees and their families, and recognize that providers should be fairly compensated. Market economics ensure that network matching will *not* lead to provider or access shortages, and because it takes place completely between providers, facilities, and payers, it can protect patients from surprise medical bills with *no government price-setting* and *minimal government involvement.* It even solves much of the "joint venture scam" in which in-network hospitals team up with private-equity-owned outsourced medical staffing firms to charge patients outrageous fees by generating surprise bills. Patients who enter in-network facilities, including the emergency room, have every reason to expect that in-network providers will care for them, at in-network rates.

Unfortunately, network matching cannot solve the problem in cases of out-of-network emergency care. For that scenario, the *No Surprises Act* nails it. ERIC and our member companies support the market-based benchmark approach, as well as others that can potentially save patients more money. For instance, most of the employer community has coalesced around proposals to set a benchmark at 125 percent of Medicare rates, which would vastly simplify the solution.

We also recently learned about proposals from the Council for Affordable Health Coverage (CAHC), and the Progressive Policy Institute (PPI), which have the potential to significantly reduce the deficit and reduce patients' health care costs, while ensuring fair compensation for providers. Those proposals would cap all out-of-network rates at around 200 percent of

Medicare, drawing down to 125-150 percent of Medicare over 5-12 years. This could potentially save billions of dollars and help to bend the health care cost curve.

ERIC also notes that some provider representatives have suggested that Congress should merely stay silent on the resolution of surprise bills – they say Congress need only take the patient out of the middle, and the free market will solve the problem. What they fail to clarify is that the resolution for this will be undertaken in courts of law, costing thousands or millions of dollars, on a case-by-case basis, and creating a patchwork of precedents in different areas. This may work in favor of providers seeking to maximize revenue, but it will harm patients who ultimately will face higher premiums to account for increased litigation and other administrative costs.

National Uniformity for ERISA Plans

It is critical that the Committee's legislation distinguishes between fully-insured health plans and those that are self-insured and thus governed by federal law – the Employee Retirement Income Security Act (ERISA) - as self-insured plans are not, and should not be, subject to state law.

Some advocates are calling for federal legislation to only take effect in states with no surprise billing laws of their own, whereas others are calling for a national "floor" – providing a baseline in all states, and giving those states the option to add even more comprehensive rules on top. This will have a profound effect on Americans enrolled in individual market plans, small employers, and families who get their insurance through a state- or local-government plan. This is because some states have enacted only half-measures, others have taken no action whatsoever, and a few have passed laws that are in fact worse than the status quo, raising costs for all patients.

In the case of self-insured plans and those governed by ERISA, it is critical that one uniform, national standard applies. These employer-sponsored plans should continue to be regulated exclusively at the federal level, unaffected by state policies and regulation. This should include the amount the plan is required to reimburse providers – while it may make sense to vary this amount based on geography, it should still be subject to one national standard. Employers with operations in many states, and their beneficiaries who work or live across the country, should be protected by the same federal standard that enables employers to sponsor nationwide health plans for their workforce. We believe this is the policy the Committee's draft lays out, and urge Congress to maintain this common-sense approach.

Mandatory Binding Arbitration: Just Say "NO"

The Committee thus far has resisted significant pressure from the provider community to punt on solving the surprise medical billing crisis, and instead impose a binding arbitration regime. For this, we salute you. The employer community stands unified in opposition to binding arbitration schemes, for the following reasons:

- These "solutions" do not end surprise billing – they merely change who is subject to paying the surprise bill. As such, binding arbitration enshrines the current strategy of certain medical providers to eschew networks and generate surprise bills. Some particularly egregious proposals put forth would require plans and plan sponsors to promptly pay reasonable market rates to providers who generate surprise bills, but then reward the provider by allowing them to take the plan into arbitration and demand more money;

- Arbitration raises costs, requiring payments to arbitrators, lawyers or other representatives to the parties, and facilities. In "*baseball style*" arbitration it mandates that sometimes the plan or plan sponsor must pay excessive "billed charges" that no competent fiduciary would ever agree to pay. These costs will be passed on directly to patients. ERIC has seen estimates such as a minimum of $1,000 per hour for representation in an arbitration proceeding, a $1,500 filing fee for each party to an arbitration dispute ($3,000 minimum per arbitration), and more. This is a recipe for the incineration of health care dollars by directing funds toward administrative and legal costs, rather than the provisioning of care; and
- In order to avoid out-of-control costs, binding arbitration would still require a benchmark payment rate for the arbitrator to consider – just as the most prominent Senate arbitration proposals do. As such, this choice should be considered less attractive to Congress than its supporters claim, because it does not actually shield Congress from making a decision about backstop payments. Instead, it merely obfuscates this decision, adding in layers of administrative costs, creating a slower and less transparent process, enshrining the current dynamics that have led to the crisis, and burdening the health care system further.

Arbitration is a backdoor way of forcing third-party payers to pay providers based on fake prices: providers' "billed charges" are no different than a branded prescription drug's "list price" or the "sticker price" at an auto dealership. Reasonable people would never agree to pay these prices, nor would the sellers expect them to – it's no different in health care, especially with the out-of-control increases in health care costs every year. Even if we could develop a method of arbitration that eliminated the vast administrative waste likely to occur, it would still be crucial to ensure that "billed charges" were not taken into account and could never be the mandated outcome in a dispute.

For these reasons, ERIC urges the Committee to continue standing strong against demands to implement a binding arbitration or other quasi-judicial regime, rather than directly solving the surprise medical billing problem.

Emergency Medical Transport

ERIC and others in the business community urge Congress not to attempt to address surprise medical billing without including ground and air ambulances. Indeed, we believe that Congress will have done a disservice to patients if they only protect them from balance bills once they enter the hospital doors, but the patient might already be bankrupted from the ride there.

Emergency medical transportation that is out-of-network should be treated exactly the same way out-of-network emergency room care would be treated. These services should be reimbursed based on a benchmark tied either to Medicare rates, or to comparable in-network rates in that of a similar geographic area. Ambulance or air ambulance providers' participation in the Medicare and Medicaid programs should be conditioned upon their agreement to abide by reasonable billing practices – thus eliminating any Congressional jurisdictional concerns that may arise. If that is not feasible, insurers and group health plans should be prohibited from contracting with or directing payments to any ambulance or air ambulance provider that does not abide by said practices – providers will quickly adopt these rules in order to maintain access to third-party payment.

We note that some medical transportation providers have opposed Congressional efforts to protect patients from *their* surprise bills. Ground ambulance providers have suggested that because they are subject to state law, federal surprise billing restrictions should not apply. ERIC notes that *all health care providers* are subject to various state laws, and that the participation of ground ambulance providers in interstate commerce (through services provided to patients and group health plans) clearly subjects them to federal jurisdiction – and that federal law can and should supersede any possibly conflicting state laws in this limited area of out-of-network billing practices. States and localities have imposed regulation on ambulances in light of a lack of consistent policy from the federal government; now is the opportunity to correct this gap, thus eliminating the need for much of this inconsistent regulation.

Air ambulance providers have stated repeatedly that they are increasingly joining insurance networks. ERIC applauds this evolution, but ERIC member companies continue to hear from beneficiaries who are saddled with devastating surprise medical bills from air ambulance providers. If more air ambulance providers are participating in networks, this should supply a robust data reference that can be used to ensure air ambulance providers are compensated fairly once they are subjected to in-network matching, or a median in-network benchmark. Increased network participation also means that federal legislation will impose minimal disruption for providers, as in-network providers already cannot generate surprise bills.

As such, the perceived impediments to including both ground and air ambulance in the Committee's surprise medical billing solution are quite surmountable – and final legislation should protect patients from surprise medical bills generated by both ground and air ambulances.

Safeguarding against Shenanigans

ERIC notes that the Committee's draft includes a provision that allows providers at an in-network facility to continue their out-of-network strategy, so long as they obtain signoff from a patient at least 24 hours prior to treatment. We are concerned that this provision, clearly designed with the good intent of preserving access, could in fact undermine the overall goals of the legislation. One of the chief causes of surprise medical billing is monopolistic behavior in various markets; effective legislative solutions will null this behavior by subjecting relevant providers to standards mutually accepted by providers and payers in other markets, and in a specific market, by the facilities where they choose to practice, and by similarly situated providers.

ERIC urges the Committee to tighten language as necessary to ensure that under no circumstance can a patient be asked (or required) to consent to out-of-network billing during an in-network visit or procedure. Otherwise, if there is no available alternative, a provider can still gouge patients – whether they obtain consent weeks in advance, or on the spot at the facility. An extremely narrow exception may be necessary, but consent should be required well in advance of any scheduled procedure, and balance billing should be outright banned in cases of an already admitted patient.

Oppose Network Adequacy Subterfuge

In communities around the country many provider specialties have adopted a business strategy not to join networks or accept health insurance. This has created significant challenges for employers who seek to create plans that can provide patients with access to quality, affordable health care. ERIC understands that representatives of such provider specialties have called upon Congress to force insurance companies to add these providers to their networks. Seeing as these providers currently choose not to participate in networks on a large scale, this request should be seen as a transparent attempt to increase their leverage to force third-party payers to pay higher prices than are reasonable in the context of a given market. In these cases, it is not about network adequacy, but tipping the scales to maximize provider revenue.

As the Committee is no doubt aware, the issue of network adequacy was addressed a decade ago as part of the Affordable Care Act. States have varying network adequacy standards, and in some cases, states that have the most draconian network adequacy requirements simultaneously have the greatest surprise billing problems. The two are unrelated, do not correlate, and as such, need not be taken up together.

Instead, the Committee should avoid relitigating the network adequacy debate – especially during the process of addressing the surprise medical billing crisis facing the more than 100 million Americans in self-insured plans. Congress has rightly recognized that network adequacy standards might make sense for products sold on a government-sponsored exchange and purchased with government-provided tax credits, but self-insured plans are not selling insurance. These plans are designed to provide adequate protection for their beneficiaries, to build networks that can handle the volume of care likely to be needed by beneficiaries, and to ensure costs are controlled to the greatest extent possible while patients are given access to providers with records of high-quality treatment. The application of network adequacy standards to self-insured plans has the potential to undermine value-driven models, eradicate centers of excellence programs, and vastly inflate health insurance premiums for beneficiaries.

At the same time, ERIC notes that providers currently abide by no network adequacy standard of their own. As a result, many providers participate in no networks at all. If providers are interested in expanding network adequacy requirements, Congress should consider whether providers should be required to participate in at least one network, to ensure no gaming of the system takes place.

Empower Patients and Payers with an All-Payer Claims Database (APCD)

Numerous states are moving forward with efforts to aggregate health claims data in their markets, and those efforts should be commended. However, states will not be able to fully achieve this goal without access to data from entities which they have no ability to regulate – namely, federal government programs, and self-funded ERISA plans. Therefore, ERIC has endorsed the creation of a national APCD that aggregates large employer claims data, as well as state-level and fully-insured data, and Medicare data, giving employers as well as researchers the opportunity to get a comprehensive view of health care markets and trends.

As outlined earlier in this testimony, self-insured plans cannot be subjected to conflicting and inconsistent regulation by the various states, and indeed the U.S. Supreme Court has ruled in *Gobeille v. Liberty Mutual* that the states cannot compel self-insured plans to report health care claims data. We believe that a national database can strike the right balance – respecting states' rights to design and administer their own databases, ensuring states get access to the multitude of data they currently do not have access to, and protecting the ability of ERISA plans to operate on a national, uniform level.

Conclusion

In conclusion, thank you for this opportunity to share our views with the Committee. The ERISA Industry Committee and our member companies are committed to working with Congress toward a bipartisan, comprehensive solution that protects patients' access to care, ends the surprise billing crisis, ensures fair provider compensation, and does so without driving up health insurance costs. We look forward to working with the Committee to enact legislation to end the surprise billing crisis.

* * *

Ms. ESHOO. Thank you, Mr. Gelfand.

Mr. Nickels, you are now recognized for your five minutes of testimony.

Statement of Thomas Nickels, Executive Vice President, American Hospital Association

Mr. NICKELS. Thank you, Madam Chair. I appreciate the opportunity. My name is Tom Nickels. I am executive vice president of the American Hospitals Association here representing our 5,000 member hospitals and health systems.

Our bottom line is that we must protect patients like Ms. Wilkes from surprise medical bills and the AHA supports Federal legislation to do so.

Congress must act, as has been mentioned, to protect the 60 percent of Americans who are in employer-sponsored plans under ERISA and those who live in states that have not enacted protections to address the issue of surprise medical bills.

Patients should not be subject to balance billing when they have access to emergency services outside their network or have acted in good faith to obtain in-network care. They also shouldn't be surprised by coverage denials from their insurers when they access any emergency services in network or out of network.

I would like to respond to a few of the ideas put forward in the Energy and Commerce discussion draft. First, we agree with that legislation should explicitly prohibit balance billing in the scenarios I just outlined and make sure that patients are kept out of the process to determine reimbursements between the payer and the provider. I would encourage you to also improve the standards for provider networks and ensure adequate oversight to prevent instances of out-of-network care.

Once the patient is protected, we believe Congress should allow providers and payers to determine fair and appropriate reimbursement.

We oppose a national rate or benchmark for out-of-network services such as a median contracted in-network rate even if geographically adjusted as it would not be able to capture the many factors that specific health plans and providers consider.

We are also concerned at setting a reimbursement standard in law would serve as a disincentive for insurers to maintain adequate provider networks.

We've already seen an increase in the use of no-network reference-based pricing models in the commercial market and this could accelerate should insurers have the option to default to a government-established out-of-network rate.

Health plans should not be absolved of their core function of establishing provider networks including negotiating rates with providers.

The committee's discussion draft provides $50 million grants for state-level all payer claims databases—APCD—that would presumably assist in determining a median contracted in-network rate.

While we appreciate the committee's efforts to develop APCDs, we do not believe that the committee should rely on them for the purposes of this policy.

While the AHA believes that hospitals and payers are able to negotiate reimbursement for out-of-network claims without government involvement, there may be a role for a dispute resolution process not for hospital services but for physician claims.

The baseball-style of arbitration similar to what New York State has implemented, which does not include hospitals, appears to be an inefficient process that places the responsibility to initiate the request with the provider or health insurer and not the patient.

Studies have shown a 34 percent reduction in out-of-network billing. Physicians have been largely split between the providers and payers, and there has not been a noticeable inflationary impact on premium insurance rates.

The National Association of Insurance Commissioners has also put forward a model act that outlines a mediation process to resolve disputes. Again, these are state-level solutions. They do not resolve surprise bills under ERISA.

However, they could be successfully deployed at the Federal level with some modification. The committee's discussion draft requires providers at the time of scheduling to give patients both oral and written notice about the provider's network status and any potential charges they could be liable for if treated by an out-of-network provider. While we believe providing the patient with this information on network status is important, it is not in and of itself a solution to surprise medical bills.

Should the committee move forward with legislative language requiring notice and disclosure, we would ask that you include physicians and insurance plans in any requirements as they also have a role to play in keeping patients informed about their status.

Lastly, I would like to address the concept of network matching, which is not in the committee's draft but has been suggested previously, in surprise medical billing. In this scenario, the facility-based practitioner will be required to contract with every plan for which the facility has a contract.

AHA opposes this approach because it would interfere with the fundamental relationship between hospital and physician partners and severely limits providers' ability to negotiate contract terms with insurers.

If you require hospitals to enforce this approach it would raise anti-trust concerns as it could be seen as an effort by hospitals to restrict the physicians' ability to practice.

Madam Chair, we have an opportunity to protect patients from surprise bills as a consensus has developed among all parties. We should not risk moving forward by adding other policies that could put passage at risk.

I look forward to working with the committee and the subcommittee to make sure that patients are protected from surprise medical bills.

Thank you very much.

[The prepared statement of Mr. Nickels follows:]

Written Testimony of Thomas Nickels, On Behalf of the American Hospital Association

Madam Chairwoman, my name is Tom Nickels, I am the executive vice president of the American Hospital Association (AHA). On behalf of our nearly 5,000 member hospitals and health systems, along with our clinician partners, I appreciate the opportunity to testify today.

Hospitals and health systems are deeply concerned about the effect of unanticipated medical bills on our patients, which could impact their out-of-pocket costs and undermine their trust and confidence in their caregivers. Protecting patients from surprise medical bills is a top priority for the AHA Board of Trustees and all of our members.

Surprise billing typically occurs when a patient receives an unexpected bill for care they thought was covered by their health plan, or when they receive a bill for out-of-network emergency services. Some forms of coverage, including Medicare and Medicaid, have strong patient protections against surprise billing. However, other types of coverage, most notably self-funded, employer-sponsored plans regulated through the Employee Retirement Income Security Act of 1974 (ERISA), do not contain the same protections. While some state governments have attempted to address this issue, only a few have passed comprehensive protections, and states have limited regulatory oversight of ERISA plans. Therefore, it is imperative for Congress to act on this issue to protect consumers from surprise medical bills in all states and in all forms of health coverage.

The three most typical scenarios for when a patient receives an unexpected bill occur when: (1) a patient accesses emergency services outside of their insurance network; (2) a patient has acted in good faith to obtain care within their network but unintentionally receives care from an out-of-network clinician providing services in an in-network hospital; or (3) a health plan denies coverage for emergency services saying they were unnecessary, including in-network emergency services. *In all of these situations, we believe it is critical to protect patients from surprise bills.*

The AHA agrees with the Committee that the patient should both be protected financially, as well as removed from the negotiating process between the health plan and the provider. Specifically, patients' cost-sharing obligations should be limited to the in-network amount. Once the patient is protected, providers and insurers can work together – without engaging the patient – to determine appropriate reimbursement, consistent with standard negotiations. *The AHA asks that the Committee preserve the ability of providers and insurers to negotiate private contracts and not establish a fixed payment amount for out-of-network services.* Arbitrary reimbursement rates could disrupt local market forces in ways that could have significant negative unintended consequences. Chief among them is the disincentive this will create for health plans to maintain adequate networks and act as good business partners to their providers. Without sufficient network adequacy requirements that address specific critical specialties and subspecialties, insurers can simply default to a benchmark payment and decline to contract with many different types of physicians. This dissolution of networks could undermine patients' ability to access care for services not protected through this draft legislation, as well as undermine efforts to enhance care coordination and improve quality through different types of value-based arrangements. Should the Committee continue to pursue some role for the government in determining reimbursement, we encourage you to consider an independent dispute resolution process in place of a benchmark rate. Our response to the Committee's request for input on their draft legislative proposal is included (see Attachment 1), and we address these and other issues below.

Issues Related to Surprise Billing

Reference Pricing

The Committee's discussion draft establishes a minimum payment standard for out-of-network emergency care and care provided by out-of-network ancillary providers during otherwise in-network care. The payment standard would be set at the median contracted (in-network) rate for the service in the geographic area in which the service was delivered. States would have the ability to determine their own payment standards for plans they regulate. We urge the Committee to reject specifying a national reimbursement rate or approach for out-of-network services.

Health plans and hospitals have a longstanding history of resolving out-of-network emergency service claims, and this process should not be disrupted. We are particularly concerned that any attempt at setting a reimbursement standard in law will have significant negative consequences, including, as referenced above, the creation of a disincentive for insurers to maintain adequate provider networks. Increases in the use of no-network, reference-based pricing models in the commercial market suggests this already is a growing strategy, and one that would accelerate if the insurer could simply point to a government-sanctioned, out-of-network rate or methodology.

The process of rate negotiation is a core function of managing a health plan. The process takes into account a number of factors that could not be accounted for in a government rate or methodology. For example, health plans and providers often consider their entire lines of business, volume, quality, partnerships on special programs or initiatives, and other factors when setting rates. In addition, providers consider other elements besides reimbursement when negotiating contracts, such as a health plan's history with respect to prior authorization and payment delays and denials, as well as other administrative burdens imposed by a particular plan. Setting a rate or methodology sufficiently simple for national use, even if geographically adjusted, would not be able to capture the many factors that specific health plans and providers consider. In addition, it would remove incentives for health plans to maintain comprehensive networks and follow fair business practices as a way of encouraging providers to enter into contracts. Health plans should not be absolved of the core function of establishing provider networks, including negotiating rates with providers.

The Committee's discussion draft provides $50 million in grants for states to develop or maintain an all-payer claims database (APCD) that would presumably assist in determining a median contracted (in-network) rate. We appreciate the Committee's efforts to develop APCDs, as we recognize the value of collecting claims for a number of different purposes, such as quality improvement activities. However, we do not believe that the Committee should rely on APCDs for purposes of setting national policy, and instead encourage consideration of funding for studies on the best way to implement these data collection entities and support such efforts at the state level.

Dispute Resolution

While the AHA believes that hospitals and payers should be left to negotiate reimbursement for out-of-network claims without government interference, there may be a role for an alternative dispute resolution process for physician claims, such as arbitration.

A number of states have passed laws to establish a dispute resolution process to mediate out-of-network claims primarily between physicians and health insurers. Prominent among these processes is "baseball-style" arbitration. In this binding arbitration model, each party must submit a proposed best and final offer to the arbitrator and the other party with the opportunity to submit a written explanation. The arbitrator must choose one of the two final offers, without modification, from those submitted. Baseball-style arbitration has some clear advantages in that it provides an incentive to the disputing parties to offer reasonable proposals to the arbitrator. It also typically expedites resolution of the dispute and significantly reduces costs as compared to traditional arbitration or litigation. The simple act of having an arbitration process incentivizes health plans and providers to resolve disputes in advance, including by coming to an agreement on in-network contract terms. In fact, in states with such processes, a very small percentage of out-of-network claims ever make it to arbitration. New York is one such state that frequently is referenced as having a successful process. One study noted that the New York law reduced out-of-network billing by 34 percent.[18] A more recent study noted that, "as of October 2018, IDR [New York's independent dispute resolution entity] decisions have been roughly evenly split between providers and payers, with 618 disputes decided in favor of the health plan and 561 decided in favor of the provider … Additionally, insurers and physicians appear to be making 'a real concerted effort' to work out their payment disputes before filing with IDR." That study also noted that, while it may be too soon to know if the arbitration process leads to higher out-of-network prices, there had not yet been an inflationary impact on insurers' annual premium rates.[19] In fact, for reasons like this, the National Association of Insurance Commissioners (NAIC) adopted a dispute resolution process as part of their 2015 Model Act on network adequacy.

For arbitration to work within the context of a federal solution to surprise medical billing, it would need to be designed effectively and accommodate existing state programs.

The key design elements should:

1. Provide for an efficient process, such as baseball-style arbitration.
2. Place the responsibility to initiate the request for arbitration with the provider or health insurer, not the patient.
3. Allow state government appointment of the arbitrator to ensure better understanding of local markets.
4. Split the cost of arbitration between the two parties in dispute to incentivize parties to resolves disputes before moving to arbitration.
5. Establish fixed timelines to ensure expeditious handling of the process.

---

[18] Zack Cooper, Fiona Scott Morton, and Nathan Shekita. Surprise! Out-of-Network Billing for Emergency Care in the United States. *NBER Working Paper No. 23623 July 2017*, Revised January 2018.

[19] Corlette, S. and Hoppe, O.; Georgetown University Health Policy Institute – Center on Health Insurance Reforms. *New York's 2014 Law to Protect Consumers from Surprise Out-of-Network Bills Mostly Working as Intended: Results of a Case Study*, May 2019. https://georgetown.app.box.com/s/6onkj1jaiy3f1618iy7j0gpzdoew2zu9.

6. Follow established procedures for documentation and claims recommended by the American Arbitration Association to include processes to reduce costs, such as allowing batching of similar claims.
7. Require that the arbitrators' decisions are confidential to not unduly influence future cases.
8. Apply arbitration to self-insured ERISA plans.

Bundling of Services

Some stakeholders are promoting the use of "bundling" of hospital and clinician services as a way to reduce the incidence of surprise medical bills. Specifically, services provided in hospitals by out-of-network ancillary providers would be incorporated into the fee that the hospital negotiates with the health plan. These providers would not be permitted to bill a patient separately. The hospital then would be responsible for compensating the provider.

This concept may seem simple and straightforward in theory; in reality, however, this approach would be administratively complex, fundamentally change the relationship between hospitals and their physician and ancillary partners, and, alone, do nothing to protect patients from surprise bills. We strongly oppose such a model.

Setting reimbursement for bundles of services involves a complex array of clinicians, statisticians, lawyers and others to define the services and duration of the bundle, to appropriately price it, and to ensure that any financial relationships between the various providers adhere to state and federal law, including the Stark law and Anti-kickback Statute. To date, the greatest success in bundling has been for services for which the clinical care is well defined and little variation is expected, such as for certain planned joint replacements. For the vast majority of these bundles, clinicians and hospitals continue to negotiate their own rates with insurers and the final bills are reconciled against a target. In other words, even in many bundled payment models, health plans are not paying a single entity, such as the hospital, a single rate for the entire course of care.

Along with all of this added complexity and cost, the act of bundling all bills into a single bill alone does nothing to stop patients from receiving surprise bills. In fact, the proponents of bundling note that in order to stop out-of-network providers from billing outside of the single bill, policymakers also must specifically ban balance billing. *In other words: The ban is the solution to surprise bills, and one that we support.* Bundling is not the solution and, therefore, appears to meet some other objective – allowing insurers to transfer to hospitals their responsibility for establishing comprehensive physician networks and managing the associated financial risk. Hospitals are not set up to manage this type of risk, and patient access to care in their communities could be threatened if they are unsuccessful.

In-Network Guarantees

One suggested solution to surprise medical billing is to have in-network hospitals guarantee to patients and health plans that every practitioner caring for the patient in the facility is considered in-network. Some health policy experts have described this approach as "network matching," where the facility-based practitioner would be required to contract with every plan for which the facility has a contract. The AHA opposes this approach because it interferes with the fundamental relationship between hospitals and their physician partners and severely limits providers' ability to negotiate contract terms with insurers. *In other words, this provision would essentially eliminate any ability of physicians to negotiate fair contract terms with health plans, including, but not limited to, their reimbursement level.*

We believe that providers and health plans should be able to develop networks that meet consumers' needs, and not be compelled to enter into contracts that could thwart the development of more affordable coverage options that support coordinated care. In addition, providers should be able to refrain from entering into contracts with health plans based on other considerations, such as whether the health plan is a fair business partner.

The approach also raises certain antitrust concerns in that it would require that a hospital compel non-employed physicians practicing in its facility to participate in the same health plan networks. It is conceivable that some impacted physicians would threaten or bring suit against the hospital, charging that such compulsion violates federal or state antitrust laws that prohibit restraint of trade in certain circumstances.

Providing an Estimate of a Patient's Out-of-Pocket Costs for Services

Some legislative proposals would require hospitals and other providers to give patients an estimate of their out-of-pocket cost obligations at the time of scheduling care. While many hospitals and health systems are working toward being able to provide this information prior to care, there are a number of reasons why they may not be able to provide an estimate at the time of scheduling for all services. First, there is an inherent uncertainty in health care that means that a course of treatment can easily change as a result of how a particular patient responds to a treatment protocol or how their unique disease or injury progresses. For many services, it simply is not realistic – and could be misleading – to give patients assurances of how their care will proceed and the associated cost. Any transparency requirement should take into account the "shoppability" of a given service or course of treatment. In addition, generating an out-of-pocket cost estimate requires that a provider communicate with a patient's insurer to obtain the individual's cost-sharing responsibilities, including where he or she is with respect to reaching annual deductible or out-of-pocket maximums defined by the insurance product. While these processes increasingly are helped by automated technologies, they still require significant engagement among hospital, health system and health plan staff to ensure accuracy. We encourage Congress to allow providers and health plans to continue their development of consumer-focused price transparency tools without inserting a potentially unworkable component as part of a surprise billing solution.

Notice and Disclosure

The Committee's discussion draft requires providers, at the time of scheduling, to give patients both oral and written notice about the provider's network status and any potential charges they could be liable for if treated by an out-of-network provider. While we believe that providing the patient with information on network status is important, it is not in and of itself a solution to surprise medical bills. Indeed, today, most hospitals have some form of notice-and-disclosure protocols in place, and a number of states have specific notice requirements. However, these have demonstrated limitations.

The nature of emergencies, and the legal requirements regarding how and when coverage may be discussed, make providing notice difficult in some of these instances. Notice may not be particularly effective in non-emergency scenarios as well. Additional paperwork often can be confusing for patients, especially in instances where they may not have another timely alternative for care. We, therefore, encourage the Committee to focus on fully protecting patients by prohibiting surprise bills rather than relying on notice as part of the solution. Should the Committee move forward with legislative language requiring notice and disclosure, we would ask that you include physicians and insurance plans in any requirements, as they too have a role to play in keeping patients informed of network status and anticipated costs.

Network Adequacy and Patient Education

Hospitals and health systems work with patients to help them navigate the health care system, including scheduling follow-up care with in-network providers. These efforts have grown commensurate with the growth in high-deductible health plans and narrow insurance networks, which demand greater patient awareness of the limitations of their coverage. Patients enrolled in these types of health plan products often lack an understanding of their out-of-pocket obligations before their coverage starts, or that their plan's narrow network limits their access to hospitals and providers.

Ensuring adequate networks and patient education about the health insurance products they purchase is critical to addressing surprise medical bills. We encourage the Committee to avoid any solution that could further erode the comprehensiveness of networks. For example, if Congress were to adopt a rate-setting methodology that enables insurers to pay providers below what they would pay as a result of negotiations with providers, insurers will be incentivized to default to building networks that meet the bare minimum standards for network adequacy, relying on the out-of-network rate for as many claims as possible. This means that patients will have access to even fewer in-network providers when they are looking to schedule care.

Air Ambulance

Some of our hospital and health system members have raised concerns about the increase in surprise billing for air ambulance services and the need for federal engagement on this issue. The Federal Aviation Administration (FAA) regulates air ambulances, and federal law preempts states from regulating rates, routes and services of air carriers. This has limited state governments' ability to address air ambulance balance billing issues. The Government Accountability Office recently released a report on air ambulance surprise bills that found that, between 2010 and 2014, the median prices charged by air ambulance providers for helicopter transports doubled, and the number of air ambulance helicopters grew by more than 10 percent.[20] In addition, the agency found that, in 2017, about two-thirds of air ambulance transports for privately insured patients were out of network, insurers typically paid only a portion of the out-of-network services, and almost all of the consumer complaints involved balance bills greater than $10,000. As required by the FAA Reauthorization Act of 2018, the Secretary of Transportation has formed an advisory committee on air ambulance patient billing. The advisory committee is directed to recommend ways to protect consumers from surprise air ambulance bills. While this issue is not in the jurisdiction of the Committee, we encourage the Congress to address air ambulance service issues while developing legislation solutions related to surprise medical billing. More specifically, we ask that the Congress extend similar consumer protections from out-of-network billing to air ambulance services and include air ambulance services in network adequacy requirements.

---

[20] GAO-19-292 Air ambulance. www.gao.gov/assets/700/697683.pdf.

Conclusion

We thank you for the opportunity to share the hospital and health system field's suggestions and concerns as they relate to surprise medical billing. We appreciate that this issue is a priority for the Committee on Energy and Commerce, as it is for our patients and members. We urge Congress to enact a legislative solution that protects patients from surprise billing without having unintended negative consequences on the health care system.

* * *

Chairman Pallone and Ranking Member Walden. on behalf of our nearly 5,000 member hospitals, health systems and other health care organizations, our clinician partners – including more than 270,000 affiliated physicians, 2 million nurses and other caregivers – and the 43,000 health care leaders who belong to our professional membership groups, the American Hospital Association (AHA) appreciates the opportunity to respond to your request for information related to the development of the No Surprises Act to protect patients from surprise medical bills. The AHA appreciates your leadership to shield patients from the financial burden of unexpected medical expenses.

Hospitals and health systems are deeply concerned about the effect of unanticipated medical bills on our patients, which could impact their out-of-pocket costs and undermine their trust and confidence in their caregivers. Protecting patients from surprise medical bills is a top priority for the AHA and our members. To that end, we have adopted the attached set of guiding principles to use as we evaluate legislative proposals, such as the one put forward by the Energy and Commerce Committee. We support a federal-level solution to protect all patients, including individuals who receive health care coverage through Employee Retirement Income Security Act of 1974 (ERISA) plans and for those who live in states that have not yet enacted comprehensive legislation to address surprise medical bills.

The AHA shares the Committee's objective of protecting patients from balance billing in certain circumstances by out-of-network providers and limiting patient cost-sharing to the in-network amount. These patient protections would apply to all emergency services or in cases where a patient cannot reasonably choose their provider. *However, we are concerned with the Committee's draft legislation's approach to determining reimbursement for out-of-network providers. The AHA believes that once the patient is protected from surprise bills, providers and insurers should then be permitted to negotiate payment rates for services provided. We strongly oppose approaches that would impose arbitrary rates on providers.* It is the insurers' responsibility to maintain comprehensive provider networks, and a default payment rate would remove incentives for plans to contract with providers.

Our specific comments to the discussion draft are as follows.

Prohibiting Surprise Medical Bills

We interpret the discussion draft to prohibit balance billing by out-of-network providers for all emergency services, as well as when the patient is treated in an in-network facility but cannot reasonably choose their provider, a position with which we agree. However, we are concerned with how the bill is drafted in that it amends the Public Health Service Act Section 2719A rather than replaces it or amends it to explicitly prohibit balance billing. We are concerned that without a specific prohibition, the draft legislation would still permit balance billing for emergency services, albeit subject to penalties discussed below. We encourage the Committee to consider adding a specific prohibition.

Enforcement of Surprise Medical Bills through Civil Monetary Penalties

The discussion draft uses civil monetary penalties to enforce its prohibition on surprise medical bills. The discussion draft seems to approach the prohibition on surprise medical bills not by directly prohibiting surprise bills but by imposing a penalty if a surprise bills is issued. It also is not clear how a violation would be triggered. Would the patient have to initiate a challenge, thus defeating the purpose of taking the patient out of the middle of provider plan payment disputes? *The AHA believes that once the patient is protected, resolution of the disputed claims should be left to the plans and providers. If a provider continues to balance bill the patient, then a penalty should be applied and civil monetary penalties would be preferable to other approaches, such as using Medicare Conditions of Participation.*

Provider and Price Transparency

The discussion draft requires providers, at the time of scheduling, to give patients both oral and written notice about the provider's network status and any potential charges they could be liable for if treated by an out-of-network provider. *The AHA supports increased transparency with regard to both in-network provider status as well as potential costs patients will face. We also believe that providing the patient with network status information is important, but is not a solution to surprise medical bills.* The best way to protect patients is by simply banning balance billing in specific circumstances. Further, the nature of emergencies and the legal requirements regarding how and when coverage may be discussed can make providing notice in some of these instances difficult. Even when scheduling care, patients can be overwhelmed. We do not think relying on notice should be part of a solution to surprise bills.

Establish Minimum Payment Standard

The discussion draft establishes a minimum payment standard for out-of-network emergency care and care provided by out-of-network ancillary providers during otherwise in-network care. The payment standard would be set at the median contracted (in-network) rate for the service in the geographic area the service was delivered. States would have the ability to determine their own payment standards for plans they regulate.

The AHA opposes setting a rate in statute, given the risk this creates for setting rates too low and compromising patient access to care. Rate setting would be nearly impossible to get right and ignores the many factors that providers and health plans consider when deciding whether or not to enter into a contract. Factors that may be relevant to one provider may not be relevant to another provider, which means that the median contracted in-network rate may not be the appropriate payment level.

Considerations include a provider's size or mix of services, such as whether a provider is the only hospital or health system in a community offering advanced trauma services, and whether a provider and payer have negotiated to enter into a value-based contracting arrangement. Providers also consider whether an insurer is a good business partner when determining when to contract. For example, does the insurer have a history of delaying prior authorization decisions or denying claims inappropriately? We should maintain the incentives on insurers to not only pay fairly but also to engage in good business practices. Rate setting, creates a disincentive for insurers, as it removes the need for health plans to form comprehensive networks and to contract and negotiate with providers.

The discussion draft also suggests a reliance on all-payer claims databases to determine the median contracted rate. We have concerns about the viability and burden associated with all 50 states establishing all-payer claims databases in a reasonable timeframe. Our recommended approach, protecting patients and then leaving providers and insurers to determine reimbursement, can be implemented immediately.

As an alternative to rate setting, there may be a role for an alternative dispute resolution process, such as arbitration or mediation in any instance of disagreement between providers and payers. We encourage the Committee to consider a "baseball-style" arbitration model in which each party must submit a proposed final offer, with the arbiter to determine the appropriate payment level. The process still would allow providers and plans to negotiate and simply would be a backstop for any claims that result in a dispute. We expect, as is the experience of states with such models today, that an arbitration backstop would create an incentive for plans and providers to come to an agreement before such a process is triggered. If arbitration is needed, the baseball-style format allows for the most expedited process at a cost that is lower than traditional arbitration or litigation.

For arbitration to work within the context of a federal solution to surprise medical billing, it would need to be designed effectively and accommodate existing state programs.

The key design elements should:

- Provide for an efficient process, such as "baseball-style" arbitration.
- Place the responsibility to initiate the request for arbitration with the provider or health insurer, not the patient.
- Allow state government appointment of the arbitrator to ensure better understanding of local markets.
- Split the cost of arbitration between the two parties in dispute.
- Establish fixed timelines to ensure expeditious handling of the process.
- Follow established procedures for documentation and claims recommended by the American Arbitration Association to include processes to reduce costs, such as allowing batching of similar claims.
- Require that the arbitrators' decisions are confidential.
- Apply arbitration to self-insured ERISA plans.

All-Payer Claims Databases

The discussion draft provides $50 million in grants for states to develop or maintain an all-payer claims database that would assist in determining a median contracted (in-network) rate. The AHA supports price transparency innovations, such as all-payer claims databases. We recognize the value of collecting claims for a number of different purposes, such as quality improvement activities. We caution the Committee against considering all-payer claims databases as a comprehensive solution to price transparency. Specifically, adoption of these databases to-date is uneven, and it has been challenging to determine the correct data to collect, to secure all of the data from all payers in a state and then determine how to use the data. For example, only 18 states have set up these systems, and many have struggled with data completeness and accuracy.

There also are issues of privacy and security and questions regarding who receives access to the data and for what purposes. At this stage, we do not believe that the Committee should rely on all-payer claims databases for purposes of setting national policy. We instead encourage consideration of funding for studies on the best way to implement these data collection entities and support such efforts at the state level.

Increasing Transparency and Ensuring Network Adequacy for Consumers

We agree with the Committee that consumers should better understand their health plans and which providers are in their network. The growth in high-deductible health plans and narrow insurance networks demand greater patient awareness of the limitations of their coverage. Patients enrolled in these types of health plan products often lack an understanding of their out-of-pocket obligations before their coverage starts, or that their plan's narrow network limits their access to hospitals and providers.

Ensuring adequate networks and patient education about the health insurance products they purchase is critical to addressing surprise medical bills. We encourage the Committee to avoid any solution that could further erode the comprehensiveness of networks. As stated earlier, by using a rate-setting methodology that enables insurers to pay providers below what they would pay as a result of negotiations with providers, insurers will be incentivized to default to building networks that meet the bare minimum standards for network adequacy, thereby relying on the out-of-network rate for as many claims as possible. This means that patients will have access to even fewer in-network providers when they are trying to schedule care.

We also encourage the Committee to strengthen existing network adequacy rules to address some of the issues of health plan participation by hospital-based specialists who practice in hospitals. This oversight would require action by the states and Congress to implement specific requirements for ERISA plans. Network adequacy will not improve without substantial oversight by both state and federal regulators.

Protecting Consumers from Surprise Bills from Air Ambulances

Our hospital and health system members have raised concerns about the increase in surprise billing from air ambulance services and the need for federal engagement on this issue. Given that the Federal Aviation Administration regulates air ambulances, state governments have limited ability to address these issues. The Government Accountability Office released a report on air ambulance surprise bills that found that, between 2010 and 2014, the median prices charged by air ambulance providers for helicopter transports doubled, and the number of air ambulance helicopters grew by more than 10 percent.[21] In addition, the agency found that, in 2017, about two-thirds of air ambulance transports for privately insured patients were out of network, insurers typically paid only a portion of the out-of-network services, and almost all of the consumer complaints involved balance bills greater than $10,000. As required by the FAA Reauthorization Act of 2018, the Secretary of Transportation has formed an advisory committee on air ambulance patient billing. The advisory committee is directed to recommend ways to protect consumers from surprise air ambulance bills. While this issue is not within the jurisdiction of the Committee, we encourage Congress to address air ambulance service issues while developing legislative solutions related to surprise medical billing.

We look forward to continuing to work with the Committee on solutions to stop surprise medical bills.

* * *

Surprise Billing Principles

America's hospitals and health systems are committed to protecting patients from "surprise bills" and support a federal legislative solution to do so. These types of bills may occur when a patient receives care from an out-of-network provider or when their health plan fails to pay for covered services. The three most typical scenarios are when: (1) a patient accesses emergency services outside of their insurance network, including from providers while they are away from home; (2) a patient has acted in good faith to obtain care within their network but unintentionally receives care from an out-of-network physician providing services in an in-network hospital; or (3) a health plan denies coverage for emergency services saying they were unnecessary. In these situations, we believe it is critical to protect patients from surprise bills.

We have developed the following principles to help inform the debate regarding surprise billing in the scenarios outlined above. In the event a patient chooses to go out-of-network for care, these principles should not apply.

- *PROTECT THE PATIENT. Any public policy solution should protect patients and remove them from payment negotiations between insurers and providers.*
  Patients, regardless of the type of health care coverage they have, should be protected from gaps in insurance coverage that result in surprise bills. Patients should have certainty regarding their cost-sharing obligations, which should be based on an in-network amount. Patients should not be "balance billed," meaning they should not receive a bill from the provider beyond their cost-sharing obligations. Patients should not have to bear the burden of serving as an intermediary between health plans and providers, rather health plans should be responsible for paying providers directly.

[21] GAO-19-292 Air ambulance www.gao.gov/assets/700/697683.pdf.

- *ENSURE PATIENTS HAVE ACCESS TO EMERGENCY CARE. Any public policy solution should ensure that patients have access to and coverage of emergency care.* This requires that health plans adhere to the "prudent layperson standard" and not deny payment for emergency care that, in retrospect, the health plan determined was not an emergency. Recent actions by some health plans to deny coverage of emergency services puts patients' physical, mental and financial health at risk.
- *PRESERVE THE ROLE OF PRIVATE NEGOTIATION. Any public policy solution should ensure providers are able to negotiate appropriate payment rates with health plans.*

  The government should not establish a fixed payment amount for out-of-network services. Health plans and providers take into account a number of factors when negotiating rates. Any rate or methodology sufficiently simple for national use would not be able to capture these factors. In addition, a fixed payment rate could undermine patients' ability to access in-network clinicians by giving health plans less of an incentive to enlist physicians and facilities to join their networks because they can rely on a default out-of-network payment rate. Providers and health plans should be able to develop networks that meet consumers' needs, and not be compelled to enter into contracts that could thwart the development of more affordable coverage options that support coordinated care.
- *EDUCATE PATIENTS. Any public policy solution should include an educational component to help patients understand the scope of their health care coverage and how to access their benefits.*

  All stakeholders – health plans, employers, providers and others – should undertake efforts to improve patients' health care literacy and support them in navigating their health coverage and the health care system.
- *ENSURE ADEQUATE PROVIDER NETWORKS AND GREATER HEALTH PLAN TRANSPARENCY. Any public policy solution should include greater oversight of health plan provider networks and the role health plans play in helping patients access in-network care.*

  Patients should have access to easily-understandable provider network information to ensure they can make informed health care decisions, including accurate listings for hospital-based physicians in health plan directories and websites. Patients also should have adequate access to in-network providers, including hospital-based specialists at in-network facilities, rather than simply a minimum number of physicians and hospitals.

  Federal and state regulators should ensure both the adequacy of health plan provider networks and the accuracy of provider directories. Health plans should be responsible for an efficient and timely credentialing process to minimize the amount of time a physician is "out-of-network."
- *SUPPORT STATE LAWS THAT WORK. Any public policy solution should take into account the interaction between federal and state laws.*

  Many states have undertaken efforts to protect patients from surprise billing, but federal action is necessary to protect patients in self-insured employer-sponsored plans regulated under the Employee Retirement Income Security Act, which cover the majority of privately insured individuals. Any federal solution should provide a default to state laws that meet the federal minimum for consumer protections.

* * *

Ms. ESHOO. Thank you, Mr. Nickels.

I know would like to recognize Ms. Thornton for five minutes for your testimony.

Statement of Jeanette Thornton, Senior Vice President, Product, Employer, and Commercial Policy, America's Health Insurance Plans

Ms. THORNTON. Thank you.

Chairwoman Eshoo and Ranking Member Burgess, and members of the subcommittee, I am Jeanette Thornton, senior vice president of product, employer, and commercial policy for America's Health Insurance Plans.

I appreciate this opportunity to testify on solutions to protect the American people from surprise medical bills. We want to end surprise medical bills so that patients like Ms. Wilkes and her family have the peace of mind in an emergency that they will not receive inflated bills from doctors they did not seek out for care.

We applaud the leaders of the House Energy and Commerce Committee for developing a bipartisan discussion draft of the No Surprises Act. This draft bill takes important steps to protect patients, ensure that doctors are paid fairly, support health plan networks, and use market-based approaches to ensure affordable high-quality care.

Our written testimony focuses on the following: a review of how surprise medical bills occur along with data demonstrating the frequency and magnitude, recommendations we support to protect patients, information on how surprise medical billing legislation will not weaken health plan networks, our concerns regarding arbitration and how this approach would increase healthcare costs for everyone, and a discussion of State laws in California, Texas, and New York that provide important lessons for Federal legislation.

We have all heard personal stories that demonstrate the need for Federal legislation to protect patients from surprise medical bills: the Yoder family whose child experienced a $142,000 snake bite at summer camp, including a $55,000 air ambulance ride; Nellie Lu, who faced a $28,000 bill for her fall on her gym's climbing wall from a hospital at which at that time did not contract with any private insurers and was her only option; Dr. Kahn, whose ride in the ATV resulted in a $56,000 air ambulance ride and a balance bill of $44,000. He was one of dozens of patients across the country who have faced air ambulance bills from $28,000 to $97,000, and we have all heard the stories of American families who are afraid to seek treatment for fear of the high bills they will experience.

These stories make it clear that surprise medical bills are creating financial hardship for the American people and that Federal legislative action is needed.

Here is what we support. First, a balance billing should be banned in situations where patients are involuntarily treated by an out-of-network provider. This includes ER services provided at any hospital, any healthcare services that are provided at an in-network hospital by an out-of-network provider, and ambulance transportation in an emergency.

Second, health insurance providers should be required to reimburse out-of-network providers an appropriate and reasonable amount in these scenarios.

Third, states should be required to establish a dispute resolution process that works in tandem with the established payment benchmark.

And fourth, hospitals and other healthcare providers should be required to furnish advanced notice to patients of the network status of treating providers.

These protections must apply for self-funded plans and for people who live in states without adequate protections. The reason surprise medical bills are a problem is not a lack of network adequacy that some may suggest.

Surprise bills are caused by a small subset of medical specialists who lack the financial incentives to participate in health plan networks.

We urge you to reject proposals that would use arbitration to determine payments to out-of-network providers. This approach imposes administrative burdens on the entire healthcare system including employers that offer self-funded coverage.

It also fails to address the root cause of surprise medical bills— exorbitant bills from certain specialty doctors.

We appreciate that the committee's discussion draft and the Trump administration have rejected arbitration in favor of a market-based approach—an in-network payment benchmark.

It is also important to look at State laws addressing this issue. Based on our analysis of laws enacted in California, Texas, and New York, we urge Congress to pursue a California style solution that both protects patients and consumers with common sense rules, does not undermine networks, and does not lead to higher cost-sharing or premiums.

I thank you for this opportunity to testify. AHIP and our member health plans stand ready to work with the committee to alleviate the financial burdens imposed by the American people by surprise medical bills.

Thank you.

[The prepared statement of Ms. Thornton follows:]

Written Testimony of Jeanette Thornton

Chairwoman Eshoo, Ranking Member Burgess, and members of the subcommittee, I am Jeanette Thornton, Senior Vice President of Product, Employer, and Commercial Policy for America's Health Insurance Plans (AHIP). AHIP is the national association whose members provide coverage for health care and related services to millions of Americans every day. Through these offerings, we improve and protect the health and financial security of consumers, families, businesses, communities, and the nation. We are committed to market-based solutions and public-private partnerships that improve affordability, value, access, and well-being for consumers.

We applaud the leaders of the House Energy and Commerce Committee for coming together in a bipartisan way to develop a discussion draft for the "No Surprises Act." This draft bill takes important steps toward ensuring that patients are protected, doctors are paid fairly, health plan networks are supported, and the free market is permitted to work to deliver affordable, high-quality care. AHIP has provided recommendations to the committee on key elements of the discussion draft, and we appreciate your thoughtful consideration of our ideas. This legislation would go a long way to protect American consumers and patients.

We appreciate this opportunity to offer our support for the No Surprises Act and other solutions that alleviate the financial burdens imposed on patients by surprise medical bills. Every American deserves affordable, high-quality coverage and care, as well as control over their health care choices. Surprise medical bills stand in the way of this commitment, which is why health insurance providers have been advocating for federal legislation that will protect all patients from these unexpected and unjustified costs.

Our member health insurance providers have come together with organizations representing American consumers, employers, brokers, and others to offer real solutions to this problem. Together we are calling for an end to arbitrary and inflated surprise medical bills imposed on patients by certain specialty doctors and emergency medical services (EMS) providers.

Our testimony focuses on the following:

- A review of how surprise medical bills occur;
- Data demonstrating the frequency and magnitude of surprise medical bills;
- Recommendations to protect patients from surprise medical bills;
- Information on the relationship between surprise billing protections and health plan networks;
- Our concern that arbitration as the primary mechanism to address surprise medical billing will increase health care costs for everyone and harm consumers; and
- A comparison of three state laws – enacted in California, Texas, and New York – that provide important lessons as we seek federal legislative solutions that will effectively protect the health and financial security of every American.

How Surprise Medical Bills Occur

Surprise medical bills occur when patients are treated by certain types of out-of-network providers under circumstances where consumers cannot reasonably plan for or avoid treatment from these providers. For example, they can occur during an emergency trip to the hospital, or when an ancillary out-of-network provider cares for a patient during a planned procedure at an in-network facility.

When patients have health care coverage and get care from doctors in their plan's network, the health insurance provider typically covers all costs beyond required cost-sharing under their health plan at a negotiated, market-based rate. However, when patients receive care from out-of-network providers – either voluntarily or involuntarily – the provider often will send patients a bill for charges for which the patient is responsible. This is because, under current law and practice, most states allow a doctor to bill a patient for any balance that may be outstanding after the health insurance provider pays the costs for which it is responsible. Unlike premiums and benefit designs regulated as health insurance under state and/or federal law, there is no oversight over or obligation to justify these charges, which means that patients may be exposed to enormous financial liability in these situations.

Patients often don't realize and have no way of knowing that many physicians are independent contractors who work *at* the hospital, but not *for* the hospital, and who independently choose whether or not to join a health plan network. That means that hospitals can have "in network" status, but the doctors delivering care to patients at that very same hospital may not. This is the type of scenario that leads to surprise medical bills, creates tremendous financial burdens for patients and their families, and can deter patients from seeking needed care.

The Frequency and Magnitude of Surprise Medical Bills

Surprise medical bills often burden patients and their families with thousands of dollars of costs—or even tens of thousands of dollars—for the care they received in, or on their way to, an emergency room or at a hospital, sometimes without even knowing or being physically seen by the doctor who treated them. This burden often comes on top of the challenges faced by patients and their families to recover from a serious health condition.

In February 2019, the USC-Brookings Schaeffer Initiative for Health Policy published a white paper[22] which reported that:

- Approximately 1 in 5 emergency department visits involved care from an out-of-network provider that could result in a surprise out-of-network bill (if not prohibited by state law).
- Among people covered in the large group market, more than 50% of all ambulance cases involved an out-of-network ambulance in 2014.
- In 15% of hospitals, the researchers reported that a patient was seen by one or more out-of-network providers in at least 80% of emergency cases.

While emphasizing that surprise medical bills "often are very large," the USC-Brookings paper explains that "out-of-network emergency physicians charged on average about eight times what Medicare pays for the same service, while in-network rates paid by commercial insurers averaged about three times what Medicare pays."

Similarly, a blog post recently published by the journal *Health Affairs* cited a study which found that mean reimbursement for the highest-level emergency physician service was 306% of Medicare's payment for the same service, whereas median reimbursement was 257% of the Medicare rate.[23]

Data clearly show that the frequency of surprise medical billing is increasing at alarming rates. Moreover, the financial burden such bills impose on both individual consumers subject to the surprise bills and all consumers who rely on health insurance to access care is enormous.

Data from the Health Care Cost Institute (HCCI) show that an increasing percentage of ER visits are being categorized as more complex based on hospital coding. From 2008 to 2017, the percentage of all ER visits categorized as Code 5 increased from 17% to 27%. At the same time, average emergency room prices increased from $549 to $1,121 for Code 5 visits, from $468 to $1,072 for Code 4 visits, and from $354 to $757 for Code 3 visits. Recognizing that

[22] Loren Adler, Matthew Fiedler, Paul B. Ginsburg, Mark Hall, Erin Trish, Christen Linke Young, Erin L. Duffy (February 2019). USC-Brookings Schaeffer Initiative for Health Policy. State Approaches to Mitigating Surprise Out-of-Network Billing. *Brookings*. https://www.brookings.edu/research/state-approaches-to-mitigating-surprise-out-of-network-billing.

[23] Loren Adler, Paul B. Ginsburg, Mark Hall, Erin Trish (May 14, 2019). Analyzing The House E&C Committee's Bipartisan Surprise Out-Of-Network Billing Proposal. *Health Affairs*.

ER visits have a high potential for surprise bills and that hospitals are paid more for complex treatments, these findings demonstrate the cost pressures that patients are facing due to rising ER prices.

The likelihood of receiving a surprise medical bill varies greatly from state to state and county to county, largely because specialists and emergency rooms in some parts of the country are markedly less likely to accept private insurance. In some regions, there is growing provider concentration on both the physician and hospital side, leading to monopolistic market power that makes it even more challenging to bring providers into an insurance network at reasonable rates in order to deliver an affordable health plan network to patients and their families. We see this in places like McAllen, Texas, and St. Petersburg, Florida, where patients had an 89% and 62% chance, respectively, of receiving surprise medical bills. Conversely, in more competitive health care markets like Boulder, Colorado, and South Bend, Indiana, researchers found the rate of surprise medical bills to be nearly zero.[24]

Even for consumers who never receive one, surprise medical bills mean higher premiums. A 2015 analysis of out-of-network charges in New Jersey[25] shows that for the largest health insurance provider in the state, out-of-network claims comprised 8% of their total commercial spending in 2013. If the plan had paid these out-of-network claims at 150% of Medicare rates, rather than the billed charges, the insurance provider would have paid 52% less for out-of-network services, amounting to savings of almost half a billion dollars ($497 million), which could have resulted in a reduction of 4.3% in total commercial claims and consumers paying 9.5% less out-of-pocket.

It is important to note that surprise billing is not an issue seen across all types of providers, however. The problem of surprise medical bills tends to be concentrated among a select number of providers from certain medical specialties often in certain geographic regions that are taking advantage of market dynamics where the patient has no choice in selecting the provider. These providers are likely to charge substantially more than similarly trained and qualified peers in other specialties. They are also more likely either to not accept private insurance or to require extraordinarily high reimbursement rates to participate in insurance networks. Studies have found that surprise medical bills are most likely to come from emergency medicine physicians, anesthesiologists, radiologists, and pathologists.[26]

For example, one study found that:

- Anesthesiologists charge, on average, 5.8 times the Medicare reimbursement rate;
- Radiologists charge, on average, 4.5 times the Medicare rate; and
- Emergency medicine physicians and pathologists charge, on average, 4 times the Medicare rate.[27]

---

[24] Cooper and Morton (2016).

[25] Avalere Health (2015). *An Analysis of Policy Options for Involuntary Out-of-Network Charges in New Jersey.* http://avalere-health-production.s3.amazonaws.com/uploads/pdfs/1427291367_AH_Analysis_of_Policy_Options WP_v3b2.pdf.

[26] Loren Adler, Paul B. Ginsburg, Mark Hall, Erin Trish (September 25, 2018) Analyzing New Bipartisan Federal Legislation Limiting Surprise Medical Bills. *Health Affairs.* https://www.healthaffairs.org/do/10.1377/hblog201 80924.442050/full/.

[27] Bai, G., & Anderson, G. F. (2017). Variation in the Ratio of Physician Charges to Medicare Payments by Specialty and Region. *JAMA*, 317(3), 315.

Since patients are subject to the "balance" of these charges in most states, these unreasonably high charges may have a devastating impact on consumers. The bottom line is that surprise medical bills create financial hardship for millions of Americans, whether or not they personally have received one. Federal legislative action is needed to address this problem for everyone, regardless of the kind of coverage they have.

Solutions for Protecting Patients from Surprise Medical Bills

Over the past year, AHIP has been advocating for federal legislation that would protect patients from surprise medical bills. Our recommendations build upon our collaboration with other leading organizations representing consumers, employers, and health insurance providers. Working with these partners, we have endorsed a set of guiding principles for federal legislation and also addressed a letter to congressional leaders, calling for meaningful steps to address surprise medical bills.[28,29]

AHIP applauds Chairman Pallone and Ranking Member Walden for developing a bipartisan discussion draft of the "No Surprises Act" and for inviting feedback and comments from consumers, health care organizations, and other interested parties. We have provided recommendations for strengthening this draft legislation, focusing on the importance of addressing surprise billing by ground and air ambulance operators, recognizing median contracted rates as an appropriate, market-based payment benchmark, and applying the median contracted rate approach to self-funded plans regulated under ERISA. We appreciate that the committee has been receptive to our suggestions.

Our recommendations for federal legislation focus on four priorities:

1. *Balance billing should be banned in situations where patients are involuntarily treated by an out-of-network provider and patients should be held harmless.*

Hospitals and other health care providers should be prohibited from billing a patient the balance in excess of any health insurance provider reimbursement for: (a) emergency health care services provided at any hospital; (b) ambulatory transportation to any health care facility in an emergency; and (c) any health care services or treatment performed at an in-network facility by an out-of-network provider not selected by the patient.

In addition, the cost-sharing that may be imposed upon an insured patient under these situations should be limited to the amount for which the patient would be responsible for a participating network provider, including for deductibles and calculating out-of-pocket maximums.

2. *Health insurance providers should be required to reimburse non-participating providers an appropriate and reasonable amount in the above scenarios.*

All health plans and health insurance issuers should be required to reimburse a non-contracted hospital or health care provider in the above scenarios an amount equal to the median

[28] https://www.ahip.org/wp-content/uploads/Surprise-Billing-Consensus-Statement-12.10.18.pdf.

[29] https://www.ahip.org/wp-content/uploads/Hill-Sign-on-Letter-Surprise-Medical-Bills-031819-2.pdf.

in-network rate for the same service under the patient's health plan contract. If no such rate is ascertainable, then the plan should be obligated to pay an amount based on Medicare Parts A and B.

These requirements should be applied to all commercial health insurance, including ERISA self-funded health plans, with the option for states to establish similar standards for reimbursement through enacted legislation, so long as the state methodology would not increase patient cost-sharing amounts or premiums.

3. *States should be required to establish an independent dispute resolution process that works in tandem with the established payment benchmark.*

An independent dispute resolution process, established at the state level, should be available when there is a dispute as to whether a reimbursement was correctly determined according to the market-based methodology we are recommending. Dispute resolution processes should not be the default or primary vehicle instead of the established payment benchmark. In addition, internal appeals processes should be exhausted prior to initiating a dispute resolution process.

4. *Hospitals or other health care providers should be required to furnish advanced notice to patients of the network status of treating providers.*

For non-emergency situations, hospitals should be required to notify patients at their first point of contact, including by a provider on a patient's behalf (e.g., scheduling surgeon), that some providers assigned to them may be out-of-network and inform them of their right to select in-network providers or decline care.

This notice should be for informational purposes only and not constitute a waiver of patient rights or a release of obligations imposed upon facilities or providers under this law. The notice should not act as a statement of consent by the patient to pay for services rendered.

Surprise Medical Billing Legislation Will Not Weaken Health Plan Networks

Provider networks are an essential part of health care coverage and the care that people receive. They help ensure that enrollees have access to a robust network of high-quality doctors and health care settings, and that these providers are held accountable to high standards for care quality at reasonable, market-driven rates. It also benefits providers and plans by reducing administrative expenses and streamlining reimbursement.

As a first step to eliminate surprise medical bills, we want providers and hospitals to voluntarily contract with health plans. This benefits everyone – both by advancing value-based payment arrangements and prompt claims payments. Early reports from the implementation of the California law which includes a benchmark is that network participation is increasing, while rates of surprise billing are decreasing. The opposite is true in states like Texas that previously enacted policies to require payments of billed charges and have proven to undermine network value.[30]

There are several circumstances under which a patient would be unable to choose whether, or from whom, to receive care. Nobody chooses which ER doctor they see when they are taken out of the ambulance, nobody makes an appointment to see their preferred anesthesiologist, or insists that their blood be examined by a particular pathologist. In these instances, the facility chooses the doctor for the patient, rather than the patient choosing the doctor. There is a clear incentive for some providers to stay out of network for financial gain, leading to surprise billing. Federal action is needed to correct this perverse incentive that leads to higher costs for all consumers.

One of the most essential roles of a health insurance provider is to offer enrollees an array of health care providers who are conveniently located, meet the needs of the patient, are affordable, and are practicing the highest quality medicine. Indeed, this is the core of the service our members provide to more than 200 million Americans. Our members and health insurance providers across this country work to ensure that when patients need to see a doctor, they can see a high quality doctor of their choosing. When an enrollee needs a primary care physician, a gastroenterologist, a dermatologist, or take their child to a pediatrician, quality provider networks make that possible. We would not and could not support any legislation or other actions that make it more difficult for quality health care providers to join networks.

While network participation is an important element of this discussion, it is important to impress upon the committee that *the reason surprise medical bills are a problem is not a lack of network adequacy that some may suggest.* Surprise medical bills are a challenge solely because a small subset of medical specialists have sufficient market power that they lack the financial incentives to participate in health plan networks since their patient volume is not driven by network inclusion unlike most other provider types. They will continue to lack an incentive to join these networks, unless legislation is enacted to truly correct this underlying market failure.

We support federal legislation that creates a competitive market environment where health insurance providers and doctors can continue to actively collaborate on offering affordable, high quality care that puts patients first. If we effectively lower costs and incentivize greater network participation by ancillary physicians, Americans will find health care more affordable and have better access to the care they need from the other providers in their health plan's network.

Arbitration Would Increase Administrative Burdens and Health Care Costs

We have serious concerns about any proposal that would use arbitration to determine payments to out-of-network providers. We appreciate that the Administration and the "No Surprises Act" have rejected arbitration in favor of a market-based approach to protecting the American people from surprise medical bills.

[30] Texas Association of Health Plans Out of Network Claims Survey, February 2019. *TAHP*. Available at: https://cdn.ymaws.com/www.tahp.org/resource/collection/16E3C8B1-6C50-4F6D-8C23-EA29F4AE4818/Texas_Findings_OOn_Claims Final_2-15-19-compressed.pdf.

The fundamental problem with arbitration is that it imposes administrative burdens on the entire health care system, including employers that offer self-funded coverage. For the 110 million Americans who receive coverage in self-funded plans, a federally-imposed arbitration process would force employers to hire staff or outside consultants to manage a complex process. Health insurance providers would need to make similar investments.

The experience of Texas, which we discuss below, shows how arbitration can slow down the claims process, increase administrative burden, exacerbate patient aggravation, and limit payment certainty. When Texas established an arbitration system to resolve surprise medical bill disputes, the number of complaints increased dramatically. In 2013, the Texas Department of Insurance received 43 requests for mediation. A year later that figure had increased to more than 600, with at least 8,000 complaints expected this year. By the fall of 2018, there was a backlog of more than 4,000 cases.[31] The administrative burdens associated with these proceedings – for all parties involved – take away resources that could be better focused on our shared goal of advancing high-quality, patient-centered health care for all Americans.

Another major concern with arbitration is that this approach fails to address the root cause of surprise medical bills: exorbitant bills from certain specialty doctors and EMS providers. Accepting their egregiously high prices as a starting point will not help to lower health care costs for Americans.

Billed charges from these specialists represent a form of price gouging. As long as the inputs into the process give credence and weight to price gouging, the end result will be payments that are excessively high – which in turn will increase premiums. And if health plans must continue paying these exorbitant bills – even if slightly reduced – everyone who buys health insurance will shoulder the burdensome costs resulting from this price gouging. Arbitration will not succeed in correcting this market failure.

Lessons to Be Learned from State Legislation

As Congress explores legislative options for eliminating the problem of surprise medical bills, it is important to look at state laws in this area. Below we review the impact of laws enacted in California, Texas, and New York.

In California, a state law passed in 2018 provides surprise medical billing protections and establishes reimbursement requirements for *non-emergency* services received from non-contracting providers at contracting facilities. This law applies to both health care service plans and health insurance providers.[32]

The new California law is not based on provider charges. Instead, it requires health insurance providers to reimburse non-contracting providers the greater of the average contracted rate or 125% of Medicare fee-for-service reimbursement for the same or similar services in the general geographic area. The methodology for determining the average contracted rate went into effect January 1, 2019. If either the non-participating provider or the

[31] Root & Najmabadi. Thousands of Texans Were Shocked by Surprise Medical Bills – Their Requests for Help Overwhelmed the State. *The Texas Tribune*. February 12, 2019. https://www.texastribune.org/2019/02/12/texas-mediation-balance-billing-faces-massive-backlog/.

[32] Health care service plans are those entities regulated by the California Department of Managed Health Care and include all HMO plans, plus some PPO and EPO plans. Health insurers are those entities regulated by the California Department of Insurance and include some PPO and EPO plans.

payor disputes whether the payment of the specified rate is appropriate, the regulator – either the Department of Managed Health Care or the California Department of Insurance – can authorize a Dispute Resolution Process. Both parties in dispute must participate, and the decision of the independent organization is binding. This significantly narrows when this approach is used.

This approach determines the reimbursement methodology based on market rates defined as what similar providers routinely accept as payment in-full for their services. As a result, it does not increase health care spending. Instead, it encourages health insurance providers and health care providers to enter into mutually beneficial contracts. If Congress chooses to implement this type of methodology to address the issue of surprise medical bills, it will allow health insurance providers to continue to manage costs through contracting with health care providers while maintaining existing incentives for contracting providers and negotiating with new providers to join networks.

By banning surprise medical billing, protecting provider networks, and not adding new costs to the system, California represents the best current approach to protecting patients. Contrary to some public reports from provider organizations, we are not aware of health insurance providers refusing to contract with doctors or dramatically reducing reimbursement rates since the law took effect. In fact, we understand that some health plan networks have increased as a result of this law and that the state is looking at how similar protections can be expanded to emergency rooms, which are not currently covered.

By contrast, existing Texas state law ties reimbursement for non-contracting providers to billed charges by requiring carriers to pay the provider's usual and customary charges. To understand the impact of this approach, we note that in Texas billed charges at the 80th percentile of FAIR Health data (usual and customary rates) for a high severity emergency department visit total $1,902. This represents a payment of 3.94 times the average negotiated rate (allowed amounts by health plans) of $483. This outcome demonstrates that linking payments for out-of-network services to unjustified provider-set charges will lead to significantly greater out-of-network charges meaning higher costs for consumers. In Texas, 65% of ER physician spending is out of network, substantially higher than all other physician specialties.[33]

Not only has this system led to higher costs, it has also done nothing to tamp down on surprise billing. In fact, Texas currently has the highest rates of surprise medical billing in the country and some of the lowest network participation by ancillary providers despite robust and stringent network adequacy requirements for plans. Put simply, the perverse incentives to remain out of network were exacerbated by the Texas surprise billing law.

Recognizing the dire need to address the market failure in the state, the Texas legislature has approved legislation to standardize consumer protections across state-regulated health plans and remove patients from billing disputes. This bill, which was signed into law on June 4 and takes effect immediately, would prohibit surprise medical billing by providers of emergency services and certain facility-based services, require carriers to reimburse providers the usual and customary rate, and transform the existing mediation system into an arbitration program between the provider and insurer only. While we appreciate that patients will be taken out of the middle, the new law will do nothing to address the perverse provider incentives to remain out of network or to lower costs for consumers.

[33] TAHP Out of Network Claims Survey, IBID.

In New York, state law provides for a "baseball style" dispute resolution process whereby providers submit a rate for consideration and health insurance providers submit their own reimbursement rate. Whichever submission the mediator finds more reasonable is determined to be the reimbursement amount for the disputed claim. The New York State system relies on a practicing physician to serve as mediator, which adds an inherent level of bias into the process. Additionally, unjustified provider-set charges are required to be a consideration in the arbiter's determination.

Costs in the New York dispute resolution system can be significant, with standard claims disputes filing fees costing plans, anecdotally, between $500-800 to resolve. For many arbitration systems, the filing fee in a two-party dispute is $1,500 per party, as identified by JAMS, a leading third-party mediation and arbitration firm, which represents a typical market rate for such services.[34] These fees do not include additional in-house or outside counsel or other costs involved in arbitration. Plans are required to factor these administrative costs into premiums, which has a direct impact on consumers and their ability to access affordable coverage.

While evidence suggests that the current system in New York reduced costs once enacted, that cost reduction is relative to an unreasonably high standard, which is what prompted the legislation in the first place. New York's previous system, like Texas, required the payment of provider-set billed charges. As a result, costs were unsustainably high.[35]

Based on the impact an arbitration system like New York's has on both market incentives and administrative costs, AHIP believes that New York's system does not deliver optimal outcomes and, if implemented nationally, would not effectively reduce costs.

Looking at the different approaches taken in these states, we urge the committee to pursue a California-style solution that protects patients and consumers with common sense rules that do not undermine networks, do not lead to higher cost-sharing or premiums, and help increase access to affordable coverage options.

Conclusion

Thank you for this opportunity to testify. AHIP and our member health insurance providers appreciate the committee's bipartisan commitment to finding solutions to surprise medical bills that will ensure quality care and lower costs for everyone. AHIP and the other stakeholders we have partnered with stand ready and willing to work with the Administration and Congress to alleviate the financial burdens imposed on the American people by surprise medical bills and make health care more affordable. By working together and putting the best interests of consumers first, we can strengthen our health care system and reduce costs for all Americans.

* * *

Ms. ESHOO. Thank you.

Dr. Vidor Friedman, you have five minutes for your testimony.

---

[34] Arbitration Schedule of Fees and Costs. *JAMS*. https://www.jamsadr.com/arbitration-fees.

[35] Lawsky, Benjamin. An Unwelcome Surprise, How New Yorkers Are Getting Stuck with Unexpected Medical Bills from Out-of-Network Providers. *NY State Department of Financial Services*. March 7, 2012, http://www.statecoverage.org/files/NY-Unexpected_Medical_Bills-march_7_2012.pdf.

Statement of Vidor E. Friedman, M.D., F.A.C.E.P., President, American College of Emergency Physicians (ACEP), Attending Emergency Physician, Florida Hospitals Celebration Health, Orlando, FL

Dr. FRIEDMAN. Thank you, Madam Chair and members of the Health Subcommittee.

On behalf of the American College of Emergency Physicians— ACEP—and our 38,000 members, I would like to thank you for the opportunity to speak with you today about this critical issue of surprise medical bills.

The reason emergency physicians like myself do what we do first and foremost is to take care of patients in their moments of greatest need. This is not the time where patients should be worrying about verifying who their provider is, are in network, or what their deductible is, or what the cost of—the total cost of treatment might be.

I care for each and every one of the patients that comes to my emergency department regardless of ability to pay. I do this not just because of the oath that I took as a physician but because it is appropriately required by Federal law.

Unlike most physicians, emergency physicians are prohibited by Federal law from discussing with a patient any potential costs of care or insurance details until they are screened and stabilized.

This important patient protection, known as EMTALA, ensures physicians focus on the immediate medical needs of patients. However, it also means that patients cannot fully understand the potential cost of their care or the limitations of their insurance coverage until they receive the bill.

We understand that this can cause frustration, confusion, and, frankly, even be scary for patients. We agree with the committee's commitments to take patients out of the middle of surprise billing disputes and I would like to emphasize 3 key principles that ACEP urges Congress to consider as it works to address surprise billing.

The first, and above all, is protecting patients. Congress should limit patients' out-of-pocket responsibility for emergency care, so they won't pay any more than the in-network amount.

Currently, this protection only applies to co-payments and co-insurance, not to deductibles. We support the committee's intent on this provision in the discussion draft but urge you to go further than simply counting co-payments and co-insurance towards any deductible or out-of-network max.

Rather, we urge you to require deductibles for out-of-network emergency services to be treated as if they were in network.

The second principle is to improve transparency. While EMTALA prohibits me from discussing potential costs of care with my patients in advance, there are other ways Congress can improve transparency for emergency patients. Insurers should more clearly convey plan details to their enrollees. This will help patients better understand the limitations of their insurance coverage and all potential out-of-pocket costs.

Insurers should also be required to explain to enrollees what their rights are under Federal law related to emergency care in easy to understand clear language.

Third, now that we have taken the patient out of the middle, Congress should ensure fair and transparent dispute resolution between physicians and insurers. The goal should be a system in which everyone is in network or essentially that.

That requires a level playing field between providers and insurers. Insurers are concerned that bench marking even median charges favors providers. Providers are concerned that bench marking the median in-network rates favors insurers. What's Congress to do?

ACEP supports a system that has already proven to be balanced between insurers and providers. That is a baseball-style independent dispute resolution process similar to that used in New York and noted in the legislative proposal put forth by Drs. Ruiz, Roe, and Bucshon.

In New York this simple and effective solution has almost completely eliminated surprise bills. It incentivizes physicians to charge reasonable rates and it also incentivizes insurers to compensate at appropriate levels. Insurance premiums and healthcare costs in New York have actually grown more slowly than the rest of the nation.

This model would be the least disruptive to the current system. It is the only model with empirical data detailing the positive impact it has had for patients and all stakeholders.

To be clear, this model has not been extraordinarily bureaucratic, costly, burdensome, or inflationary. More must be done to protect patients and their families from unexpected medical bills, and we stand with you in this regard.

On behalf of the 150 million Americans my members care for every year, I thank you for your consideration and the opportunity to speak with you today.

[The prepared statement of Dr. Friedman follows:]

Written Testimony of Vidor E. Friedman, M.D.

Introduction

Thank you Mr. Chairman and members of the Health Subcommittee. On behalf of the American College of Emergency Physicians (ACEP), our 38,000 emergency physician members, and the more than 150 million Americans we treat on an annual basis, I would like to thank you for this opportunity to testify before your committee today on the issue of surprise medical bills.

In a medical emergency, getting treatment as soon as possible is the number one priority – not verifying which providers are in-network, figuring out how much your deductible is, or worrying how much treatment will cost. These are important considerations to be sure, but the reason my colleagues and I do what we do for a living is, first and foremost, to take care of our patients. Responsibility for their well-being is our top priority, but there are aspects of what we do that make us unique, and this sometimes causes frustration when a patient receives a bill for services rendered that they thought would be covered by their insurance.

Unlike most physicians, emergency physicians are *prohibited by law* from discussing with a patient any potential costs of care or insurance details until they are screened and stabilized. This important patient protection enacted in 1986 under the Emergency Medical Treatment and Labor Act (EMTALA) ensures emergency care focuses on immediate medical needs. However, it also means that patients often do not fully understand the potential costs that could be involved in their care or the limitations of their insurance coverage until they receive their bill.

ACEP, and most of the groups represented at this table and around the room today have been working with lawmakers on this issue for nearly a year. The early discussions focused more on education about how the system currently operates, what Congress could and should do to address this important issue, and evaluating what states have already enacted. As these discussions progressed and we began to see the initial proposals from various Members of Congress, ACEP announced and put forward a framework of the three key principles that Congress should consider as earlier proposals were refined and new ones introduced:

Protect Patients

Take patients out of the middle of billing disputes. Establish caps on patient responsibility for unanticipated emergency medical care so that patients won't pay more out-of-pocket (i.e., co-insurance, co-pay, ***and*** deductible) than they would have paid if their emergency care were provided in-network. This is an important distinction because these protections currently only apply to co-insurance and co-payment amounts.

Level the Playing Field

ACEP would strongly urge Congress to limit the scope of their proposal as much as possible to avoid unintentionally providing an advantage to one party over another when there is a disputed claim for out-of-network care, provided the patient has already been removed from such discussions as I previously mentioned. For this reason, we would urge the committee to reconsider using an independent, "baseball-style" arbitration process. This process is a simple, efficient solution that incentivizes providers to charge reasonable rates and insurers to compensate at reasonable rates. For example, in New York, where this process was enacted in 2014 and which became effective in January 2015, this model has almost eliminated surprise medical bills. Meanwhile, insurance premiums and health care costs in the state have grown more slowly than the rest of the nation. This model would be the least disruptive to the current system and is the only one with empirical data detailing the positive impact it has had for patients and stakeholders alike.

Improve Transparency

To ensure patients better understand the limitations of their insurance coverage and all potential out-of-pocket costs each time they seek care, insurers should more clearly convey beneficiary plan details to their customers. This should include printing the deductible on each insurance card; clearly explaining their rights related to emergency care in easy-to-understand, clear language; and maintaining up-to-date lists of in- and out-of-network providers that are easily accessible.

ACEP appreciates the work the committee members and their staffs have already done to protect patients and their families from unexpected medical bills. It is my sincere hope that my testimony will further help you understand the complexities of this issue, which are not readily apparent upon first glance, as well as illustrate the intended and possible unintended consequences of various surprise medical bill legislative proposals. We all have the same objective: protect patients and ensure their continued access to all types of physicians and specialists so they can get the care they need and deserve.

What Is EMTALA and What Does It Do?

Essentially, the Emergency Medical Treatment and Labor Act (EMTALA) is a federal law that requires anyone coming to a hospital emergency department to be stabilized and treated, regardless of their insurance status or ability to pay.

In 1986, EMTALA went into effect as part of the Consolidated Omnibus Reconciliation Act (COBRA) of 1985. It was designed to prevent hospitals from transferring uninsured or underinsured patients to public hospitals without, at a minimum, providing a medical screening examination (MSE) to ensure they were stable for transfer, and if needed, stabilization care. There are three main obligations associated with this law:

1. For any person who comes to a hospital emergency department, there is an affirmative obligation on the part of the hospital and its physicians to provide that patient with an MSE to determine whether an emergency medical condition (EMC) exists.
2. If an EMC exists, the hospital (through the services of emergency and other on-call physicians from other specialties) must stabilize the medical condition provided within its facility or initiate an appropriate transfer to a facility capable of treating the patient. Hospitals are required to maintain a list of these on-call physicians who can provide the treatment needed to stabilize an EMC.
3. Hospitals with more specialized capabilities are obligated to accept appropriate transfers from hospitals that lack the capability to treat unstable EMCs.

While EMTALA only applies to hospitals that participate in the Medicare program, in practical terms, this means that it applies to virtually all hospitals in the United States and the obligations associated with EMTALA apply to all patients, not just to Medicare patients.

Under the EMTALA statute (42 U.S.C. 1395dd) an EMC is defined as a medical condition manifesting itself by acute symptoms of sufficient severity (including severe pain) such that the absence of immediate medical attention could reasonably be expected to result in –

1. Placing the health of the individual (or, with respect to a pregnant woman, the health of the woman or her unborn child) in serious jeopardy,
2. Serious impairment to bodily functions, or
3. Serious dysfunction of any bodily organ or part, or
4. With respect to a pregnant woman who is having contractions, that there is inadequate time to effect the safe transfer to another hospital before delivery, or that the transfer may pose a threat to the health or safety of the woman or her unborn child.

As is the case with the term EMC, the EMTALA statute defines when a patient is "stabilized," but this determination is ultimately a matter of clinical judgment on the part of the medical professional assessing the patient.

Violations of EMTALA can subject the hospital and/or physician to a fine of up to $104,826 per violation (hospital over 100 beds) and up to $52,414 per violation (under 100 beds).

How Does EMTALA Affect Physician-Insurer Contracts

EMTALA ensures that emergency departments, emergency physicians, and other on-call specialists have a "safety-net" of care so that anyone in the nation which requires emergency medical treatment will receive it. However, because the federal government mandates that these services be provided, regardless of insurance status or ability to pay, it means two things. First, the services rendered by the hospital and its providers often go unreimbursed. Second, because insurance companies know their beneficiaries will receive care in the emergency department regardless of whether the company has a contract for these services or not, there is less incentive for insurers/plans to negotiate for these services and bring emergency physicians in-network.

This, unfortunately, means the claims of physicians who provide emergency care for commercially insured services are often paid by health plans at rates that are substantially below the usual and customary value of these services. In the recent past, most plans based the allowed benefit for these services on the 70th or 80th percentile of usual and customary charges. But, as was the case with Ingenix in New York[36,37] the database used for this purpose underrepresented these charges. In response to successful legal challenges to such flawed databases, some insurers/plans have established out-of-network benefit rates that are still substantially below usual and customary payments.

The lack of a system to ensure fair benefit reimbursements has allowed insurers/plans to underpay the fair value of emergency services, which has created an imperative to preserve balance billing, or at the very least establish a corresponding fair and independent mechanism to resolve provider-insurer reimbursement disputes. This is vital to ensuring the financial viability of the nation's emergency care system. If an emergency department cannot keep its doors open, then the community it serves loses access to these lifesaving services, and that affects the insured and uninsured equally.

Improving Transparency for Consumers

While patient cost-sharing as a part of health insurance benefit structure can help incentivize patients to make better and lower-cost decisions when seeking scheduled health care, there are significant limitations to its effectiveness in an emergency. As noted earlier, emergency physicians and hospitals are prohibited under EMTALA from discussing with the patient any potential costs of care or details of their particular insurance coverage until they are screened and stabilized. This is an important patient protection that helps ensure their care stays focused on their immediate medical needs. But it also means that patients may not fully understand the costs involved in their care or the limitations of their particular insurance coverage until they get the bill.

Often any bill following emergency care is, therefore, a surprise to the patient, who assumed that their insurance coverage would only be subject to the (for example) $150 copay that is listed on their benefits card. ACEP proposes insurers be required to include the policyholder's in- and out- of-network deductibles for care on the benefit card, to at least make it clearer to that policyholder what the limits of their insurance coverage really is, and the amounts of cost-sharing they will be personally liable for should they require emergency or other care.

Plans or issuers must specify their insurance product on the patient's member ID card so that it is clear to both the patient and treating providers. For scheduled care, this information can greatly facilitate providers being able to assist patients at the point of care with navigating

---

[36] https://www.lexisnexis.com/legalnewsroom/insurance/b/medicalinsurance/posts/final-approval-granted-in-350-million-settlement-with-united-in-reimbursement-dispute.

[37] https://www.nytimes.com/2009/01/17/opinion/17sat1.html.

their coverage and benefits and more specifically provide out-of-pocket pricing estimates. As well, for both emergency and scheduled care, having this information recorded in a patient's record can help the provider resolve billing issues and potential disputes on the patient's behalf, keeping the patient out of the middle.

Furthermore, plans or issuers must provide their enrollees with meaningful and simple explanations regarding coverage for emergency care that they are guaranteed under federal law. This includes informing them of the federal Prudent Layperson Standard, which requires coverage for patients who seek emergency care for "acute symptoms of sufficient severity (including severe pain) such that a prudent layperson, who possesses an average knowledge of health and medicine, could reasonably expect the absence of immediate medical attention to result in the following:

- Placing the health of the individual (or, for a pregnant woman, the health of the woman or her unborn child) in serious jeopardy.
- Serious impairment to bodily functions.
- Serious dysfunction of any bodily organ or part."

While this requirement is in federal law for all commercial plan types, over the past year insurers such as Anthem, United, and Blue Cross Blue Shield of Texas have all implemented policies that to varying degrees can retroactively deny a range of emergency care for policyholders who seek it for symptoms that turn out to be non-emergent.

ACEP is particularly concerned about the lack of transparency around out-of-network rates for services. ACEP has pushed for years to have these rates be determined through a transparent process, using publicly verifiable data. However, regulators have allowed a lack of enforceable and transparent standards for out-of-network benefits in legislation and regulations governing health plan coverage for emergency care services. Many insurers use the usual, customary, and reasonable ("UCR") amount to determine their out-of-network rates. We strongly believe that when determining UCR insurers should use a database of geographically comparable usual and customary charges maintained by an independent non-profit organization that is not affiliated, financially supported, and/or otherwise supported by an issuer or by a supplier. This type of database, such as FAIR Health as one example, should be transparent, statistically valid, and protected against conflict of interest.

Ensuring Network Adequacy

In many parts of the country, insurers have near-monopolies (if not full monopolies) of market share; there are numerous examples of a single plan controlling more than half of the market. Such market power allows insurers to offer take-it-or-leave-it contracts and narrow their physician networks, which just further exacerbates issues of out-of-network care and the unexpected bills that can sometimes result. In fact, according to the Kaiser Family Foundation, the top three insurers in the large group market had a market share of at least 80 percent in 43 states in 2017.[38]

---

[38] https://www.kff.org/other/state-indicator/market-share-and-enrollment-of-largest-three-insurers-large-group-market.

Emergency physicians *want* to contract with insurers and provide in-network care. Physicians accept low-discounted contract rates with private payors because being in-network provides long-term certainty of a contract, allows for better projections of future business needs, and provides additional assurance of reimbursement directly from the insurer, rather than shifting the responsibility so that physicians must seek it from patients following their care. While all physicians enjoy benefits from being in-network, this last point is especially relevant to emergency physicians. Unlike many physicians of other specialties who practice in the community and can collect patient payment up-front before the patient is even allowed into a treatment room, EMTALA forbids emergency physicians from such practices.

While many states (and even federal law under the Affordable Care Act) require insurers to have adequate networks, these standards are vague, qualitative, and not being enforced. For example, a 2016 survey of physicians in Texas by the Texas Medical Association found among physicians who approached a plan in an attempt to join its network, *35 percent received no response from the plan*—this was an increase of 6 percentage points from a survey in 2014, and a 13-point increase from 2012.[39]

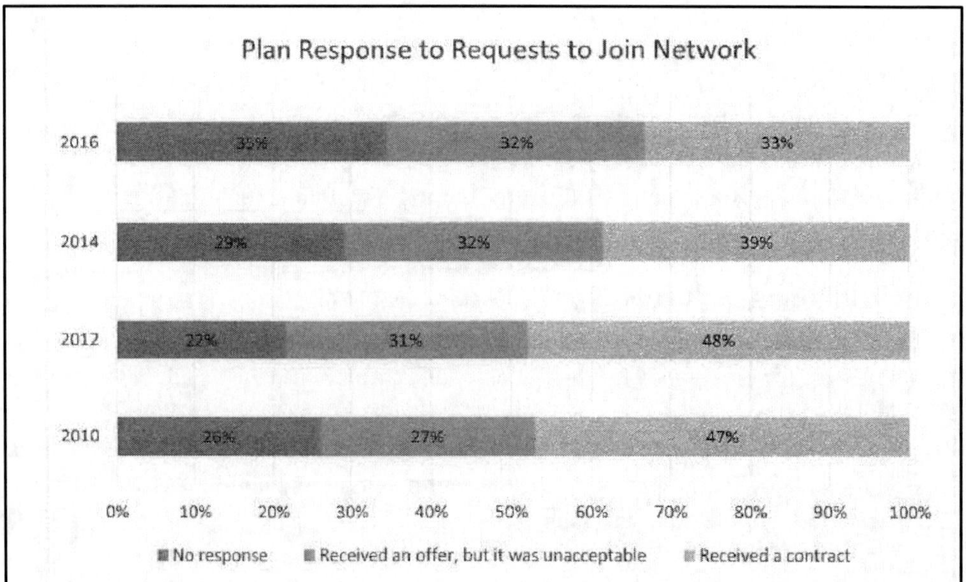

As can be seen in the chart above, the percentage of surveyed physicians who received a contract correspondingly decreased over the same years, yet the percent who received an offer from the insurance plan but found it unacceptable (i.e., turned it down) remained stable. From this, we can conclude that the majority of physicians are continuing to make good faith efforts to be in-network, but are being met with growing resistance from the insurance plans.

Similarly, in California, there are numerous reports of insurers refusing to renew long-standing contracts (that paid more than the benchmarked under law out-of-network rate of 125% of Medicare). Some insurers are terminating contracts unless physicians accept payment reductions as substantial as *forty percent*. Other payors are reportedly closing their networks to new physicians, and most are reducing their physician networks overall to eliminate historical contracted rates from the industry benchmarking database to avoid having them serve as a basis

---

39 *Texas Medical Association*, "Survey of Texas Physician 2016: Research Findings," available at: https://www.texmed.org/uploadedFiles/Current/2016_Advocacy/2016_Physician_Survey_Findings.pdf.

for establishing the state contracted rates in the future. And overall, California premiums continue to rise.

At a minimum, Congress should seek to establish a federal patient emergency care access standard and ensure a corresponding enforcement mechanism. This would require health plans or issuers of all commercial products (including ERISA) to demonstrate to their State Insurance Commissioner that their plans ensure patient access to emergency care for an emergency medical condition. The standard should include consideration of time, distance, and provider capacity within the relevant geographic area, and an endeavor to support such access through good faith, comprehensive efforts to contract with emergency treatment providers at reasonable/adequate rates and under timely payment terms.

Therefore, we ask the committee to include specific language in any legislation considered that insurers be required to maintain adequate provider networks. The legislation should require the Secretary of Labor, in consultation with the Secretary of Health and Human Services, to adopt quantitative standards that insurers must meet in order to ensure access to a sufficient number of contracted physicians (specialists, subspecialists, and primary care) and other health care providers in each geographic region who have the requisite training and expertise to provide that care, and in sufficient numbers, so patients may obtain timely access to all necessary medical care from in-network providers when possible.

Special consideration should be given to hospital-based physicians who provide emergency medical care under the federal EMTALA mandate as they cannot refuse treatment of any patient who presents themselves to the hospital emergency department. Without such consideration, insurers would have no incentive to contract with these providers. Additionally, the network adequacy standard must be approved by the Secretaries of Labor and Health and Human Services before each plan may be offered in the market.

Developing an All-Payer Claims Database

ACEP supports the development of robust all-payer claims databases (APCDs) that mandate the collection of claims from all payers. While this may provide informative data for research purposes, if the APCD is used to calculate out-of-network reimbursement rates, then only data derived from commercial plans should be used for that purpose. Fifteen states have APCDs in place, and numerous others are either considering or in the process of, implementing APCDs. States can mandate the submission of some data by state law, resulting in consistent, uniform data.

In all, there are examples of strong state APCDs that collect claims data from all payers, such as Oregon, and others that are not as robust and only collect some data from those payers that voluntarily participate. Virginia's APCD falls in the latter category; although it collects claims from almost every payer, it does not mandate collections, so insurers can pick and choose what data to submit and thus leave room for data manipulation. See Appendix B[40] of a report prepared by the University of Chicago's NORC for a summary of APCD features by the state as of May 2017.

However, per the U.S. Supreme Court's ruling in *Gobeille v. Liberty Mutual Insurance Co.*, the Court held that states may not require plans regulated under the Employee Retirement

[40] https://endinsurancegap.org/wp-content/uploads/2017/01/NORC-Revised-Final-5-24-17-2.pdf.

Income Security Act (ERISA) to submit their data to the state's APCD (though such data may still be submitted voluntarily). Given that ERISA plans can represent more than 50 percent of employer-sponsored coverage in many parts of the country, APCDs in such states will have limited data that is not representative of the entire population.

As the House Energy and Commerce Committee considers creating a grant program to fund state efforts to implement new, or maintain existing, APCDs, the committee should specify certain criteria for APCDs that states must agree to adhere to to receive the funding. *States that are awarded the grants to develop new APCDs must, on condition of receiving the grant, mandate participation from all payers, including ERISA plans.* The current discussion draft released by the committee does not include any such requirements or even provide guidance for states to consider when implementing new APCDs or maintaining existing APCDs. Furthermore, the draft does not specify the purposes for which states can use the APCDs developed using the grant funding, which would impact how the state decides to structure the APCD. If a state's APCD is used for the eventual purposes of creating an established payment amount that would be paid to out-of-network providers (as allowed under the discussion draft's newly added Section 2719A(b)(2)(H)(i) of the Public Health Service Act), it is even more important for the APCD to include claims data from all payers so that the payment amount determined by the state is accurate and not biased. *In short, any federal legislation that mandates the use of a state APCD as a transparent database from which to benchmark out-of-network payments must also provide a corresponding federal requirement that ERISA plans contribute data to it as well.*

An additional technical issue with the current discussion draft relates to the appropriations language. The Committee should clarify that the $50 million appropriations must be used solely for the actual grants to states. By stating that the appropriation would be used to "carry out this subsection," the Secretary of the Department of Health and Human Services (HHS) could use some of the funding for administrative purposes to establish the grants. Furthermore, the discussion draft should include a deadline by which the HHS Secretary would be required to make the grants to states, or at least issue the funding opportunity announcement. This would ensure that grants are awarded to states in a timely manner.

We believe the changes highlighted above will strengthen the current section in the discussion draft on APCDs and ensure that the grants are used effectively to create APCDs that contain accurate data that is representative of the entire state population.

Using a Benchmark Rate to Determine Reimbursement Disputes

ACEP has previously stated that payment disputes that can sometimes arise between insurers and out-of-network providers should be resolved in a manner that takes the patient completely out of the middle, is transparent, and does not increase federal healthcare expenditures. However, we have strong concerns and oppose the use of a benchmark for establishing out-of-network (OON) payment amounts. We noted previously that emergency physicians want to contract with insurers and accept low-discounted contract rates with private payors in exchange for certain benefits – such as business certainty, reduced administrative burdens, and more efficient reimbursement.

Allowing insurers to access a discounted contract rate (via benchmarked OON payments) without providing the benefits of contracting in exchange will discourage contracting and result in narrower networks of physicians and less patient choice. Discounted OON payments will severely harm emergency physician's ability to cover even just their practice costs and serve patients, given the additional challenges they face as safety-net physicians who must absorb significant amounts of under- and uncompensated care as a result of the EMTALA mandate.

Insurance design changes in recent years have raised deductibles to amounts far beyond what the average American can pay. As noted recently by the Kaiser Family Foundation[41] (emphasis added),

> …from 2006 to 2016, average payments for deductibles and coinsurance among people with large employer coverage rose considerably faster than the total cost for covered benefits; however, the average payments for copayments fell during the same period. As can be seen in the chart below, over this time, *patient cost-sharing rose notably faster than insurer payments for care as health plans have become a little less generous in this regard.*

This exponential skyrocketing of deductibles (top, or green, line in the graph below) has resulted in a corresponding increase in the amount of bad debt that emergency physicians incur.

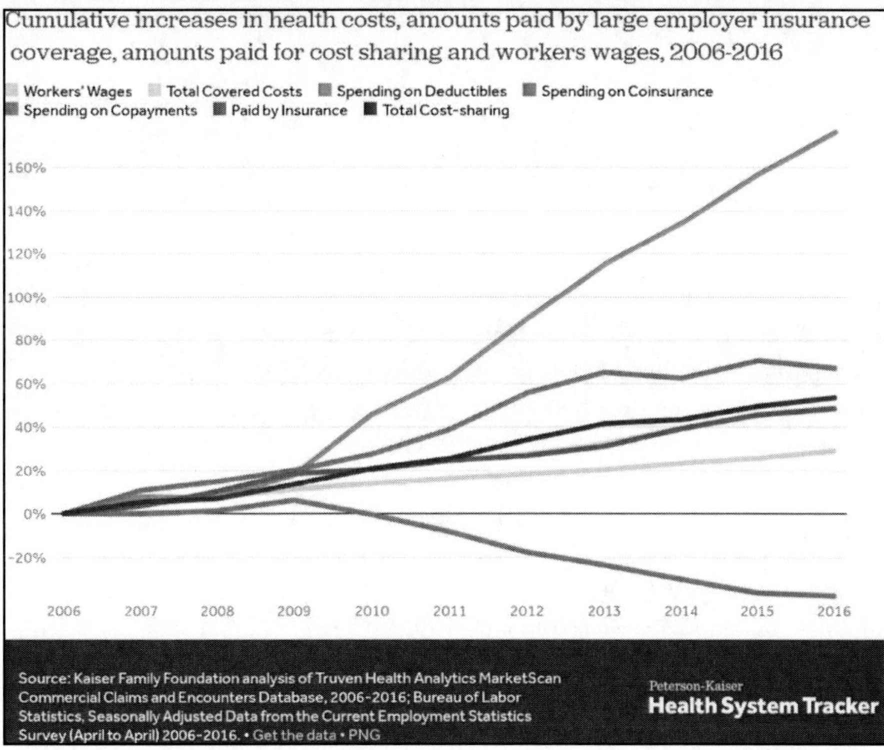

Accompanied by the further decline in Medicare reimbursements since then, as well as Medicaid expansion in many states that greatly increased the proportion of Medicaid patients, such losses continue to grow. Emergency physicians are the only safety net for many in our country, including vulnerable uninsured, Medicare, Medicaid, and pediatric patients. Should commercial insurance reimbursement rates be further scaled back, it will be very difficult to

---

[41] https://www.healthsystemtracker.org/brief/increases-in-cost-sharing-payments-have-far-outpaced-wage-growth/#item-start.

keep the doors open 24 hours a day, seven days a week, and 365 days a year in many emergency departments, especially those in rural or urban underserved areas.

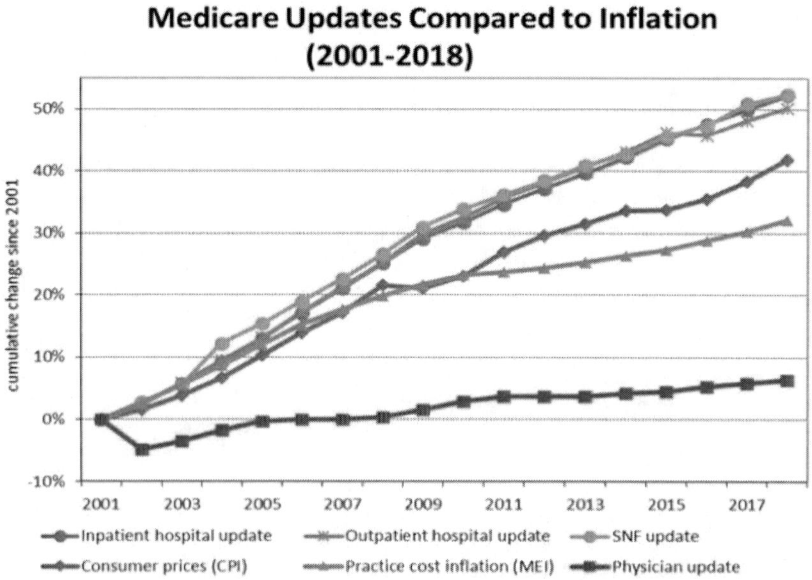

Sources: Federal Register, Medicare Trustees' Reports and U.S. Bureau of Labor Statistics.

A benchmarked payment based on commercial in-network rates (such as the Energy and Commerce Committee draft calls for) will also have a ripple effect on future contracts, since the out-of-network payment rate becomes the new natural "high" in a geographic area, and future in-network contracts will always be lower. As this continues year-over-year, there will be a downward spiral with unintended consequences for maintaining patient access to emergency care. Sites with high-acuity, complex patients, including emergency departments in rural areas (where it is harder already to recruit physicians) may especially be put at risk with such a benchmark cap on out-of-network payments.

It is important to note that a benchmarked payment based on a percentage of Medicare rates (rather than in-network contracted amounts) is also flawed, because:

- Medicare rates were never intended to reflect market rates and have not kept pace with inflation. According to data from the Medicare Trustees, Medicare physician pay has barely changed over the last decade and a half, increasing just 6 percent from 2001 to 2018, or just 0.4 percent per year on average. In comparison, Medicare hospital pay has increased roughly 50 percent between 2001 and 2018, with average annual increases of 2.5 percent per year for inpatient services, and 2.4 percent per year for outpatient services. The 2019 Medicare Trustees Report[42], specifically states that annual Medicare updates for physicians do NOT keep pace with the average rate of physician cost increases. The Trustees believe that absent a change in the delivery system or future legislative update to physician rates, access to Medicare-participating physicians will become a significant issue in the long term.

---

[42] https://www.cms.gov/Research-Statistics-Data-and-Systems/Statistics-Trends-and-Reports/ReportsTrustFunds/Downloads/TR2019.pdf.

- Medicare does not accurately reflect practice costs. Medicare physician pay has declined 19 percent from 2001 to 2018, or by 1.3 percent per year on average.
- Medicare rates were never designed for the general population but rather an age-specific group (e.g., does not include pediatrics or obstetrics).
- Medicare is shifting toward a value-based payment approach, and it is unclear how it could be used as a basis for determining a benchmark rate in future years.

In California, for example, where out-of-network payments are based on an average in-network contract rate somewhat similar to the committee's discussion draft, many insurers have decided they don't need contracts because they can simply pay the lower rates established in the new law and refuse to contract. This has resulted in even further narrowing of networks and reduced access to care.

We are also concerned with the discussion draft's definition of how such in-network rates are set. Experience has shown that when criteria are set in state or federal law for out-of-network emergency service payment, insurers frequently fail to adhere to these criteria, and regulators have failed to enforce such adherence adequately.

For example, as you may know, Congress enacted a provision in the Affordable Care Act forbidding insurers from imposing coverage limitations on out-of-network emergency services that are more restrictive than any limitations imposed on in-network emergency services[43]. In 2010, the Obama Administration issued an interim final rule (IFR) to implement this provision. Since the statute did not ban balance billing, the IFR established a "reasonable payment" for out-of-network emergency services. This payment amount was necessary because, otherwise, insurers might establish extremely low payment rates, thus subjecting patients to very high balance bills. The IFR established for this payment a "greatest of three" (GOT) methodology in which the insurer must pay the greatest of the following:

- The insurer's in-network amount;
- The amount calculated by the same method the plan generally uses for out-of-network services, such as the usual, customary, and reasonable ("UCR") amount; or,
- The Medicare amount.

Unfortunately, the GOT policy did not have its intended effect of being a reasonable and objective payment standard, and we have repeatedly voiced concern with the second of the GOT standards since the IFR was promulgated in 2010. The UCR amount is subject to insurer manipulation unless it is in some way objectively verifiable, and the term "usual, customary, and reasonable amount" is not an objective standard for calculating out-of-network payments because it is not defined. Accordingly, we have recommended that the data supporting the calculation be subject to independent verification.

In the end, because the underlying statute did not provide an appropriate amount of specificity surrounding payment, we find ourselves in a situation where the regulation that was necessary to fill in the missing details represents a substantial threat to the financial viability of the emergency medicine profession and patient access to qualified emergency physicians and emergency department on-call specialists. Not surprisingly, emergency physicians have seen

[43] Section 2719A(b)(1)(C)(ii)(II) of the Public Health Service Act as added by Section 1001 of the Patient Protection and Affordable Care Act.

payments for out-of-network services drop significantly since the GOT regulation was issued in 2010.

For these reasons, we strongly oppose the use of any payment benchmark for setting out-of-network payments in emergency care. Should one be used, it must at least include the following provisions:

- Be directly tied to an independent, transparent, and robust national database such as FAIR Health.
- Data used to determine allowed amount benchmarks should include both in-network and out-of-network claims, from both ERISA and non-ERISA private, commercial plans alike, and include the co-pay and co-insurance. Given the variability that can exist in the payment amounts from a single insurer to a single provider across its products (i.e., out-of-network ERISA vs. small group vs. individual market), we are concerned the benchmark estimates will be distorted downward.
- Be anchored to a specific year, with a medical cost of living inflation index added each year, to alleviate the "downward spiral" on future contracting described earlier, as well as possible insurer manipulation of the benchmark through contract eliminations.

Preferred Approach to Resolve Reimbursement Disputes

To prevent significantly distorting negotiations between insurers and providers and wholesale disruption, *we strongly recommend the committee adopt the proven and successful approach used in New York State instead.* The bi-partisan legislative proposal, the "Protecting People from Surprise Medical Bills Act,"[44] that is soon to be introduced by Reps. Raul Ruiz (D-CA) and Phil Roe (R-TN) specifically use this successful state solution as the federal approach to protecting patients and resolving out-of-network reimbursement disputes.

Under the New York law, which incorporates an independent dispute resolution (IDR) process wherein the provider and insurer participate in arbitration, patients are no longer required to pay out-of-network provider charges for surprise out-of-network services that are higher than the patient's standard in-network co-payment, deductible, or co-insurance amounts. Since enactment, New York successfully reduced the rate of out-of-network patient billing for emergency department services from 20.1% in 2013 to 6.4% in 2015, a near 70 percent reduction.[45] This New York law has since been repeatedly hailed as an example for the rest of the country among the health care community, and provides an effective, balanced solution, while still adhering to free-market principles.

Not all claims are included in the IDR process. Smaller claims for emergency services that are currently less than $683.22 (annually adjusted for inflation) and do not exceed 120 percent of "usual and customary cost" (UCR) are automatically exempted. UCR is defined as the 80th percentile of all charges for a health service rendered by a provider in the same or similar specialty and provided in the same geographic region as reported by a benchmarking database maintained by a non-profit organization. New York identifies the FAIR Health charge database

[44] A section by section summary of the "Protecting People from Surprise Medical Bills Act" is available at: https://ruiz.house.gov/media-center/press-releases/reps-ruiz-roe-release-outline-bipartisan-legislation-reps-morelle-taylor.

[45] Cooper, Z.; Morton, F. S.; and Shekita, N. (2017). Surprise! Out-of-Network Billing/or Emergency Care in the United States. *National Bureau of Economic Research*, https://www.nber.org/papers/w23623.pdf.

as an independent entity that can calculate UCR. Effectively, these claims are automatically paid if they conform with this standard. Otherwise, it would potentially cost more to arbitrate these low-dollar claims than the value of the services, and it helps reduce the number of instances when arbitration may be necessary.

Under the established IDR process for emergency services, the arbitrator picks either the charge set by the provider or the allowed amount offered by the insurer, without modification. The party whose amount is not chosen must pay for the cost of the arbitration (estimated by the State of NY to range from $225 to $325 per appeal), as well as any outstanding amounts as a result of the decision. The FAIR Health database rates are benchmarks to *guide* final payment, *but they do not constitute government rate-setting*. Both insurers and physicians can submit additional information as outlined in the law to substantiate their payment position.

This "loser pays" baseball-style arbitration process has proven to be an effective way of incentivizing providers to charge reasonable rates, while at the same time encouraging insurers to pay appropriate and reasonable amounts. Since both parties have this powerful incentive to act fairly, most claims do not even need to go into the IDR process. As seen in the chart below, out of the approximately 7 million visits to the emergency department each year in New York[46], only 849 emergency claims went to arbitration. As well, the decisions rendered on these were evenly split, further demonstrating that the system is working.

Emergency Services

Total received	849
Not eligible	162
Still in process	139
Decision rendered	548
Health Plan payment more reasonable	143
Provider charges more reasonable	176
Split decision	165
Settlement reached	64

The New York law has preserved access to emergency care and has not led to significant increases in insurance premiums. The Kaiser Family Foundation has shown that premiums in New York have grown more slowly than rates for the rest of the nation over the last five years.[47] Physician networks are stable and not declining. New York insurers reported to Georgetown University researchers[48] that the law had incentivized insurers to have networks of physicians as "expansive as possible." Further, a FAIR Health report[49] shows that the "billed charge" payment rates have declined by 13 percent since enactment.

It is clear that the New York law has been a success, minimizing disruption, constraining costs, keeping premiums stable, and, most importantly, protecting consumers. *We therefore*

---

[46] https://nyshc.health.ny.gov/web/nyapd/emergency-department-visits-in-new-york.

[47] Kaiser Family Foundation (2015-2019): "Marketplace Average Benchmark Premiums," https://www.kff.org/e4f94bd/.

[48] Corlette, S.; Hoppe, O. Georgetown University Health Policy Institute: Center on Health Insurance Reform, "New York's 2014 Law to Protect Consumers from Surprise Out-of-Network Bills Mostly Working as Intended: Results of a Case Study," (May 2019). https://georgetown.app.box.com/s/6onkj1jaiy3f1618iy7j0gpzdoew2zu9.

[49] The New York State Health Foundation, "Issue Brief: New York's Efforts to Reform Surprise Medical Billing," (February 2019), https://nyshealthfoundation.org/wp-content/uploads/2019/02/new-yorks-efforts-to-reform-surprise-medical-billing.pdf.

strongly urge the committee to use this approach rather than the one proposed in the discussion draft.

Other Recommendations

There are also aspects of the committee's draft legislation that ACEP believes should be included or modified. First, the draft proposal should be more explicit regarding patient protection from high out-of-network deductibles. The legislation should go further than solely counting cost-sharing payments (defined as copayments and coinsurance) towards any deductible or out-of-network maximum, and instead require deductibles for out-of-network services to apply the same as if those services were provided in-network. Specifically, the legislation should amend Section 2719A(b)(1)(C)(ii)(II) of the Public Health Service Act (42 U.S.C. 300gg-19a(b)(1)(C)(ii)(II)) by inserting ", deductible amount," after "copayment amount."

Second, the committee should include a timely payment requirement (applicable to ERISA plans, at minimum) for the automatic payment that requires insurers to have the provider receive payment within 30 days from receipt of the claim. Failure to provide the proper reimbursement amount or to comply with the prompt pay timeline would trigger a civil monetary penalty (CMP) for the insurer/plan.

Concerning CMPs, we believe that the committee should not penalize providers who may have unknowingly violated the new requirements outlined in the proposal. The CMP applied to providers in the discussion draft who balance bill patients for services in the emergency department or independent freestanding emergency department (IFSED) should only apply if there has been a pattern of behavior and/or willfulness, rather than a single, unknowing instance.

Finally, ACEP appreciates that the discussion draft updates the definitions listed under Section 2719A(b)(2) of the Public Health Service Act to include IFSEDs. ACEP agrees that IFSEDs should be held to the same standards and requirements as both on-campus and off-campus hospital-based emergency departments. We believe that all emergency departments should meet certain criteria – including being available to the public 24 hours a day, seven days a week, 365 days per year; have policy agreements and procedures in place to provide effective and efficient transfer to a higher level of care if needed; and follow the intent of the federal EMTALA statute. This would ensure that all individuals presenting at an IFSED would be provided an appropriate medical screening exam and, if necessary, be provided with stabilizing treatment within the facility's capability or transferred to an appropriate another facility for definitive care. IFSEDs should also have equivalent standards as hospital-based freestanding emergency departments for quality improvement and governance as hospital-based emergency departments.

Conclusion

As stated previously, ACEP fervently agrees that more must be done to protect patients and their families from unexpected medical bills and provide greater transparency in these encounters when time permits, and it is appropriate to do so. I would like to thank you again for your work in this regard and, based on my personal experience, I am encouraged that you continue to keep an open mind about the best way to protect these patients and resolve reimbursement disputes between physicians and insurers in a fair, reasonable manner that minimizes federal intrusion into the private marketplace. Fortunately, all parties involved in this debate have expressed their desire to accomplish the goal of taking patients out of the middle. For what remains of the outstanding balance for these services, I encourage you to modify your current draft legislative proposal to use a baseball-style arbitration approach that has proven to be a successful approach to resolving these disputes.

Thank you again for your consideration and for the opportunity to speak to you today on behalf of nearly 40,000 emergency physicians nationwide and the 150 million Americans we treat each year.

* * *

Ms. ESHOO. Thank you, Doctor.

Now I have the pleasure of recognizing Ms. McAndrew for five minutes for your testimony.

Statement of Claire McAndrew, M.P.H., Director of the Campaigns and Partnerships, Families USA

Ms. MCANDREW. Chairwoman Eshoo, Dr. Burgess, and members of the subcommittee, I am Claire McAndrew, the director of Campaigns and Partnerships at Families U.S.A., where I lead the organization's work on surprise billing.

For nearly 40 years, we have served as a leading voice for healthcare consumers and our mission is to ensure that every individual can access the healthcare and the best health in order to ensure that no matter where you live or who you are you can have the life that you need to—based on achieving the best health and healthcare.

And so high and rising healthcare costs are truly an affront to our mission as they are forcing people to choose between getting the healthcare they need and affording their other most basic necessities, and we heard about that from Ms. Wilkes.

Surprise bills are a particularly egregious form of healthcare costs because families who are doing everything, they can to navigate our overly complex healthcare system, working to go to only in-network providers, going to only in-network facilities are still receiving these egregious bills.

And, unfortunately, these bills are incredibly common. One in five emergency visits results in a surprise bill. But these bills are also occurring outside our emergency situations.

For examples, families who welcome a new baby, ensuring that they're getting an in-network OB/Gyn in an in-network facility are still getting surprise bills 11 percent of the time.

So, what's causing these bills? Surprise bills are the result of a systemic problem in our healthcare system placing families directly in the middle of a tug of war between healthcare providers and health insurers fighting over the price of services.

While health systems and insurers are vying for leverage including because of consolidation, consumers are completely trapped between these industries.

What does not cause surprise bills, despite claims by some stakeholders, evidence does not conclude that narrow networks are a driving factor behind surprise bills.

We know that people who are covered in plans that tend to have narrower networks and people covered in plans that tend to have broader networks are actually getting surprise bills at about the same rate.

And so, I want to be clear that Families USA does support network adequacy standards. It is something we have advocated for. But we understand that in this particular situation around surprise bills network adequacy standards aren't going to solve the problem alone.

Another common misperception I want to raise that we heard about from Ms. Wilkes is the fact that this is not a new problem. Consumers have been subjected to unexpected and unaffordable costs from surprise bills for literally decades, and the proof is real for us because Families USA has been working on this for decades.

We actually joined with other stakeholders in 1997 recommending banning surprise bills in emergencies as part of President Clinton's efforts around the Consumer Bill of Rights. So this is a very longstanding problem and for far too long it's warranted congressional action.

Only Congress can fix this, because even when states address this problem, many consumers are left out because they are in ERISA-regulated plans.

So we commend the Energy and Commerce Committee for responding to this urgent need with the release of the No Surprises Act. This legislation takes really important steps.

It holds consumers harmless from surprise bills and it sets a reasonable benchmark to pay providers from insurers at a rate that's not inflationary so that families don't experience increased premiums.

We support the No Surprises Act, but we are concerned. So much of this debate has been about making insurers and providers happy based on a payment rate. This legislation is supposed to be about consumers.

And so, we want to ensure that this discussion is not consumed about what makes powerful industries happy and that the needs of consumers are not lost, and the pace of this legislation is not slowed based on appeasing insurers and providers.

And so we want to make two recommendations about the needs of consumers. First, we urge the subcommittee to broaden the scope of the providers included in the legislation so that no loopholes remain.

We want to make sure that there's not just a discrete set of providers and facilities subject to the legislation but that any facility or provider that could incur a surprise bill is included.

And second, we urge the subcommittee to strengthen the bill's notice requirements. We are concerned that just 24 hours' notice could be too short for a consumer to find out that nonfacility-based providers are out of network.

We would urge looking at more like a week because if you have scheduled medical leave, if you're about to undergo an important medical procedure, 24 hours might be too short of a time to learn that you have to find another option.

We are so grateful to the subcommittee for taking on this issue. This is such an important hearing. We urge Congress to very swiftly take action. Our number-one recommendation is not to wait.

This legislation must pass this year. I really appreciate what you said, Chairwoman Eshoo. If stakeholders can't agree, Congress has to solve the solution because consumers cannot wait any longer and Families USA is with you to help you solve this problem in any way possible.

Thank you very much.

[The prepared statement of Ms. McAndrew follows:]

Written Testimony of Claire McAndrew, M.P.H.

Chairwoman Eshoo, Dr. Burgess, and members of the House Energy and Commerce Committee, Subcommittee on Health: Thank you for the opportunity to speak with you today. I am Claire McAndrew, the Director of Campaigns and Partnerships at Families USA. For nearly 40 years, we have served as one of the leading national voices for health care consumers both in Washington, D.C. and on the state level. Our mission is to allow every individual to live to their greatest potential by ensuring that the best health and health care are equally accessible and affordable to all.

Testimony Summary

My testimony seeks to convey a number of key points for the Subcommittee's consideration. Specifically:

- Surprise bills are a significant and longstanding problem, causing economic insecurity and stress for millions of families each year.
- Surprise bills are the product of distorted market incentives in the negotiation between health plans and providers. In surprise bill situations, consumers are caught in the middle of these powerful industries with no recourse.
- Surprise bills occur across health care settings and must be dealt with holistically.
- While Families USA supports committee's bipartisan legislation, several changes are needed to ensure the bill protects all consumers affected by surprise bills.
- Only Congress can fully protect consumers against surprise billing. The time for bold action is now.

The Larger Context of Health Care Costs for Families

High and rising health care costs place an untenable burden on millions of families across America – even those with health insurance. Four in ten people with employer coverage have difficulty affording health care costs.[50] Additionally, a startling 30 percent of people in our nation report that health care costs are interfering with their ability to meet the most basic necessities of their life, like securing food, heating, or housing.[51]

---

[50] Hamel, Liz, Cailey Munana, and Mollyann Brodie. "Kaiser Family Foundation/ LA Times Survey of Adults with Employer-Sponsored Health Insurance." *KFF*. May 2019. http://files.kff.org/attachment/Report-KFF-LA-Times-Survey-of-Adults-with-Employer-Sponsored-Health-Insurance.

[51] NORC at the University of Chicago and West Health Institute. "Americans' Views of Healthcare Costs, Coverage, and Policy." *NORC at the University of Chicago*. 2018, https://www.westhealth.org/wp-content/uploads/2018/03/WHI-Healthcare-Costs-Coverage-and-Policy-Issue-Brief.pdf.

The United States is one of the wealthiest nations in the world and we spend twice as much as other high-income nations to provide health care.[52] People across the country should not have to live in fear of getting sick and facing a sudden, crippling financial burden. And, yet, this what so many American families experience every day.[53] In fact, a larger percentage of the population actually fear medical bills from a serious illness more than the serious illness itself (40 percent vs. 33 percent).[54] What's more, according to the American Psychological Association, the stress associated with medical bill anxiety can actually make them sicker.[55]

The Cost and Frequency of Surprise Medical Bills

Surprise bills— also known as out-of-network "balance bills"— are a particularly egregious health care cost, as they are unpredictable for families and occur despite every effort consumers make to avoid them. Surprise medical bills occur when consumers are charged for care from out-of-network providers that they receive due to no fault of their own. Families who make their best attempt to navigate the health coverage and care system by identifying in-network facilities and providers still receive surprise medical bills that can amount to hundreds, thousands, and even tens-of-thousands of dollars.[56]

Surprise medical bills are incredibly common. One-in-five emergency department visits results in a surprise medical bill.[57] Surprise medical bills also occur even when families do their very best to go to an in-network provider and suddenly, after-the-fact, discover ancillary services like anesthesiology, radiology, lab, or ambulance fall outside of their provider network.[58] For example, more than one-in-five lab claims (22.1 percent) for inpatient hospital care in an in-network hospital were billed as out-of-network.[59]

Allow me to highlight the experience of Nicole Briggs, from Morrison, Colorado. Nicole woke up in the middle of the night with intense stomach pain. After first visiting a freestanding ER, she was told she needed an emergency appendectomy, and she went to the local hospital. She did her due diligence to confirm repeatedly that the hospital and its providers accepted her insurance. However, months later, she received a surprise bill from the surgeon for $4,727. While the hospital was in-network, the surgeon was an independent, out-of-network provider.

---

[52] Papanicolas, Irene, Leana Woskie, and Ashish Jha. "Health Care Spending in the United States and Other High-Income Countries." Journal of the American Medical Association. *JAMA*. 2018. https://jamanetwork.com/journals/jama/article-abstract/2674671.

[53] American Psychological Association. "Stress in America: Uncertainty about Health Care." *APA*. 2018. https://www.apa.org/news/press/releases/stress/2017/uncertainty-health-care.pdf.

[54] NORC at the University of Chicago and West Health Institute, op. cit.

[55] American Psychological Association, op. cit.

[56] New York State Department of Financial Services. "How New Yorkers Are Getting Stuck with Unexpected Medical Bills from Out-of-Network Providers." New York State. 2012. http://www.statecoverage.org/files/NY-Unexpected_Medical_Bills-march_7_2012.pdf; Cooper, Zack and Fiona Scott Morton. "Out-of-Network Emergency-Physician Bills — An Unwelcome Surprise." *New England Journal of Medicine*. 2017. https://www.nejm.org/doi/full/10.1056/NEJMp1608571.

[57] Cooper, Zack and Fiona Scott Morton. "Out-of-Network Emergency-Physician Bills — An Unwelcome Surprise" *New England Journal of Medicine*. 2017. https://www.nejm.org/doi/full/10.1056/NEJMp1608571.

[58] Kennedy, Kevin, Bill Johnson, and Jean Fuglesten Biniek. "Surprise out-of-network medical bills during in-network hospital admissions varied by state and medical specialty, 2016." *Health Care Cost Institute*. 2019. https://www.healthcostinstitute.org/blog/entry/oon-physician-bills-at-in-network-hospitals; Garmon, Christopher and Benjamin Chartock. "One in Five Inpatient Emergency Department Cases May Lead to Surprise Bills." *Health Affairs*. Vol 36. No. 1. 2017. https://www.healthaffairs.org/doi/10.1377/hlthaff.2016.0970.

[59] Kennedy, Kevin, Bill Johnson, and Jean Fuglesten Biniek, op.cit.

Nicole explained the situation to the insurer, but they continued to demand payment. She declined to pay the bill, and within two years, a credit agency representing the surgeon took her to court, and won the full amount, including interest. As a result, a lien was placed on her home, and the collection agency garnished her wages by 25 percent each month. This came right as she was pregnant and about to go on maternity leave.[60]

Air ambulance services are particularly likely to lead to surprise medical bills. Nearly 70 percent of air ambulance patient transports that people often require in life-or-death situations are out-of-network, and balance bills from these air ambulance providers are rarely below $10,000.[61]

Surprise Bills Occur Across Health Care Settings

Surprise bills do not just occur in emergency situations. Families can schedule medical procedures far in advance and still be vulnerable to surprise billing. For example, Pennsylvania Insurance Commissioner Jessica Altman has described multiple people in her state receiving surprise bills after visiting their in-network OB/GYN's office because their mammograms were sent to out-of-network labs for review.[62] One recent study found that people who selected in-network facilities and in-network providers for the delivery of their babies still had surprise bills from ancillary providers 11 percent of the time.[63] Families may schedule a procedure with an in-network surgeon weeks or even months in advance, only to end up with a surprise bill because, unbeknownst to them, an out-of-network assistant surgeon or anesthesiologist participated in their care.[64]

The Cause of Surprise Bills

Surprise out-of-network bills are a terrible example of how distorted economic incentives in the health care sector are overwhelming the interests of patients. They are the result of a systemic problem in our health care system that places families directly in the middle of a tug-of-war between health care providers and insurers over the price of services.[65]

---

[60] Bomnin, Lindsey and Stephanie Gosk. "Surprise Medical Bills Lead to Liens on Homes and Crippling Debt." *NBC News*. 2019. https://www.nbcnews.com/health/health-news/surprise-medical-bills-lead-liens-homes-cripplingdebt-n984371.

[61] U.S. Government Accountability Office. "Air Ambulance: Available Data Show Privately-Insured Patients are at Financial Risk." *GAO*. 2019. https://www.gao.gov/assets/700/697684.pdf.

[62] Remarks from Pennsylvania Insurance Commissioner Jessica Altman. "Emerging policy solutions to surprise medical bills- A USC-Brookings Schaeffer Initiative for Health Policy Event." *C-SPAN*. 2019. https://www.c-span.org/video/?459049-1/surprise-medical-bills-policymakers-panel&start=2764.

[63] Chartock, Benjamin, Christopher Garmon, and Sarah Schutz. "Consumers' Responses to Surprise Medical Bills in Elective Situations. *Health Affairs*. March 2019. https://www.healthaffairs.org/doi/abs/10.1377/hlthaff.2018.05399.

[64] Fuse Brown, Erin C. "Consumer Financial Protection in Health Care." 95 *Wash. U. L. Rev*. 127. 2017. http://openscholarship.wustl.edu/law_lawreview/vol95/iss1/7.

[65] Adler, Loren, Matthew Fiedler, Paul B. Ginsburg, Mark Hall, Erin Trish, Christen Linke Young, and Erin L. Duffy. "State Approaches to Mitigating Surprise Out-of-Network Billing." *USC-Brookings Schaeffer Initiative for Health Policy*. 2019. https://www.brookings.edu/wp-content/uploads/2019/02/Adler_et-al_State-Approaches-to-Mitigating-Surprise-Billing-2019.pdf.

The rate negotiated between providers and insurers for services is at the center of their business models. Larger hospital systems have significant leverage, allowing them to command top dollar for in-network rates. Insurers are often forced to pay their high charges for in-network status, or insurers may simply walk away from the negotiation.[66] On the other hand, when hospitals are smaller, insurers hold the leverage. Those hospitals must choose between accepting lower negotiated rates than they desire, or walking away from the negotiation and providing care out-of-network.[67] These distorted market incentives frequently lead to out-of-network provider status and ultimately, harmful surprise bills for families. In general, compared to in-network providers, out-of-network providers charge nearly three times as much for care.[68] This leaves families with balance bills that average over $600, but can exceed $20,000.[69]

One driver of this problem is the movement by hospitals to offload staffing requirements for their emergency departments to third-party management companies. These companies have no responsibility to ensure hospital-based providers are in the same networks as the hospitals themselves.[70] In fact, two-thirds of hospitals in the U.S. outsource the staffing of their emergency departments to third-party physician management firms.[71] Research shows that out-of-network claims are higher in hospitals that contract with common staffing companies.[72] All too often, these firms use a business model that leverages the higher prices that can be charged with an out-of-network status.[73] As a result, a patient with a medical emergency, who rightly thinks they are going to an in-network hospital, often receives professional services from an out-of-network physician. This is inexcusable behavior on the part of the hospital, doctor, and health insurer. They each know or should know that patients have no real way of understanding the financial trap they have walked into. In these surprise bill instances, we and many believe it is the providers and payers who should bear the burden of settling on a fair payment.[74]

Despite claims by some stakeholders,[75] evidence does not conclude that narrow networks are a driving factor behind surprise bills.[76] People covered by plans that tend to have broad provider networks are nearly as likely as those in plans with typically narrower networks to receive surprise bills.[77] Families USA strongly supports network adequacy requirements. We

---

[66] Berenson, Robert, Paul Ginsburg, Jon Christianson, and Tracy Yee. "The Growing Power Of Some Providers To Win Steep Payment Increases From Insurers Suggests Policy Remedies May Be Needed." *Health Affairs*. 2017. https://www.healthaffairs.org/doi/full/10.1377/hlthaff.2011.0920.

[67] Commonwealth of Massachusetts Health Policy Commission. "Community Hospitals at a Crossroads: Findings from an Examination of the Massachusetts Health Care System." *Commonwealth of Massachusetts*. 2016. https://www.mass.gov/files/documents/2016/07/xf/community-hospitals-at-a-crossroads.pdf.

[68] Cooper, Zack and Fiona Scott Morton, op. cit.

[69] Ibid.

[70] Cooper, Zack, Fiona Scott Morton and Nathan Shekita. "Surprise! Out-of-Network Billing for Emergency Care in the United States." December 2018.

[71] Ibid.

[72] Ibid.

[73] Ibid.

[74] Adler, Loren, Matthew Fiedler, Paul B. Ginsburg, Mark Hall, Erin Trish, Christen Linke Young, and Erin L. Duffy, op. cit.

[75] American Medical Association. "Issue Brief: Balance Billing." *AMA*. 2016. https://www.ama-assn.org/sites/ama-assn.org/files/corp/media-browser/balance-billing-issue-brief-final.pdf.

[76] Linke Young, Christen, Loren Adler, Paul B. Ginsburg, and Mark Hall. "The relationship between network adequacy and surprise billing." *USC-Brookings Schaeffer on Health Policy*. May 2019. https://www.brookings.edu/blog/usc-brookings-schaeffer-on-health-policy/2019/05/10/the-relationship-between-network-adequacy-and-surprise-billing/.

[77] Gunja, Munira Z., Sara R. Collins, Michelle M. Doty, and Sophie Beutel. "Americans' Experiences with ACA Marketplace Coverage: Affordability and Provider Network Satisfaction." *The Commonwealth Fund*. July 2016.

have advocated for such standards at the state and federal level for years, as well as standards to improve provider directory accuracy.[78] We also criticized recent actions that relaxed network adequacy and provider directory requirements for plans in the federally facilitated marketplaces.[79]

However, broadening network adequacy will not, by itself, solve the problem of surprise bills. Network adequacy standards are designed to ensure that a health plan has a sufficient number and variety of network providers to deliver the benefits the plan covers to its enrollees. For example, network adequacy standards ensure there are a sufficient number of primary care doctors and specialists in a plan's network relative to the number of enrollees in the plan. These standards ensure enrollees will not have to wait unduly long or travel unduly far for appointments.[80] They do not, however, guarantee that any particular provider or facility is in a plan's network. Requiring a plan to include each provider and facility as a participating provider would defeat the cost-control purpose of having a network.[81] Since surprise bills occur when a consumer ends up at a *particular* out-of-network emergency or at an in-network facility where a *particular* provider is out-0f-network, they require targeted protections.

The History of Surprise Medical Bills

Another common misconception is that surprise bills are a new phenomenon. That is false. Consumers have been subjected to these unexpected and unaffordable costs for decades. Early discussions of protecting consumers from surprise billing occurred in response to the "managed care revolution" of the 1980s and 1990s. The revolution occurred when health insurers began shifting more risk to providers with the creation of networks, as opposed to bearing that risk through fee-for-service models.[82] Under fee-for-service models common previously, insurers would simply reimburse the usual and customary rate (UCR) for services to the provider, except for a share paid by the enrollee.[83] However, consumers could still be balance billed for provider charges that exceeded the UCR.[84] Insurers played little role otherwise, and enrollees could see any doctor of their choosing, with no network structure in place.[85]

From 1980 to 1999, network-based managed care plans grew enormously in efforts to help employers contain rising health care costs. In 1980, 5 percent of Americans were enrolled in

https://www.commonwealthfund.org/sites/default/files/documents/media_files_publications_issue_brief_2016_jul_1883_gunja_americans_experience_aca_marketplace_affordability_v2.pdf.

[78] Claire McAndrew. "Standards for Health Insurance Provider Networks: Examples from the States." *Families USA*. 2014. https://familiesusa.org/product/standards-health-insurance-provider-networks-examples-states; Claire McAndrew. "Improving the Accuracy of Health Insurance Plans' Provider Directories." *Families USA*. 2015. https://familiesusa.org/sites/default/files/product_documents/ACA_Provider%20Directory%20Issue%20Brief_web.pdf.

[79] Parcham, Cheryl and Claire McAndrew. "Final 2019 Marketplace Rules from the Trump Administration Will Harm Consumers." *Families USA*. April 2018, https://familiesusa.org/product/final-2019-marketplace-rules-trump-administration-will-harm-consumers.

[80] Claire McAndrew. "Standards for Health Insurance Provider Networks: Examples from the States," op. cit.

[81] Linke Young, Christen, Loren Adler, Paul B. Ginsburg, and Mark Hall, op. cit.

[82] Fuse Brown, Erin C., op. cit.

[83] Gaynor, Martin and Tami Mark. *Physician Contracting with Health Plans: A Survey of the Literature*. June 2, 1999. https://www.andrew.cmu.edu/user/mgaynor/Assets/mdcontractingfinal3.pdf.

[84] U.S. Congress, Office of Technology Assessment. *Benefit Design in Health Care Reform: Background Paper-Patient Cost-Sharing*. U.S. Government Printing Office. September, 1993, https://ota.fas.org/reports/9310.pdf.

[85] Gaynor, Martin and Tami Mark, op. cit.

health maintenance organizations (HMOs). By 1999, 30 percent of Americans were HMO enrollees. Other forms of managed care grew at this time as well, such as preferred provider organizations (PPOs). By 1998, less than 15 percent of people with employer-based coverage in the United States had traditional fee-for-service plans.[86]

With the advent of networks, surprise billing became more apparent. Now that care from certain providers could expose families to much higher out-of-network costs compared to the same care from other providers, families could find themselves in situations where they received out-of-network care due to no fault of their own.

Throughout the 1980s and 1990s, states began to work to address surprise bill problems for managed care enrollees. States first took measures to ban participating providers from balance billing HMO enrollees, and some extended these protections to non-participating providers.[87] Some states later expanded these laws to other types of managed care plans, and slowly continue to expand these protections today.[88]

Even at the federal level, Families USA and other stakeholders discussed the need for surprise bill protections as early as the 1990s. The Advisory Commission on Consumer Protection and Quality in the Health Care Industry, appointed by President Clinton on March 26, 1997, to "advise the President on changes occurring in the health care system and recommend measures as may be necessary to promote and assure health care quality and value, and protect consumers and workers in the health care system," made recommendations to prevent surprise billing in emergency situations.

The Consumer Bill of Rights that President Clinton asked the Commission to draft recommended that:

> Health plans using a defined network of providers should cover emergency department screening and stabilization services both in network and out of network without prior authorization for use consistent with the prudent layperson standard. *Non-network providers and facilities should not bill patients for any charges in excess of health plans' routine payment arrangements.*[89]

Families USA served on this 34-member advisory panel in 1997 and contributed to its recommendations on surprise billing.[90] However, our work on surprise bills began before then, as we assisted states in their efforts to pass protections on the issue even earlier.[91] As Families USA and others[92] have fought to protect consumers from surprise bills for over two decades,

---

[86] Ibid.

[87] Hoadley, Jack, Kevin Lucia, and Maanasa Kona. "State Efforts to Protect Consumers from Balance Billing." *Commonwealth Fund*. January 18, 2019, https://www.commonwealthfund.org/sites/default/files/2019-01/To_the_Point_BalanceBilling.pdf; Gordon Feinblatt. "Can an HMO Be Billed for the Balance?" *GFR Law*. September 22. 1999, https://www.gfrlaw.com/what-we-do/insights/can-hmo-be-billed-balance.

[88] Hoadley, Jack, Kevin Lucia, and Maanasa Kona, op. cit.; State of Colorado, House Bill 19-1174, https://leg.colorado.gov/sites/default/files/documents/2019A/bills/2019a_1174_rer.pdf.

[89] Advisory Commission on Consumer Protection and Quality in the Health Care Industry, "Consumer Bill of Rights and Responsibilities Report to the President of the United States." November 1997, http://www.csun.edu/~hfdss003/atacp/supplements/fph9.html.

[90] Pear, Robert. "Clinton Names Panel to Draft Health Consumer Bill of Rights." *New York Times*. March 27, 1997, https://www.nytimes.com/1997/03/27/us/clinton-names-panel-to-draft-health-consumer-bill-of-rights.html.

[91] Dallek, Geraldine. "HMO Consumers at Risk: States to the Rescue." *Families USA*. 1996.

[92] Teisberg, Elizabeth, Michael E. Porter, and Gregory B. Brown. "Making Competition in Health Care Work." *Harvard Business Review*. July-August 1994, https://hbr.org/1994/07/making-competition-in-health-care-work.

we strongly urge this Subcommittee and Congress to wait no longer to pass comprehensive legislation on this critical issue for families.

It is Past Time for Congress to Address Surprise Bills

The ubiquity of surprise medical bills in all types of health plans and in all states warrants immediate federal action. Current federal law provides limited protections for families who receive out-of-network care in emergency situations.[93] Specifically, the ACA limits copayments and coinsurance charged by an insurer to in-network amounts when families receive services from an out-of-network emergency provider.[94] Despite these protections, however, providers may still balance bill families for additional out-of-network costs. Furthermore, insurers are not required to count copayments or coinsurance paid by a family toward in-network deductibles and out-of-pocket caps.[95] Thus, current federal law leaves families with considerable financial exposure for surprise out-of-network bills for emergency services and no protections for other categories of surprise out-of-network bills.

Across the country, some states have stepped up to address this problem for their residents in the absence of federal protection.[96] However, state protections are patchwork, as only 10 states have comprehensive protections in place for plans that fall under state regulatory authority.[97] Even in those states, many residents are left unprotected, as states do not have meaningful authority over ERISA-regulated self-insured plans.[98] A large majority of working families across the nation— 61 percent— are enrolled in ERISA health insurance products.[99] These families are no less likely to receive a surprise bill than those in fully insured group or individual plans.[100] With so many states and families left unprotected from surprise medical bills, people across the country are looking to this Subcommittee and Congress for action.

Legislation under the Committee's Consideration

Families USA commends the Energy and Commerce Committee for the release of its draft "No Surprises Act." This legislation would both 1) take important steps to hold families harmless from surprise bills and 2) ensure that payments between insurers and out-of-network providers are not inflationary, so that families do not experience increased insurance premiums.

---

[93] 29 CFR § 2590.715-2719A(b). https://www.law.cornell.edu/cfr/text/29/2590.715-2719A.

[94] 29 CFR § 2590.715-2719A(b)(3). https://www.law.cornell.edu/cfr/text/29/2590.715-2719A.

[95] Ibid.

[96] Hoadley, Jack, Kevin Lucia, and Maanasa Kona, op. cit.

[97] State of Colorado, House Bill 19-1174, https://leg.colorado.gov/sites/default/files/documents/2019A/bills/2019a_1174_rer.pdf; Hoadley, Jack, Kevin Lucia, and Maanasa Kona, op. cit.

[98] Pierron, William and Paul Fronstin. "ERISA Pre-Emption: Implications for Health Reform and Coverage." *Employee Benefit Research Institute*. 2008, https://www.researchgate.net/publication/5554287_Erisa_Pre-Emption_Implications_for_Health_Reform_And_Coverage.

[99] Claxton, Gary, Matthew Rae, Michelle Long, Anthony Damico and Heidi Whitmore. "Employer Health Benefits 2018 Annual Survey: Section 10." *Kaiser Family Foundation*. 2018, http://files.kff.org/attachment/Report-Employer-Health-Benefits-Annual-Survey-2018.

[100] Adler, Loren, Mark Hall, Caitlin Brandt, Paul B. Ginsburg, and Steven M. Lieberman. "Stopping surprise medical bills: Federal action is needed." *Health Affairs*. 2017, https://www.healthaffairs.org/do/10.1377/hblog20170201.058570/full/.

Specifically, the bill includes important provisions that:

- Protect families from paying more than they would pay in cost-sharing if they received in-network care during surprise bill situations. Further, it specifically ensures that these payments count toward in-network deductibles and out-of-pocket maximums.
- Establish a benchmark payment rate such that in a surprise bill situation, insurers will pay out-of-network providers median contracted rates.
- Provide grants to states for the establishment of All-Payer Claims Databases.

Protecting Families from Out-of-Pocket Expenses beyond In-Network Cost-Sharing

To providing meaningful protection from surprises bills, the No Surprises Act explicitly ensures that families in surprise bill situations will pay no more than they would if they received care from an in-network provider. This recognizes that families should not be left holding the bag when they do everything they can to obtain care from an in-network provider, but still receive out-of-network care due to no fault of their own. *We strongly support that the No Surprises Act protects families from paying more than they would in-network and explicitly states that these payments count toward in-network deductibles and out-of-pocket maximums.*

Establishing a Benchmark Payment Rate between Insurers and Providers

Families USA believes that the payment mechanism between insurers and providers in a surprise billing situation is a consumer issue: If payments are unduly high, they will be passed on to consumers in their insurance premiums. *We therefore strongly support the establishment of a benchmark payment rate, which will prevent nontransparent and fluctuating payments that may lead to inflationary costs.*

In particular, we support the benchmark of median in-network rates because it avoids tying payment to billed charges. Billed charges are set based on the rates providers want to get paid, not on the rates they actually get paid by insurers. Therefore, they vary widely and are determined arbitrarily. Furthermore, charges are highest for the very providers most likely to send surprise bills: While provider charges generally are about two times Medicare rates, anesthesiologists and emergency doctors charge five times what Medicare pays.[101] Including billed charges in any payment methodology for resolving surprise bills, including a benchmark rate or an arbitration system, would inflate costs and ultimately harm consumers.

Providing Funding for the Creation of All-Payer Claims Databases

We support incentives for the creation of All-Payer Claims Databases (APCDs) in states. APCDs can assist in addressing surprise billing, network adequacy, and a host of other issues related to costs and access. For example, Colorado recently passed the tenth comprehensive state law to protect consumers from surprise medical bills. The state has an APCD, and it is using that database as the source of information on in-network rates for its out-of-network provider payment formula in the law.[102] This allows the state to use a payment rate that is based on what all insurers in the state reimburse providers, instead of using separate rates for each

[101] Loren Adler. "Policy Approaches to Addressing Surprise Out-of-Network Billing." *USC-Brookings Schaeffer Initiative for Health Policy*. March 2019, https://www.brookings.edu/wp-content/uploads/2019/01/Surprise-Billing-2-20-event-presentation_Adler.pdf.

[102] State of Colorado, House Bill 19-1174, https://leg.colorado.gov/sites/default/files/documents/2019A/bills/2019a_1174_rer.pdf.

insurer. This will protect against some insurers paying unduly high rates or some with great market power paying unduly low rates, creating a more level, competitive playing field among insurers.[103]

However, *Gobeille v. Liberty Mutual Insurance Company* restricted the ability of state APCDs to require self-insured, ERISA-regulated health plans to participate in APCDs.[104] It would therefore be beneficial for Congress to develop strategies to obtain claims information from self-insured plans, such as through the creation of a database at the federal level.

Families USA supports the No Surprises Act, though we recommend three significant changes to better protect consumers from egregious and unpredictable surprise bills:

1. Expansion of consumer protections to ensure all provider and facility surprise bills are captured
2. Establishment of federal surprise billing law as a protective "floor," so that states cannot implement weaker laws that undermine it
3. Improved consumer notice requirements

Surprise Bill Protections Should Include All Providers and Facilities

Families USA recommends modifying the No Surprises Act to ensure that families are protected from surprise bills in all facilities and from all providers that can expose them to involuntary out-of-network bills. The draft legislation uses a list of "participating facilities" and list of "facility-based providers" to establish the scope of surprise bill protections. We are concerned this approach will fail to capture all of the locations and providers from which families may experience surprise bills, and therefore will still leave them exposed to unfair balance bills.

Rather than creating discrete facility and provider lists to which surprise bill protections apply, we recommend that the legislation take an approach that defines a surprise bill situation. Specifically, protections should apply to:

- Emergency services provided by an out-of-network health care professional or at an out-of-network facility;
- Health care services provided:
  - At an in-network facility (including use of equipment, devices, telemedicine services, or other treatments or services); and
  - By an out-of-network health care professional; and
- Additional health care services required for an enrollee who initially entered a hospital through the emergency department but then receives non-emergency services from an out-of-network provider or at an out-of-network hospital or facility after the enrollee has been stabilized, unless the enrollee can safely travel to an in-network hospital. (And for which in-network medical transportation is available, if necessary.)

Whether in this bill or in future legislation, federal protections should hold consumers harmless from paying more than in-network cost-sharing for both ground and air ambulance

[103] Adler, Loren, Matthew Fiedler, Paul B. Ginsburg, and Christen Linke Young, op. cit.

[104] Gobeille v. Liberty Mutual Insurance Company. No. 14–181, 577. Supreme Court of United States. March 1, 2016, https://www.scotusblog.com/case-files/cases/gobeille-v-liberty-mutual-insurance-company/.

transport when they have no option for in-network ambulance transport. Additionally, federal preemptions that prohibit state regulation of air ambulance rates and networks should be eliminated.

Without these modifications, consumers will still be vulnerable to surprise bills from providers who are not currently listed in the draft legislation, such as lead surgeons and labs to which they are referred by in-network providers.[105]

Congress should Prevent State Law from Undermining Federal Protections

Families USA believes states should have the opportunity to develop innovative solutions to providing surprise bill protections for their residents. However, these solutions must not undermine federal surprise billing protections such that consumers in some states are afforded fewer rights than federal law provides nationally. If federal law does not provide a floor of consumer and cost protections, state laws could swiftly undermine federal efforts to protect consumers and improve cost stability for the health care system.

Families USA recommends permitting states to apply their own surprise bill laws, if state law is equally or more robust than federal law, in terms of both consumer protections and a payment rate between insurers and providers that holds costs down. We are concerned that the draft legislation currently would allow state laws that have less robust protections than federal law to preempt federal law. *We recommend clarification in the No Surprises Act that federal law applies unless state law is equally or more robust.*

Consumer Notice Requirements Must Provide Sufficient Protection

The No Surprises Act allows out-of-network providers to balance bill as long as providers deliver 24-hours' advanced notice of their network status to consumers. Families USA believes that permitting a non-participating provider to balance bill when a consumer has received only 24 hours' notice of the provider's network status and estimated out-of-network charges is an insufficient protection. If a consumer is scheduled for surgery, or a C-section delivery, or another critical procedure that requires the care of anesthesiologists, surgeons, or other highly-specialized providers, rescheduling care that is to occur in just over 24 hours may put their health at risk. Even if it does not jeopardize health, it may require rescheduling medical leave or making burdensome choices between families' wellbeing and large financial burdens. People should not receive a mere 24 hours' notice to choose between hundreds or thousands of dollars in out-of-network costs or delaying an important medical procedure.

We therefore recommend revising the No Surprises Act to provide no less than 7 days' notice to consumers regarding the participation of any out-of-network providers in their care. If any provider or facility does not give a consumer at least 7 days' notice that a specific non-participating provider will be involved in their care, along with estimated charges from that provider, the provider must not be allowed to balance bill. We also recommend clarifying that a general notice about the possibility of an out-of-network provider is not sufficient notice: Notices must be specific to an individual care episode and mention the provider or service that will be out-of-network by name with a corresponding cost.

---

[105] Sarah Kliff, "A spinal surgery, a $101,000 bill, and a new law to prevent more surprises." *Vox*. 2019, https://www.vox.com/health-care/2019/3/19/18233051/surprise-medical-bills-arbitration-new-york; Schulte, Fred. "An Out-Of-Network Lab, An Elaborate Urine Test And Then A Surprise Bill." *NPR WAMU*. 2018, https://wamu.org/story/18/02/16/an-out-of-network-lab-an-elaborate-urine-test-and-then-a-surprise-bill/.

Without such modifications, notices may be used by facilities and providers to waive their liability for balance billing and not to provide consumers with useful information.

A Call to Action

Families USA is grateful to the subcommittee for holding this important hearing today. For decades, families have been trapped in the tug-of-war between providers and payers that leads to surprise medical billing, and without your action it will only get worse.

The public has identified health care costs as a top priority for action this Congress.[106] Addressing surprise billing is a chance to demonstrate real bipartisan leadership to our nation. Families USA urges Congress to swiftly take advantage of this opportunity and to pass legislation to protect consumers from surprise medical bills this year.

* * *

Ms. ESHOO. Terrific. Thank you very much to each one of our witnesses. So now we have concluded all the statements and move to members' questions.

Each member will have five minutes to ask questions of our witnesses and I will begin by recognizing myself for five minutes.

To the panel, does everyone here agree that patients should not receive surprise billing? Is there anyone that disagrees with that?

A hundred percent. Well, that's a good beginning.

Mr. Nickels, are there hospitals in your association that send patients surprise medical bills and, if so, why?

Mr. NICKELS. The statistic that we like to quote the most is most of our member hospitals are in network. The Federal Trade Commission did a study recently that showed——

Ms. ESHOO. Well, do you have any hospitals in your association that send surprise medical bills, yes or——

Mr. NICKELS. You mentioned one a little earlier, I believe—San Francisco General.

Ms. ESHOO. Yes.

Mr. NICKELS. To the best of my knowledge, they are the only ones who were doing what you described.

Ms. ESHOO. And how many hospitals do you represent in the country?

Mr. NICKELS. Five thousand.

Ms. ESHOO. Five thousand. So 4,999 do not send any surprise bills?

Mr. NICKELS. Where the hospital services—the facility charge, no, they do not, and coming to one of our——

Ms. ESHOO. Do you have any hospitals that have—well, you're saying that 4,999 of your hospitals have successfully stopped sending surprise billing?

Mr. NICKELS. For the facility—for the hospital facility fee, that is correct.

Ms. ESHOO. What does that mean, what you are saying? I don't get it.

[106] Kirzinger, Ashley, Bryan Wu, and Mollyann Brodie. "KFF Health Tracking Poll – November 2018: Priorities for New Congress and the Future of the ACA and Medicaid Expansion." *Kaiser Family Foundation*. 2018, https://www.kff.org/health-reform/poll-finding/kff-health-tracking-poll-november-2018-priorities-congressfuture-aca-medicaid-expansion/.

Mr. NICKELS. Well, the examples that have been given have been physician examples and we are not absolving ourselves from responsibility here. These are physicians who practice in our institutions.

Ms. ESHOO. Well, using your own words in the way you describe your systems—your hospitals—how many actually do surprise billing?

Mr. NICKELS. If you're saying are there—are you asking if there are physicians in our facilities who are surprise billing?

Ms. ESHOO. You're representing hospitals.

Mr. NICKELS. Right. Hospitals——

Ms. ESHOO. Hospitals are a part of the problem, right?

Mr. NICKELS. Well, the——

Ms. ESHOO. We have hospitals, we have insurance providers, we have physicians. You're 1 of the stakeholders. So I don't want to spend all of my time questioning you, but it doesn't seem to me that you can give me—perhaps you can give me a better answer in writing.

Mr. NICKELS. Sure.

Ms. ESHOO. Let me go to Dr.—to the Drs. Zaafran and Dr. Friedman. Have you or any physician you know billed a patient with what we would consider a surprise bill——

Dr. ZAAFRAN. So the company that I work——

Ms. ESHOO [continuing]. And why, if you have?

Dr. ZAAFRAN. The company that I work for has a policy of not sending surprise bills. What I will tell you, though, is that in instances where we don't know that we are actually out of network, and that's one of the things that I wanted to make sure that I brought up is that this out-of-network providers concept is a little bit of a misnomer.

I may be in network with every single insurance carrier out there but happen to be out of network with one plan of one carrier, and in many instances, I may not know that.

And as much as we try to know if we are out of network with that specific plan, we may not know that right away and we may actually inadvertently send a bill.

But once the patient contacts us, we take care of that right away. So that's where there's some discrepancy as far as whether we know we are actually in network or not out of network with a specific plan of a specific carrier.

Ms. ESHOO. I can't help but wonder what Ms. McAndrew and Ms. Wilkes are thinking so far in terms of the question I asked and the answers we have gotten. Think about it for a moment.

To Ms. Thornton, I want to ask you the same question. Are there any health plans in your association that where patients are not protected from surprise billing and, if so, why?

Ms. THORNTON. Yes. So patients who receive coverage through their employer through a self-funded plan are not protected by the various State laws that are out there.

Ms. ESHOO. Which is one of the main reasons that Congress has to act. Right. But there is surprise billing, though, in terms——

Ms. THORNTON. Yes. There have been widespread reports. Yes.

Ms. ESHOO. Yes. Right. So I want to go to the patient advocates. Tell us what you think—I think I know what you think but it's worth stating it for the record. We've heard a lot of testimony. They're all stakeholders. These are all good people with a system that's really messed up.

So what would you like to tell the committee? You want us to do it pronto. We all agree with that. Patients are being subjected to absurdities. What else would you like to say, having heard everyone else's testimony?

Ms. WILKES. Well, I believe that, as I said, insurance is very, very difficult to navigate. My husband and I consider ourselves to be pretty health literate and we still don't understand our insurance plan.

So in the case of an emergency, that's not your first thought. Your first thought is take care of my baby—take care of myself, and I feel like it should just be go to your doctor, get the care that you need, and not have to worry about the business side of things.

Ms. ESHOO. Right. Ms. McAndrew?

Ms. MCANDREW. I think the data speaks for itself. This is happening in urban areas, rural areas, non-profit hospitals, for-profit hospitals. Everyone agrees the patient should be held harmless, but the patient isn't being held harmless. This is not going to stop unless we have a policy solution.

So I understand that everybody, you know, wants to stop this problem. But there's money involved. There's not going to be any voluntary cessation of this problem unless we have a congressional solution.

Ms. ESHOO. It is always about money. That's just the way it is.

I now would like to recognize the ranking member for his five minutes of questioning, Dr. Burgess.

Mr. BURGESS. Thank you, and Ms. Wilkes, let me just say your testimony was very compelling this morning and it underscores why not just this discussion this morning is important but we are also having discussions on drug pricing.

I guess the good news in the realm of illnesses such as your son's is there are some very promising therapies right on the horizon with gene therapies. These may be single administration therapies that produce long-term benefits, and we have no frame of reference on how to price.

And the work we are doing on drug pricing becomes so important because everyone on this committee voted for a bill called CURES for the 21st Century. We want those cures to be put in the hands of doctors. They don't do any good if no one can afford them when they arrive.

So the work that this subcommittee does, yes, on this issue is important and on the larger issue of drug pricing in general and how do we—how do we price these new breakthrough therapies—hemophilia, sickle cell disease, spinal muscular atrophy. All of these are big deals that are happening, and we are grateful that they're happening.

They're happening largely because of work done in this subcommittee. We've got to be—the same type of forward-leaning thought that went into CURES for the 21st Century also needs to be there on the pricing of those therapies.

So, Dr. Zaafran and Dr. Friedman, let me just talk to you all for a moment. Now, I had a medical practice. I didn't use a billing service in my medical practice. I just billed through—we had our own billing department.

I never turned anyone over to collections because you never knew down the road when someone's going to have a problem and if they got a bill the same day they would say, hey, it's your fault, and being an OB I practice defensive medicine as one of my specialties.

But you have—Dr. Zaafran, I am going to assume that you're— you have got a big anaesthesia group—you have a billing service, correct?

Dr. ZAAFRAN. Correct.

Mr. BURGESS. And, Dr. Friedman, in your ER group?

Dr. FRIEDMAN. That's correct.

Mr. BURGESS. So are you doing anything with the billing services that you employ to at least begin to mitigate this issue or do you have a patient ombudsman who will look into these things if they're brought to your attention?

Dr. ZAAFRAN. Dr. Burgess, we have a customer service line to make sure that if Ms. Wilkes ever received a bill that she was not expecting that we would work with her directly to make sure that if it was an out-of-network bill, for example, in the very, you know, small percent of cases where it might be the case that we would— that we would not let her have to get involved in that.

There are other instances where because, again, of high deductible plans where if we happen to be 1 of the first ones who have billed and the patient's responsibility for the deductible is the entire amount that's there, there may be some difficulties there.

And part of the problem is that physicians are responsible, or hospitals, are responsible for having to collect those deductibles and co-pays, and as those numbers have been increasing, as those deductibles have been increasing to, in many instances, more than $5,000, it has put a significant burden on us having to work with patients to collect that.

I mean, I think since it's a contract between the payer and the consumer, it would be better for the payer to collect what they contractually agreed to collect and not have to put that burden on us where I may not have any idea at what portion of the deductible that patient has been paid.

Mr. BURGESS. Yes. You never want to be first. That's right.

Dr. Friedman?

Dr. FRIEDMAN. Yes. The companies that I've worked for—and I've worked for 3—we have all had customer service folks that will work with people when they get an out-of-network bill.

One of the things that I want to emphasize to the committee I happen to work in Orlando, Florida at the hospital closest to Disney World.

Forty percent of my patients come from out of the state.

Mr. BURGESS. Sure.

Dr. FRIEDMAN. So 40 percent of my patients are out of network.

Mr. BURGESS. And can you just comment a little bit on EMTALA and how that intersects with all of this discussion, having——

Dr. FRIEDMAN. Well, as I mentioned in my testimony, both my written and my oral, EMTALA prohibits us from discussing anything about payment.

In my 30 years of practice as an emergency physician, I've never asked a patient if they have insurance. I take care of the patient.

I get them to the place they need to be, whether that's home or admitted to the hospital or an observation unit, and then afterwards they get a bill.

But I don't know if they're in network. I don't know if they even have insurance, and that's the way we operate in emergency medicine.

And one of the concerns that we have is that while folks have talked about the fact that high deductibles may not be the root cause of this, high deductibles, unfortunately, give an incentive for insurers to not negotiate in good faith with emergency providers.

They know we are going to take care of their enrollees. We are obligated by Federal law to do that.

Mr. BURGESS. And you do obligate then the downstream—the cardiologist, the OB/Gyn to whom you refer—they also are obligated under those—without having a contract?

Dr. FRIEDMAN. The boundaries in EMTALA are a little bit——

Ms. ESHOO. Please wrap up. The gentleman's time has expired. Just quickly.

Dr. FRIEDMAN. Oh, OK.

Mr. BURGESS. Please answer the question.

Dr. FRIEDMAN. The boundaries of EMTALA are complicated. It would make it a lot simpler if it was when the patient was discharged from the hospital that EMTALA ended.

Mr. BURGESS. All right. Thank you.

Ms. ESHOO. The gentleman yields back.

I now would like to recognize the chairman of the full committee, Mr. Pallone, for his five minutes of questions.

Mr. PALLONE. Thank you, Madam Chair.

Healthcare costs are one of the top issues on the minds of all our constituents and this discussion has really highlighted the shocking costs people are dealing with, and when you look at some of these bills they're very unclear about what services were provided and why the services cost as much as they do.

So I wanted to ask some questions. Ms. Wilkes, when you received that $50,000 bill, was it easy to understand what you were being charged for and were you able to compare costs and determine if you were being billed fairly?

Ms. WILKES. No. The bill was not itemized at all. It just was a dollar amount.

Mr. PALLONE. You know, I have to say, you know, this is, totally anecdotal but a few years ago—it might be, like, 15 years ago—I remember talking to one hospital administrator who told me that, you know, that basically they just assign costs, you know, on a bill without any reference to what the actual cost is.

And so that's why you can have an ice bag that's, you know, $150 at one place and $15 at another because it's really not based on the actual cost.

But who knows? You know, hopefully that's not true.

Dr. Zaafran or Dr. Friedman, could you briefly explain who determines provider charges and how they are set? Start with Dr. Zaafran.

Dr. ZAAFRAN. Thank you, Mr. Pallone.

Our charges are based on an aggregate cost of what it costs us to deliver service. So in anaesthesia it's a little unique because it's time based. So we charge based on a unit of time for every 15 minutes.

So it's not an arbitrary cost. We know exactly how much we are billing, depending on whether the surgeon takes 15 minutes or an hour or hour and a half.

We, from our standpoint, because we try to focus on quality care, our expenses include nursing, having an opioid-free type of perioperative type of environment because we know it reduces overall cost. So all of that is built into how much we charge per unit of time.

Mr. PALLONE. And it's not broken down?

Dr. ZAAFRAN. Actually, if a patient calls us and asks us what that is, we do break it down because, again, it's based on the specific type of surgery. We can tell them exactly——

Mr. PALLONE. They'd have to ask you?

Dr. ZAAFRAN. We can provide it, and if it's on a piece of paper it may not make sense because we don't know how long a surgery is going to take. But we tell them that it took about an hour and a half, it was this kind of surgery, it was this many units and this much unit per time, and this is what the total cost was.

Mr. PALLONE. OK.

Dr. Friedman?

Dr. FRIEDMAN. So in emergency medicine, Chairman, it's a little bit different. We bill typically by what's called E&M codes, which are levels of service.

There are five E&M codes from a level one, which is we hardly ever use—it's basically a suture removal or recheck on something minor—up to a level 5, which would be someone that would be going to a critical care unit.

Maybe you are having a heart attack. You're receiving significant amounts of care. And then we can also bill a critical care charge, which would supersede that if you do receive critical care treatment in the emergency department.

Mr. PALLONE. All right. Thanks.

Now, we have all heard stories about patients being billed for hospital fees. One Vox article tells a story of a man who took his one-year-old daughter to the emergency room after a minor accident, as many worried parents do. For five minutes of the provider's time, water, gauze, and a Band-Aid for his daughter's finger, led to a $629 bill from the hospital's emergency department.

So I am going to go back to Dr. Nickels. But, again, I use the example where, you know, a few years ago a hospital administrator told me, you know, we just assign these things—they're not actually referencing, you know, actual costs for the—you know, in this case for the Band-Aid or the gauze or the water or the provider's time.

You know, could you give us a sense, Mr. Nickels, of how much hospitals charge and facility fees on average and what are hospitals doing to make these fees more transparent?

And, you know, maybe if you want to dispute what I just said, you know, like in this case would they actually figure out how much it costs for these different things, or not?

Mr. NICKELS. Yes. I mean, the charge system is obtuse, to be kind, and I think it's a broken system. We are trying to work—we have a committee.

We are working with the Trump administration. We need to figure out a way to fix it. But most people, almost anyone who is insured is not paying charges. The Government doesn't pay us charges. We negotiate with insurers. They don't pay charges——

Mr. PALLONE. Well, I only—30 seconds. So it's very possible that in this case, or using my example, you know, there's really no breakdown for those five minutes of the provider's time, the water, the gauze, the Band-Aid. It is not done that way.

Mr. NICKELS. Correct. It may be but it may not, if that's——

Mr. PALLONE. Right. So very possible that what I talked about, you know, 10 or 15 years ago, we just assign things—very possible.

Mr. NICKELS. Yes.

Mr. PALLONE. All right. That's pretty sad, Madam Chair.

But thank you.

Ms. ESHOO. Thank you, Mr. Chairman.

I now would like to recognize my friend, the ranking member of the full committee, Mr. Walden, for his five minutes of questions.

Mr. WALDEN. Thank you, Madam Chair, and we have this other hearing going on upstairs I had to go up to on FERC—Federal Energy. So we are back.

Ms. Thornton, the comments submitted to the committee as well as Dr. Zaafran's testimony providers have argued that California's benchmark has led to payers refusing to renew long-standing contracts or offering lower rates.

But in your testimony you mentioned that California's benchmark has led to an increase in network participation and the Blue Shield of California has told us that current State laws on network adequacy still apply and, in fact, since their surprise billing law went into effect they have increased their number of contracted physicians by five percent overall and six percent specifically at acute care hospital facilities.

Can you help this committee better understand what's taking place in California by sharing a bit more about those preliminary reports? And what about other states such as mine, Oregon, with benchmark solutions? What can you tell us about that?

Ms. THORNTON. Thank you. So yes, so there's been a lot of debate around the California law, and the California law just took effect in January of 2019. So it's very new.

Mr. WALDEN. Right.

Ms. THORNTON. And so we have been talking with our plans and their experience with implementation of the law and they have not reported to us that they've seen, you know, decrease in network participation.

In fact, as you have mentioned. One of our plans has actually seen an increase in providers participating. So I don't think the California law can be used as a reason why we'll see decreasing networks. We want strong networks for our members.

Mr. WALDEN. And have you seen something similar in Oregon?

Ms. THORNTON. No, I have not.

Mr. WALDEN. OK. So you don't have any data on what's happening in Oregon? All right. Doctor, do you want to address this from your point of view?

Dr. ZAAFRAN. Yes, sir. Thanks, Mr. Walden. We know of actually 2 of the largest groups in California. One of them who has been in network for many, many years have not had actually any kind of cost of living increase or anything like that.

We were told point blank that they're going to have to take a big cut or they can simply just go out of network and they'll be paid a very low benchmark based on Assembly Bill 72.

We also know of a very large group in the northern part of California where they have not been in network, have wanted to be in network, have been told that they have no desire to be allowed to be in network and, again, that they would be paid a very low benchmark based on Assembly Bill 72.

Again, I know that it's a new law that just started in January. But the anecdotal evidence that we have from the groups that are being affected by this is that they've been impacted.

Mr. WALDEN. And who is telling them that?

Dr. ZAAFRAN. The specific insurance carriers that they're negotiating with to try to be in network.

Mr. WALDEN. I suppose you don't really want to identify those specific insurers here before us today?

Dr. ZAAFRAN. I would rather just talk in general statements, but yes.

Mr. WALDEN. Uh-huh. All right. Several stakeholders suggest requiring plans to update their provider network directories in a more timely manner. Seems pretty practical. I think Texas was working on—oh, you're no longer from Texas.

[Laughter.]

Mr. WALDEN. You're changing out on me. I know Texas was working on some of that disclosure language as well. I don't know where that ended up through the system.

But how regularly do plans update their directories right now? And I've heard from people that go, great, I signed up for the plan. I am in the system. The provider is in the system.

Then something changes and I can't change my insurance and now I am stuck in a plan that my provider used to be in and now they are not. Now I am out of network. Now I am going to get one of these nutty bills. That is not putting the consumer first. Ms. Thornton, can you address this, please?

Ms. THORNTON. Sure, of course, and I think one of the things I first want to set aside is that in an emergency situation we don't want anybody to have to worry about the provider directory. We want the patients to be protected in that situation.

But I will say to your question it is very important to our plans that we have accurate and reliable data for consumers for—in the provider directories when they are seeking care, scheduled care, et cetera, and are working very hard to make sure that that occurs. Mr. WALDEN. Can you put all of that online on a regular basis? How do these directories work? Do I have to get a printed copy sent to me in the mail?

Ms. THORNTON. Oh, they're all online. You can also call our plan's customer service to get information via the phone if you don't have access online.

Mr. WALDEN. Do you notify policy holders when things change?

Ms. THORNTON. If a patient has been seeing a particular provider there is also often a notification that takes place.

Mr. WALDEN. Often. All right. Because I think you ought to be notified. I think you ought to—how do you know? How do you keep up with this stuff? You think you're covered. I am just telling you that you're headed to a big train wreck here.

Ms. THORNTON. Information changes daily. I understand.

Mr. WALDEN. And you know it because you know how to send a bill out. The consumer ought to know it because they're the ones getting the surprise bill.

That's where I am coming from here, as a consumer and representing consumers. How do we know? I will tell you 1 quick story, and I know I am going to go over. Just a second, Madam Chair, with your indulgence.

A guy at a think tank here—this is second hand—who goes in for a colonoscopy, is on the table prepped and ready to go—and those of you who are old enough to have been through this you understand what's at stake here—asked the doc, is the anesthesiologist in my network. I don't know. Well, before I sign this I need to know.

Well, I can't tell you—I don't know. Do you want the procedure today or not, because I've got five more of these to do? The guy signs it, goes under, boom, done. Is that what we are doing to consumers? I think this is nuts.

Ms. THORNTON. I mean, that's horrible and that's why we need this legislation.

Mr. WALDEN. And this is going on every day in America and it shouldn't be. You forgot who you serve and it's the consumer.

Thank you, Madam Chair, for your indulgence.

Ms. ESHOO. Thank you for your important questions. I don't know—I just want to throw something out here. This business of notification, and you just put a spotlight on it. Who's going to be notified when, and then what the heck do they do once they're informed?

What, you're in labor and then you find out that the—whomever, the anesthesiologist is—exactly—well, I will hold on to this child and try to get to another place. I don't know what this notification—most of this is in an emergency room setting, at least that's what the statistics show.

So I don't know if it's really very smart to be focusing on notice. Yes, people should be noticed. But let's use some common sense about how notice is—how effective, quote, "notice" is going to be.

I mean, given the settings, it's not making too much sense and it's making it sound as if we throw that in there that it's, boy, is this really going to do something. So I am not—you can tell I am not convinced.

All right. With that, I would like to recognize a total gentleman from North Carolina—yes, it's you. It is you. Mr. Butterfield for five minutes of his questions.

Mr. BUTTERFIELD. I will wake up, Madam Chair. Thank you. Thank you so very much for those kind words. Thank you for convening this very important hearing today.

Thank you to the eight witnesses for your testimony. Like Mr. Walden said, I've been bouncing between hearings today and knew that my time was coming up pretty soon and so I am back here with you.

While I am on the thank you trail, let me also thank Mr. Pallone and Mr. Walden for their bipartisanship in putting forth this discussion draft. I think it's going to lead to good legislation which is ultimately going to protect every consumer in America.

Let me begin with Mr. Nickels. Mr. Nickels, I represent a very low-income district in eastern North Carolina. It is not unlike any other rural community in America. We face unique challenges when it comes to healthcare.

In some areas in my district there isn't a hospital for many, many miles, and you have heard that before and it's not a surprise. These markets have little competition. Residents have few facilities to choose from.

The small hospitals that do serve these areas are often operating at a loss or near loss and they rely on reimbursements as their primary revenue source.

In your opinion, how would the imposition of statutory rates impact small rural hospitals?

Mr. NICKELS. Yes. We do worry about, as you said, the imposition of those kinds of rates. One-size-fits-all won't work because there are unique circumstances——

Ms. ESHOO. Can't hear you.

Mr. NICKELS. OK. I certainly agree with what you're saying there. One of the reasons we don't like national rates is because they don't take into consideration local conditions like the ones you describe and it's really important that that be more of a function of negotiation between the hospital and the insurer who will be, hopefully, persuaded of the importance of those facilities. And there is a crisis in rural America. There's a crisis of rural hospitals. It is a whole different issue but it's another one that we need to solve.

Mr. BUTTERFIELD. We have competing interests here between small rural hospitals and the need to protect the consumer, and as legislators we have got to work through that tension and find a good solution.

Mr. Friedman, can you help me with that a little bit?

Dr. FRIEDMAN. Well, I would agree with you that there is a conflict there. But I would suggest that one of the things that the Congress consider is that access is vital.

If you have a mechanism that goes into place, as you suggested, that would decrease access, particularly in rural communities, that doesn't serve consumers either.

If they can't get—they don't get a surprise bill but there's no provider or hospital to provide that service, we have done them a service.

Mr. BUTTERFIELD. Ms. McAndrew, can you help us with this?

Ms. MCANDREW. I would just call attention to the fact that the reason we are having this discussion right now is that this is already a problem in rural areas. I actually pulled some data in advance of this hearing and I just want to draw attention to how many consumers are already suffering because there are not in-network providers and consumers are getting surprise bills in rural areas.

I looked at your State of North Carolina and already consumers are—in-network hospital admissions are getting out-of-network claims more than 10 percent of the time. So what that tells me is that providers are staying out of network already and consumers are suffering.

So while I acknowledge the fact that we want to study this as we move forward on the legislation, I would urge against hesitating because consumers are suffering from this problem in rural areas. So we already know status quo this is a problem.

And so while we can worry about unintended consequences, we know the current consequence is that consumers are getting out-of-network bills in rural areas. That's also true more than 10 percent of time. Consumers in in-network hospitals are getting out-of-network claims and rural states like Indiana, Kentucky, Oklahoma are represented on this committee so I would not hesitate to solve this problem because of unintended consequences in this.

Mr. BUTTERFIELD. Well, you know, I've seen both consequences. I've seen rural hospitals close for lack of revenue. That's at one end of the debate. I've seen consumers go bankrupt because of their inability to pay those statements when they arrive. I've seen it from both extremes and, as legislators, we have got to reconcile those two interests.

Ms. Thornton, let me—let me conclude with you. What role does the lack of network adequacy play in the occurrence of surprise bills?

Ms. THORNTON. Thank you. So health plans need networks to function. We want our members to have access to a large and high-quality network.

However, you cannot control when you have an emergency, you know, where you are across the country. And so we really don't think the network adequacy is directly related to the issue of surprise billing.

Claire—Ms. McAndrew, excuse me—mentioned that you're just as likely to experience a surprise medical bill if you're in a large employer plan with a broad network in a narrow—more narrow network individual market plan.

Mr. BUTTERFIELD. Thank you.

Madam Chair, I yield back and right on time. Thank you.

Ms. ESHOO. I thank the gentleman.

I recognize the gentleman from Illinois, Mr. Shimkus, for his five minutes of questioning.

Mr. SHIMKUS. Thank you, Madam Chairwoman.

Madam Chairwoman, I also asked—I was happy that you asked about Ms. Wilkes' son. I am sure he's very proud of you today, and if he's not had him talk to me because you did a wonderful job.

I would also like to ask unanimous consent that this letter sent to me on June 10th by the Illinois Hospital Association be submitted for the record.

Ms. ESHOO. Without objection, so ordered.

[The information appears at the conclusion of the hearing.]

Mr. SHIMKUS. Thank you, Madam Chairman.

You know, a lot of this debate and a lot of testimony referenced specific State attempts to address this issue and baseball, apparently, and we are getting close to the congressional game so a lot of us are focused on baseball.

For example, Illinois does use the baseball-style arbitration method in the event a dispute arises between providers and health plans. Each party must submit a proposed best and final offer to the arbiter who then chooses one of the two without modification, thus keeping the consumer out of that fight. You really have different sizes of big versus the small individual in that process.

However, these State laws don't apply to self-insured ERISA plans, as has been highlighted by the testimony, used by, roughly, 100 million Americans.

I was also interested to hear a number of witnesses mentioned another Federal law involved in this debate, the Emergency Medical Treatment and Labor Act—EMTALA.

I talk about it quite a bit because it—we all need them. We all use emergency rooms. Cost shifting at the hospitals to help pay for the emergency room, and what's occurred, as you all know because you live in this world, is that we are really pushing our citizens and constituents to go to urgent care centers, you know, if they're not emergent.

We need emergency rooms, but we need—we need to encourage that.

But EMTALA, the Federal law right now is unique to emergency care and it's an important element of our nation's safety net.

But in choosing to require providers to treat patients regardless of their ability to pay presents unique challenges of its own in some States like Texas and Colorado through free-standing emergency center operations with a State license, not a Federal license.

So, Dr. Zaafran, in states with free-standing emergency centers do those facilities have to abide by a similar standard to EMTALA since they're not Federally licensed?

Dr. ZAAFRAN. If they are licensed as an emergency center, they do. Urgent care centers, of course, have a little bit of a different definition. They're not necessarily looked at as emergency centers by that definition so they wouldn't fall under that category.

Mr. SHIMKUS. Yes, and I am following guidance by staff and I talk about urgent care centers, but I really was interested about state-licensed emergency centers not under the Federal guidelines and that's what I am trying to get to.

Dr. ZAAFRAN. State-licensed emergency centers are—they have to abide by EMTALA. That's correct.

Mr. SHIMKUS. You also referenced the difference between hospital-based physicians and physicians not bound by EMTALA. Can you please walk the committee through the justification for having one resolution process for facilities and another for providers?

Dr. ZAAFRAN. Yes, sir. One of the things that EMTALA does very specifically is that it asks for emergency room physicians to make sure that they have to see every patient regardless of costs or anything like that.

But, again, you have a patient who may come in and the emergency room physician decides that this person needs to be seen by a surgeon because they have an infected appendix.

Well, that person is going to have to have surgery by the surgeon. They're going to have to have anaesthesia by the anesthesiologist and, you know, they many not necessarily be specifically bound by EMTALA but once you're admitted into that hospital and you're in an emergency setting where it is impractical, unreasonable, and unsafe to transfer that patient, all the physicians that are on call during the time period where that physician has been admitted and has to be treated in a very short fashion by all those different providers, all those different physicians have to be—it has to be done in a timely fashion.

So even though EMTALA may not directly apply to them, we have to take care of them and the way we operate as anesthesiologists is you're taking care of many of these facilities 24 hours a day, 7 days a week, regardless of whether they have insurance, don't have insurance. We don't even ask.

Mr. SHIMKUS. So my final question for you—in supporting a benchmark concept with an arbitration backdrop you mentioned that four recent State adoptions enjoyed the support of providers, insurers, and patients.

So I want to clarify if your hospital partners supported these State efforts, too.

Dr. ZAAFRAN. So yes, they did. In Texas, specifically, which the bill recently passed several weeks ago, all the stakeholders—emergency room physicians, Texas College emergency physicians, the Texas Medical Association, the Texas Society of Anesthesiologists, the Texas Association of Health Plans, the consumer advocacy groups including AARP—all supported the bill.

It was a consensus bill. It was an excellent bill that was passed that involves baseball-style arbitration with specific guardrails to make sure that costs were contained within that framework.

Mr. SHIMKUS. Thank you, Madam Chairman. I yield back my time.

Ms. ESHOO. The gentleman yields back.

The gentlewoman from California is recognized for five minutes for her questions—Ms. Matsui.

Ms. MATSUI. Thank you very much, Madam Chair.

I thank you all for being here today. This is a very important issue. I kept hearing about it in my roundtables back home.

As you may know, my home State of California already has some of the country's most robust protections against balance billing patients for certain procedures.

In my district, I've already heard from many hospitals that in an increasingly fragmented healthcare system there is concern that a Federal policy that may further discourage contracting between insurers and providers will have the unintended consequence of decreasing innovation and partnerships that are facilitating better and more coordinated care and reducing costs.

As Congress considers solutions modelled after California law, I would like to discuss how our State effort is working to influence market dynamics between healthcare purchasers and providers and how those changes are ultimately impacting patients.

Specifically, the reimbursement model in California benchmarks payments for out-of-network physicians at the greatest of 125 percent of Medicare, or the average contracted rate.

Dr. Zaafran, can you discuss how using a median in-network rate as a benchmark may put downward pressure on future contracted rates offered by insurers?

Dr. ZAAFRAN. Yes, ma'am. Thank you for that question.

So median, by definition, means that you have certain contracts that are above that number and certain contracts that are below that number, and there's a reason for that.

As I have mentioned in my testimony, there's a differentiator for why certain physicians have contracts that pay more than others. In fact, in Washington State my specific company, Blue Cross Blue Shield, actually put out a press release touting a value-based contract that they signed from the standpoint that they're paying a premium, but they understand that the overall cost of care is actually less.

So the ability to make sure that you're able to differentiate based on quality metrics that a higher payment is due is something that has to be preserved. If you keep everything at the median and not allow for those differentiators to exist, you're essentially kind of bringing everybody down to that number.

And the other problem is, is that as new contracts are negotiated, if they're negotiated in a downward fashion, that median actually starts going down also.

Ms. MATSUI. OK.

Dr. Friedman and Mr. Gelfand, from each of your perspectives, if Congress were to establish a Federal default fixed rate, what benchmark metric should we consider that would preserve the incentive for future contracting between plans and providers?

Dr. Friedman? Mr. Gelfand?

Dr. FRIEDMAN. Yes, thank you for the question, Congresswoman Matsui. We firmly believe, as I pointed out in our testimony, that it would be virtually impossible to find the perfect rate, one that both providers would be happy with and insurers would be happy with, and that's why we think that going back to an independent dispute resolution to work out agreements between providers of care and the insurers—the payers of care is the most cost effective and evidence-based model that we have.

Ms. MATSUI. Mr. Gelfand?

Mr. GELFAND. Congresswoman, we support the California model. The perfect should not be the enemy of the good. The data bears out that the California model is working and, in the end, a benchmark that works is a benchmark that is rarely used because it brings parties to the table to get in network and that's our goal.

Ms. MATSUI. Mr. Nickels, from the hospital perspective, is setting a default rate for emergency and other services necessary to stop patients from being balance billed?

Mr. NICKELS. Yes. I mean, I think there should be no balance billing in the emergency department. There should be no balance billing when a patient in good conscience and knowledge comes in to an in-network facility. They should not get anything from an out-of-network physician where they don't have to pay any more than their in-network co-insurance.

Ms. MATSUI. OK. What effect might a Federal fixed payment rate have on a hospital's ability to ensure adequate staffing and patient access to care?

Mr. NICKELS. Yes, we are not supportive of any kind of benchmark or any kind of rate like that, and I think it would have all the negative consequences that were outlined already.

I mean, our members negotiate with insurers. We talk quality. We talk volume. We talk all kinds of things that, I think, would— especially with innovation would be really hindered by kind of a one-size-fits-all approach.

So we do not support that. If Congress is going to do anything, we do think that the baseball-style arbitration approach is the best one. But let's let, you know, the negotiation between us and the insurers continue.

Ms. MATSUI. OK. Probably I am running out of time here to ask the next question, but I wanted to ask about ERISA. You know, states like California are taking on important steps to address surprise bills.

Congress needs to enact a Federal solution to expand these protections to all privately-insured patients. But some 25 states have already enacted some form of balance billing protections at payment dispute resolutions.

And I am running out of time, but when crafting a Federal balance billing solution how should Congress consider existing State laws for determining out-of-network payment for surprise bills? Should State law always supersede a new Federal law? And I am out of time.

Anyone want to comment on that in one second?

Ms. MCANDREW. So we do acknowledge that some states have done a good job, including California, of enacting comprehensive legislation. However, there are consumers who would be left out.

We also worry that if laws that are less comprehensive were to be allowed to supersede Federal law, you will have a race to the bottom. You pass a comprehensive law here in Congress, you will see a flood of lobbyists trying to pass less comprehensive laws in the State if they are to supersede it. So we recommend that Federal law take precedent unless a State law is more comprehensive. Also, Federal law wraparound to cover ERISA when State law cannot.

Ms. MATSUI. Thank you very much, and thank you, Madam Chair.

Ms. ESHOO. Thank you.

Pleased recognize the gentleman from Kentucky, Mr. Guthrie, for his five minutes.

Mr. GUTHRIE. Thank you very much, and it's—thanks for everybody being here. Thanks to Ms. Wilkes for being here with your story.

And, you know, it's kind of frustrating. It gets to kind of a larger thing. I am on Oversight investigations. We are looking at insulin pricing and it kind of looks at the difference in net price and list price, and it seems here—I have an incidence—we all have instances in our area. Emergency situation wasn't emergency room physicians where a person in my district who's actually an insurance broker so he's very sophisticated—talk about insurance literate. Had an emergency situation with his son and was billed over $30,000 for a service, and if he had an insurance that had been in network it would have been less than $10,000. And he actually sat down—he wanted to. They would refuse to do it.

He said, if you will sit down with me and show me your price and your charge and some kind of reasonable return, I would pay it. But they wouldn't sit down and go through the pricing charged.

So that's just a big issue. He said, I will write you a check today if you will let me—if you can show to me that it's really part of it, and that's the source of the problem that we are getting at, just the overall system here.

Mr. Gelfand, getting back to the notice of out of network, in your testimony you mentioned the need to tighten the requirements in the discussion draft on patient consent for out-of-network procedures.

Could you elaborate what you think this should be?

Mr. GELFAND. Yes. We associate ourselves with the remarks of Families USA in that you cannot simply give 24 hours and allow the physician to surprise bill as long as you have 24 hours' notice that a surprise bill is coming because oftentimes you may be going to a facility but you literally have no choice about some of those ancillary providers that will be present at that facility.

Mr. GUTHRIE. So I guess to Ms. Thornton, Ranking Member Walden said that a person asked about is the anesthesiologist, before I sign this form, in network and the provider there didn't—I am sure it was the gastroenterologist or whoever is doing—didn't know.

I mean, how do the health insurance plans fit into notice? How— we are trying to figure out how this would work. Somebody walks in, I need service. If they're out of network, how do we know and how would the health insurance plans be involved in this?

Ms. THORNTON. So in the first place, it's important—when you have an emergency or you're at an in-network facility patients are protected, right. The Federal —this Federal law would sort of swoop in.

So you wouldn't have situations where consumers are getting that bill because they would be protected by the payment benchmark that we are talking about today.

Now, in scenarios that aren't covered by the bill we do think there is an important role to get notice, to be able to call the health plan and say, hey, I've got this procedure next week—can you let me know, you know, what the network status of my provider will be, and we think that process can work for more things that are scheduled in advance, and not emergency care when you have no control over who's going to see you and you're in no position to have that discussion.

Mr. GUTHRIE. Well, it couldn't be just in the emergency room because Ms. Wilkes wasn't in—she was in a labor and delivery room, I assume, and next thing you know you're in a NICU. So, I mean, it's not just EMTALA type of situation.

Ms. THORNTON. No, exactly.

Mr. GUTHRIE. I understand that, you know, we talk about just don't look at unintended consequences—we just have to move forward. But it is an issue with emergency room physicians because they have to take care. They can't talk about price, and that is different than other things, moving forward.

I do have a question, Ms. Thornton. You're subject to the medical loss ratio requirements, and those are requirements that require a minimum percentage of premium dollars taken to be spent on paying claims.

Can you speak to how an arbitration system might have an impact on MLR requirements?

Ms. THORNTON. Sure, happy to do that.

So there are two different components of a medical loss ratio— sort of what we are spending on medical care and what we are spending on administrative costs.

On the medical cost side, it's really important here that any solution that we are talking about to end surprise billing does not increase medical spending. That $30,000 bill that you mentioned, right, that's reflected in people's premiums that they pay every month for coverage. So that's sort of one piece.

But on the other side, if you're taking kind of a bureaucratic process and inserting it into the healthcare system—Dr. Friedman mentioned 150 million ER visits a year. Even if you took a percentage of those and threw that to arbitration with those administrative costs, that would be adding a lot of costs to the system.

Mr. GUTHRIE. So we would have to—your argument would be that we'd have to take that out of the medical loss ratio calculation?

Ms. THORNTON. It would be administrative costs borne by the health plan, yes.

Mr. GUTHRIE. OK. So this really isn't for everyone but I just have a few—less than a minute. But so once a bill is put into place, there's a Federal —if there is becomes a Federal arbitration system, what do you think congressional oversight should be and I don't know if that would be something Ms. Wilkes wants to talk about or——

Ms. WILKES. Well, I've been sitting here listening, thinking, I pay my insurance premiums. I do my part and I expect the bill to be paid. I mean, there's only so much I can do to control that.

I don't really care how the reimbursement works and, quite frankly, I think the insurance industry is doing probably better in their bottom line than my bottom line. I want to go to the best provider possible and I want the best care. I don't really care how the payment works.

Mr. GUTHRIE. OK. Thanks. And I won't go on down the list because my time has expired. But I do hope things are going well, and the other part of our area we are looking at genetics and things like that and some really great things that are happening in hemophilia. So, hopefully, your son will qualify for those as well as they—his genetics will qualify, not just your insurance. Your genetics will qualify is my point.

Thanks. Appreciate it.

Ms. ESHOO. The gentleman yields back.

I now would like to recognize the gentlewoman from Florida, Ms. Castor.

Ms. CASTOR. Well, thank you, Madam Chair, for holding this important hearing and thank you to the witnesses for your expert recommendations to the committee.

Ms. Wilkes, thank you so much for sharing your personal story. My home State of Florida adopted a balance billing law in 2016 and my understanding of the law is that first and foremost it works to protect the patient and then establishes a process for the payer and the provider to resolve a payment issue.

So that if a patient receives care from a provider that is out of network, the patient will only be responsible for in-network cost sharing and then providers and the insurance plans have to go through a State-arranged voluntary dispute resolution process where a penalty is assessed to the party that refused to accept an offer that was close to the final arbitration order.

And I understand that the negotiation is based on the usual and customary rate in that particular geographic area and then it binds the parties, going forward.

Florida's law is relatively new; but I wanted to see if any of the witnesses have feedback on how my State is doing.

Dr. Friedman, you practice in the State of Florida. What's your view?

Dr. FRIEDMAN. Yes, thank you for the question, Congresswoman Castor.

It is untested, frankly. The history of balance billing in Florida and dispute resolution in Florida is not necessarily one that is particularly good and the pervious—we have had a balance billing for a long time for HMO products in Florida and there was an attempt to—some time ago to add PPO products to that.

The dispute resolution process as the State used turned out to be very insurer friendly and providers refused to use it after a while. So this new law has been tweaked and we hope that it will be more provider friendly and it will be one that both providers and insurers are happy to use.

It has not been tested yet. I know that within the emergency medicine community at least it is due to be tested very shortly and we look forward to seeing the results of that experiment.

Ms. CASTOR. So what will happen if the Pallone bill with Mr. Walden passes in my—

Dr. FRIEDMAN. Some of that refers to the earlier question around Federal pre-emption of State law and we believe, first of all, that the Federal law should apply if the State law does not have at least the same level of protections, certainly for patients, but also for the providers' system.

We have to support our providers that are taking care of patients.

Ms. CASTOR. Ms. McAndrew, what's your view of the—a dispute resolution process versus bench marking?

Ms. MCANDREW. Thank you very much for your question, Congresswoman Castor.

At Families USA our preferred approach would be the benchmark approach. I think the initial reports on a CBO score of the various approaches were quite telling—that the benchmark approach is—produces the largest cost savings, and cost savings that come from these various approaches trickle down to consumers.

The reason that we think this matters to consumers is that when we have any surprise bill law that could potentially result in any inflationary costs within the system, those will trickle down to consumers in their premiums.

So our goal is to have a payment rate that is as least inflationary as possible. However, I will say, you know, at the end of the day what matters most to us is the consumer protection part of this.

And so while we prefer the benchmark rate, when it comes to discussing an arbitration system, the devil is in the details. The bottom line for us is that billed charges, should not be considered in this.

Ms. CASTOR. So how do we—how do we ensure that what we do to protect patients from surprise medical bills doesn't cause higher premiums?

Ms. MCANDREW. Well, I think that goes back to what's considered in the payment rate. So at the end of the day, whatever the system is as long as it's not based on billed charges I think that's what matters most because as some discussion has alluded to before, charges can be quite arbitrary. Sometimes I compare them to, like, the list price of a prescription drug. Nobody really pays it, as Mr. Nickels said before. So we wouldn't want to bake it into our system.

Ms. CASTOR. Does anyone else want to comment on dispute resolution versus bench marking?

Dr. ZAAFRAN. I would. So, you know, we have data in New York already as to how this has been proven and the premium increase in New York has been actually very commensurate with the premium increase in California.

So, you know, you have bench marking in one area. You have dispute resolution in the other, and the premium increases have not been any different.

But you have a decrease in New York from the standpoint of how many out-of-network providers you have from 20.1 percent down to a 6.4 percent.

What I do want to emphasize, though, because cost has come up here several times, in New York the average cost of a dispute resolution process is about $300. It takes an average of two weeks. It is all entered in electronically, and the resolution is adjudicated within those two weeks. It is a very seamless, quick, and easy process and it has worked.

What I would say also from the standpoint of bench marking versus a dispute resolution is it is not a one-size-fits-all. My company invested a tremendous amount of resources to make sure that we do opioid-free anaesthesia so that we don't have folks who are on opioids a year later after they've had surgery or that they don't have surgical site infections that have them to be readmitted back into the hospital after they've been discharged. Those actually decrease the cost of care, and as referenced earlier, we have insurance carriers who are willing to pay us a premium because they understand; and they know that the overall cost of care does down.

Ms. ESHOO. I thank you. Your time has concluded, Doctor.

Ms. CASTOR. Thank you.

Ms. ESHOO. I thank the gentlewoman yielding back.

I now would like to recognize Dr. Bucshon from Indiana.

Mr. BUCSHON. Thank you, Madam Chairwoman, and I was a cardiovascular surgeon prior to coming to Congress and I think we can all agree it's about patients here.

That said, the current draft of the No Surprises Act, although well intended, in my view is not completely the right solution.

Again, we can all agree that we—the liability of surprise out-of-network bills should not be on the patient. We need a solution. However, in my view, the draft legislation would lead to a reimbursement race to the bottom.

It would encourage narrow networks and lower provider reimbursement, limiting patient access, and ultimately is going to continue to result in further physician shortages.

Since the late 1980s, physician provider reimbursement has continually been cut in an attempt to control healthcare costs—and you can see that hasn't worked—while other areas of the healthcare system including large publicly-held companies continue to earn record profits.

The draft legislation would ultimately, I believe, ask again for providers to shoulder the financial responsibility of a healthcare system that costs too much. As long as we have a system that allows the business side of medicine to march on while cutting reimbursement to those who are actually providing patient care, our problem doesn't go away.

An approach similar to the State of New York or a hybrid combination of bench marking and arbitration, in my view, could help solve the problem and not lead to a reimbursement race to the bottom.

So with that said, Dr. Friedman, based on my experience, physicians who accept lower in-network payment rates may get additional benefits from the health plans, preferred—preferential referrals, things like that. Considering that there still could be an incentive to take a lower rate offered by an insurer, can you talk about what reasons a physician may not be part of an insurance network?

Dr. FRIEDMAN. Well, I think, you know, from the standpoint of my members, we want to be in network. We actively try to contract with insurers. The only time that an emergency—most of the emergency physicians that I know and most of the groups that are part of my organization are out of network is when we cannot reach a reasonable negotiated rate with an insurance company or the example that I used before where I work in Florida and I take care of a lot of folks from out of State because those contracts are regional. They're not national, even for the ERISA plans.

So I think that we want to—as providers, we want to be in network. We want to be in contract. We don't want to be sitting here talking about patients that have been harmed by out-of-network billing.

Mr. BUCSHON. Right, and that's the point I wanted to get at is that physicians—we want to be in network. We don't want patients to not be in network, and that's why my concern about setting a benchmark could lead to an incentive from the plan's perspective just to not renew contracts, and we have heard that from Dr. Zaafran today—and make everybody out of network and then we have this lower benchmark and then, of course, as the higher contract—reimbursement contracts all of a sudden go away, the benchmark lowers and then you get this race to the bottom in provider reimbursement, which is—which is, I think, the concern the State of New York had when they put in an arbitration model, which is working. We've heard from people from the State of New York.

So that's my main concern. So that's what I wanted to get at. Providers want to be in network. We don't want people to be stuck with these bills.

So in Indiana, in the largest group market last year the largest insurer had 65 percent of the market share. The next largest at 21 percent and the third only five percent. Considering the limited competition, what leverage do physicians have when negotiating reimbursement rates with insurers? And I guess, Dr. Zaafran, you might comment on that.

Dr. ZAAFRAN. Well, again, as Dr. Friedman said, we always try to negotiate and be in network. But in many instances when a large carrier does not necessarily need to because they're narrowing their networks, they just simply won't negotiate.

And that's why, frankly, network adequacy standards are so important. I understand that some folks may not. But I can give you a very specific example in Texas where it was extremely important.

We had one specific carrier a year ago between February and August essentially drop all the anaesthesia groups in the state—mainly, the five largest cities—out of network. These are all mid-contracts. These were not being in the midst of renegotiating contracts. They just dropped them.

The medical associations and societies found this out. They realized it. They took it to the Texas Department of insurance and based on network adequacy laws, the Texas Department of Insurance brought this carrier in, found out that they were not meeting those standards, put a fine on them of $700,000 and a rule that within 90 days that they have to make sure that they bring back their network into adequacy, and it did.

Mr. BUCSHON. Thank you very much. My time has expired.

Ms. ESHOO. The gentleman yields back.

The gentleman from New Mexico, Mr. Luján, is recognize for five minutes for his questions.

Mr. LUJÁN. Thank you, Madam Chair, and I thank you and the ranking member for bringing us together today on an important issue facing our constituents all across America.

Mr. Sherlock, can you explain to me what the average charge per air ambulance service is?

Mr. SHERLOCK. Excuse me. Thank you for the question.

According to a study conducted by Xcenda in 2017, the median charge for a helicopter or medical transport is $10,199.

Mr. LUJÁN. So can I ask a follow-up there? In your testimony you described the $10,199 amount as the median cost. Is the median cost and the average charge the same thing?

Mr. SHERLOCK. No, they're not. When you look at——

Mr. LUJÁN. So the question that I ask you was what is the average charge today of an air ambulance.

Mr. SHERLOCK. The charges are not—I don't know that there is an average charge.

Mr. LUJÁN. So the——

Mr. SHERLOCK. The charges—when you look at the fact that 70 percent of our patients are covered by Medicare, Medicaid, or are uninsured and the fact that Medicare, according to the same study, reimburses at less than $0.60 of those charges—of those costs, rather—Medicaid is always less and the uninsured virtually pay, you know, $350. Yet that cost of uncompensated care is what needs to maintain network adequacy because——

Mr. LUJÁN. So if I may, Mr. Sherlock, what the study is that you quoted in your report by Xcenda in 2017 states that the median cost of providing one helicopter transport is $10,199.

What the Government Accountability Office found in 2017 is that the median price charged is $36,400. A study that was conducted in the State of New Mexico showed that in 2015 the average amount charged per flight was $45,000.

I think it's an increase of about 300 percent from 2006 to 2015 in the State of New Mexico alone. I am just trying to get my hands around why this is costing so much and why so many of my constituents are hit with surprise bills when it comes to air transport across the country.

What is it that is—is it in fact that you agree that the average cost then is $10,199 for an air transport?

Mr. SHERLOCK. The median cost. If you look at the fact that some——

Mr. LUJÁN. Let me ask the question differently then. I apologize.

We don't have so much time. What's the break-even point?

Mr. SHERLOCK. The break-even point, depending on the—on the area of the country is based on the fact that you have Medicare that reimburses at less than $0.60 to the cost of providing the services, Medicaid that reimburses at less than $0.35 on the dollar to the cost of providing services, and uninsured.

That cost of uncompensated care then raises the cost of transports in order to be able to maintain access to healthcare for millions of Americans who would not be able to get to a level 1 or level 2 trauma center in an hour or less——

Mr. LUJÁN. Are you able to give me the cost breakdown, exclude Medicaid and Medicare, what the cost breakdown is for an hour transport for that aircraft? Could I submit that to you, and you get that to me?

Mr. SHERLOCK. Yes. The transport is also based on the fact that our members, our programs, are ready to respond 24 hours a day 7 days a week.

Mr. LUJÁN. Well, whatever it may be—whatever it may be, Mr. Sherlock, I just want you to give me that breakdown, because in your testimony you argue that there has not been a study looking at the breakdown of costs.

I just would argue that when the median cost is $10,199, GAO says that the average charge is $36,000, in the State of New Mexico they say the average charge is almost $46,000, something is broken. There is something that's terribly off there.

But I want to go to someone else. I think we need to rein this in and the concern that I have in this area is that the Airline Deregulation Act of 1978 pre-empts states' ability to regulate air ambulance services. We need to do something about this, and I hope the Act that we have does.

My next question, though, is for Jeanette Thornton. Ms. Thornton, who gets to make decisions about medical necessity? Insurance companies or medical doctors? Who makes that decision?

Ms. THORNTON. Thanks for the question. It typically is a joint discussion between——

Mr. LUJÁN. Shouldn't my medical doctor make the decision about what's medically necessary for me when I am in a hospital room as opposed to some insurance company say, I am sorry, but your doctor didn't mean to fix our heart—we are not going to cover that cost—they should have only fixed your toe?

Ms. THORNTON. Sure. We want our members to have really high-quality care and a lot of times things like medical necessity and prior authorization are really getting at safety issues related— opioid prescriptions is a great example of that. And so, you know, we welcome that conversation.

Mr. LUJÁN. Madam Chair, as my time has expired, I would like to ask unanimous consent to submit into the record a few pieces of information, the first being a study by the New Mexico Super-intendent of Insurance on air ambulance information, and the second an article by Larry Barker, published February 21st, 2019, about medical emergency could end in bankruptcy, which also talks about medical necessity and who's making those decisions.

Ms. ESHOO. So ordered.

[The information appears at the conclusion of the hearing.] Mr. LUJÁN. Thank you.

Ms. ESHOO. The gentleman yields back.

I would like to recognize the gentleman from Florida, Mr. Bilirakis, for five minutes for his questions.

Mr. BILIRAKIS. Thank you. Thank you, Chairwoman. I appreciate it very much. Thanks for holding this hearing as well. Thanks to the ranking member.

Ms. Thornton, I believe it's safe to say that we would all like to see patients held harmless in any final proposal on surprise and balance billing.

A question—we have heard a lot about the merits of various proposals. Could you discuss the key differences between New York and California—their models?

Ms. THORNTON. Thank you. Happy to do so.

So the different proposals out there are really aligned based on either having a payment benchmark. So in one of these situations where someone does see an out-of-network provider in an emergency where they're at an in-network facility, there would be a quick and easy way to determine what payment should be for that out-of-network provider.

We want that to be fair and reasonable, based on what similar providers are paid in that geographic area. So that's sort of the benchmark approach and that's been implemented in California at the beginning of this year, as I mentioned.

The contrasting approach that's been mentioned on our panel is arbitration and this is where different parties come to the table if they disagree with the payment that was made and produce information as to why they should be paid a different amount, and that goes to an independent person.

Our concern with that—and this has been used in New York, as was mentioned—our concern with that is it gives equal weight to these excessive charges that have been talked about at the hearing today as well as information from the health plan and it adds unnecessary administrative costs to the system.

Mr. BILIRAKIS. OK. Thank you.

Dr. Zaafran, what could be the potential long-term consequences of reducing the number of physicians in network—if you could maybe describe what the consequences would be long term. I will give you some time to elaborate too because that's so important.

Dr. ZAAFRAN. Thank you. You know, access to care would be significantly affected. I mean, number one, first of all, when you're out of network, your cost sharing is much higher.

So even though my charge or rate may be the same, the patient's responsibility for a deductible and co-pay is much higher in an out-of-network setting versus an in-network setting. So that right away would put the patient at a disadvantage.

Again, there are costs to providing care, and if there is a race to the bottom, that access to care is going to be affected because if you have to have a physician open an office and be able to deliver that high-quality care that's going to be affected.

And, again, from the standpoint of not a one-size-fits-all thing that I really want to talk about—we talked about opioids a second ago—and other types of things that provide high-quality care, if a physician is providing that high-quality care it has to be—it has to be taken into consideration.

One thing that, like I said, we did in Texas, which I would call New York 2.0—New York's law was absolutely fantastic and we just tried to take it 1 step further, which, again, brought the health plans along and actually agreed to the bill, is that we wanted to reference previous history of in-network contracted rates in the arbitration criteria along with charges.

So the arbitrator would be able to look at a contract that may have just been terminated and said, well, you know, you just terminated a contract that was in existence for the last 10 years—at least give the contracted rate that was there for those last 10 years, and from that standpoint the score of the bill actually decreased significantly because what you're trying to do is preserve the 90 to 95 percent of the in-network market that already exists and not break that while at the same time addressing the 5 to 10 percent that is out of network and fix that and not have the unintended consequence of pushing those in-network providers into a situation where they're having to be paid less and not be able to deliver the kind of care that they expect to be able to deliver.

Mr. BILIRAKIS. Very good. Again, you touched on this, but have any states tried to create standards for network adequacy and track plan performance? If so, what has the result been for patients in those states?

Dr. ZAAFRAN. So, again, I referenced earlier the State of Texas has excellent network adequacy laws. We strengthened it in this last legislative session by changing it from a self-reporting mechanism to an automatic audit by the Texas Department of Insurance every 2 years to make sure that they are actually able to look at the networks.

I gave the example of a year ago where one particular carrier essentially took all the anaesthesia companies, and this is not 1 company. This is a variety of different companies—small groups, big groups—and put them out of network in existing contracts.

And if it wasn't for that network adequacy law where the Texas Department of Insurance Commissioner was able to hold that carrier accountable, the conversation between that carrier and the providers would have never happened because, essentially, they just refused to talk to the providers and say, you're out of network—that's it—end of story. The network adequacy law basically forced them to create an adequate network again and those conversations happened.

Mr. BILIRAKIS. Very good. OK. I yield back, Madam Chair. Thank you.

Ms. ESHOO. The gentleman yields back.

I now would like to recognize the gentleman from Oregon, Mr. Schrader, for his five minutes of questions.

Mr. SCHRADER. Thank you, Madam Chair.

Dr. Zaafran, curious about evidence with the frequency of surprise billing. I mean, is it a big chunk of the marketplace reimbursement or is it a small piece of the reimbursement puzzle, and does it—does it vary dramatically from network to network and does it vary geographically? We've heard some testimony.

Dr. ZAAFRAN. Thank you for that question and, you know, first of all, one out-of-network bill to Ms. Wilkes is one too many, and that's why we have to address that.

But the overall incidence of out-of-network providers is actually fairly low. It is in the 5 to 10 percent range. I think nationally, if you look at all the different services provided, it's 80 to 95 percent. So there's a little bit of variation there.

But, again, going back to the point of preserving the in-network providers or physicians that are already in network, we don't want a system that's going to disincentivize carriers or incentivize carriers not to continue those networks.

Again, we started to anecdotally see that happen in California. We've seen the exact opposite happen in New York where you had 20 percent of emergency rooms physicians out of network and it went down to 6.4 percent.

So the evidence that is out there shows that with a good arbitration style that is fair and expedited you actually can have the effect maintaining that in-network market but adjudicating out-of-network market in a fair manner.

Mr. SCHRADER. Mr. Nickels, would you agree with those comments in the relative states and the results we are seeing?

Mr. NICKELS. Absolutely, and I would throw Oregon into the mix, too, which, as you know, the law is new there and also, I think it's reflective of what New York set up, what Texas have. They're all a little different.

Ms. ESHOO. Could you bring your microphone closer?

Mr. NICKELS. Sorry. I keep doing that. So I think the arbitration model, again, the data coming out of New York is very persuasive that it works.

I don't think it's going to be the situation where there is some, like, really high amount and some reasonable amount, and to think that the really high amount is going to win, no arbiter is going to pick the really high amount.

The reason we have arbitration in New York that's successful is it brings people toward the middle. A lot of people settle them beforehand anyway. So I think those approaches are the best and I know our members were supportive of the Oregon law. I know its brand new. More data needs to be—you know, come—more data needs to come forward.

Mr. SCHRADER. Ms. Thornton, Dr. Zaafran talked about the incidence of surprise billing and certainly one is too much. I get that. But I want to get a feel from an economics standpoint, you know, what percentage of the insurance industry's healthcare business is resulting in paying these surprise billing.

Ms. THORNTON. Sure, not a problem.

And back to network adequacy, I just wanted to mention that Texas has one of the largest rates of surprise billing in the country, even though it has a robust network adequacy provision.

But back to the economic impact, I included some data in our testimony that was put together by Avalere as New Jersey was considering what changes to make as part of its changes to its out-of-network billing law and it really shows there is quite a large economic impact.

It could be as high as—and the study showed four percent of claims could be as a result of a benchmark that is based on billed charges and is a higher amount than some of the other proposals that are out there. So definitely hitting consumers in their pocketbook in terms of economic impact.

Mr. SCHRADER. So it seems to me like there's this dynamic tension between making sure that we have a robust provider network, the insurers are encouraged, frankly, to reach out to providers, and at the same time make sure that providers don't get to raise rates so that the consumers at the end of the day end up paying higher.

So there's going to be this dynamic tension because in the long run. The more robust provider network, in my opinion, market forces will driver those costs down. But we have got to make sure we don't injure the consumer here in the near term.

The other big piece that's out there is transparency. I mean, it'd be interesting to get real good data, and I would ask you, Ms. Thornton, to talk with your insurance plans and get back to me and the committee on what percentage of, you know, your business is surprise billing—you know, are there different subsets. Some people testified that there may be certain specialties that is occurs more frequently with—some testimony would indicate that while, no, it's all pretty equal. It would very helpful for the committee, I think, to get that information so we can get perspective on that.

My standpoint, I think the solution is pretty—a lot simpler than what we are making it out to be where you can encourage a robust network and make things happen.

Take the patient out. Everyone agrees with that. Ms. Wilkes shouldn't have to deal with these issues. This is an insurer, you know, provider issue and, you know, I think it you just have the insurers providing a little extra—making sure that they have a robust network we are not going to have this problem at the end of the day.

So appreciate everyone being here and I yield back.

Ms. ESHOO. The gentleman yields back.

I now would like to recognize the gentleman from Oklahoma, Mr. Mullin, for his five minutes of questioning.

Mr. MULLIN. Thank you, Madam Chair.

I want to talk a little bit more about—Ms. Thornton, about the surprise billing. Can we get a little bit more specific about what the surprise billing ratio is in rural parts of the country, specifically, maybe in Oklahoma?

And Ms. McAndrew, I saw you just kind of wiggle in your seat like you might have some of that information too. So I don't care which one wants to answer that.

Ms. MCANDREW. Thank you for the question.

Yes, over 10 percent of in-patient admissions in Oklahoma result in a surprise bill and that's the case too for other rural states represented on the committee like North Carolina, like Kentucky. And so I think it is important to recognize that already there are instances in rural states where we have out-of-network providers.

And I think, you know, we talked a little bit about how providers want to be in network. But there's not, you know, an equal incidence of surprise bills across——

Mr. MULLIN. What's the biggest issue with the out of network? I mean, we have seen this huge increase of out-of-network billing over the last years. One, what's caused that and what's the biggest issue on that?

Ms. MCANDREW. Well, I guess what I was going to say is that we have talked about how providers want to be in network, but I think for certain types of providers, people want to be in network but not as much as they want to get paid far more than——

Mr. MULLIN. Well, the point is people want to be in network only if the provider provides what I am asking for them to pay me back. And then they have another choice——

Ms. MCANDREW. Providers—certain providers want to be in network only if they can make very high rates.

Mr. MULLIN. Right, and then they have a choice, well, I don't have to be in network because I can still—I can still have access to the hospital. So why do we see that big increase now? Why are we seeing this big increase on surprise billing?

Ms. MCANDREW. So I would say that we haven't always had great data on surprise billing. So the data I have seen hasn't necessarily indicated an increase because the data we have on the surprise billing problem tends to be newer data in general.

And as I indicated, this is a problem that we have been working on for many years, and so it has been a long-standing problem.

Mr. MULLIN. Well, let's talk about the data. You were talking about one size doesn't fit all and Mr. Nickels, you're kind of echoing that, too.

I do agree with that to some degree. But I do also understand job costing and as small as my company is, I can still go back through it and find out what my average costs are on certain jobs, because some of them are repetitive.

Is that information not out there? I am not a big—I am not big into arbitration for sure but there should be a fair road someplace.

I think Ms. Thornton or, Mr. Nickels, you talked about in the middle with arbitration finding out where it is. Maybe that's the legislation that we are looking for that we can provide that data. If you can't provide the data, we can provide the data and say, I know what the average costs of a hip replacement is. I know what the average cost of getting two stents put in.

I understand there's special circumstances that take place. I understand what the average costs of delivering a child is. I've got five of them.

I can get those average costs, and is that the starting point of coming up to where the network and the provider should find? Somebody?

Mr. NICKELS. I will take a stab at that first. I think that there are some instances where getting the average cost is easier. Hip replacement—if there are no complications——

Mr. MULLIN. No, I get that. There're standard operations. There're nonstandard operations. There're standard jobs that my company does. There's standard jobs that they don't do. I get—I get the per hour costs and I also get the idea about bidding jobs.

Mr. NICKELS. Right.

Mr. MULLIN. And that is called flat pricing—up front pricing. You can't tell me we don't have an average cost of what it takes to do as many surgeries as we do inside this country on as many different parts of the body—you can't tell me we can't come up with an average cost on that.

Mr. NICKELS. Yes. In most instances, we can.

Mr. MULLIN. OK. Those are the most instances we are talking about. The special cases are special cases on themselves. We can solve the most cases, though.

For instance, this finger right here—not that I am doing anything bad—all fingers are up—it just happened to be this finger right here.

In Louisiana, I cut this finger. Eleven thousand dollars is what it cost me to get stitches put in that finger. This thumb right there, $150 at my local emergency room. Can somebody explain to me the differences in that? Both of them were, by the way, by a knife, which is why I don't carry one.

Dr. ZAAFRAN. Well, I can tell you that from the physician's standpoint—for emergency room physicians, for example, the average weighted cost of every visit is about $150. That's the average across the board for all services provided and as was indicated——

Mr. MULLIN. OK. There's our—then that's our starting point.

Dr. ZAAFRAN. So you had your——

Mr. MULLIN. So why is it that we can't find an average when we start negotiating prices?

Dr. ZAAFRAN. My point is, though, it is not—it's not as high as folks think it is.

Mr. MULLIN. Listen, your point I get. But the billing says it is. So your point—you can say whatever you want to about your point. The fact is the bills that come in our mailboxes say they are very expensive.

So I think it was Dr. Burgess that said if you don't fix it, we will, and you guys probably won't like it, and that's the road that we are going down because we can get access to that data. We can find that average cost. And if you all don't want to solve it then we are going to. All we are saying is is do it. Solve it.

With that, I yield back.

Ms. ESHOO. The gentleman yields back.

We have a vote that we need to go to the floor to take. But before we recess, I want to recognize the gentleman from California, Mr. Ca´rdenas, for his five minutes of questions.

Mr. CÁRDENAS. Thank you very much, Madam Chair, and I appreciate the witnesses sharing your perspectives and, Ms. Wilkes, your personal story. Thank you so much. I am glad to hear that your son got the critical need that he needed in that very moment.

I do have a question for you, Ms. Wilkes. When that provider group sent you that $50,000 bill, was it easy to understand what you were being charged for?

Ms. WILKES. No. As I mentioned earlier, it was just a dollar amount. There were no specifics as to what services were provided. Mr. CÁRDENAS.T1 OK. AND WHAT WAS THE PROCESS THAT YOU FELT WAS AVAILABLE TO YOU OR HOW DID YOU FIGURE OUT HOW TO DEAL WITH THAT AND WHAT OPTIONS YOU HAD?

Ms. WILKES. So we called the billing—the person that was giving us the bill—the entity that was giving us the bill, and they were not willing to work with us on a payment plan. It was—it was an all or nothing situation, and as we began asking questions that's how we found out that they were a third-party provider that was out of network in the facility that was in network.

So it really just was butting heads. We never could come to a solution to be able to even begin to think about paying that off.

Mr. CÁRDENAS.T1 OK. I Mean, I Have Grandchildren and I still have children on my plan at home, and I was thinking maybe we need to make t-shirts that we need to put on our loved ones whenever they go to the emergency room or to the doctor or what have you and it says "Only in-network provider! By the way, please don't let me die, happy face."

I am not trying to be funny. What I am saying is Americans should expect when they go see a provider, whether it's an emergency basis or not—I have a son who's on my plan and he went out of network. We knew it. I, as a policy maker, didn't know to ask more tertiary questions about how much each one would be.

Luckily for me, it was associated—in this case, I think it had to do with associated with a local university that one of my fine colleagues had been to, et cetera, and, you know, it was another $500 here, another $500 there. Thank God there were no more zeroes on that. My son had already met the deductible for the year.

So that was over and above what my plan had said, OK, you're doing with your deductible—every time you go in plan then you're going to be OK, family Ca´rdenas.

What bothers me, and you're hearing my colleagues, Republicans and Democrats, saying we need help to understand what's going on out there in the real world; otherwise, we are going to provide a solution and you're not going to like it.

Legislators, collectively, aren't necessarily known—our track record isn't that great of hitting the nail on the head when it comes to fixing big problems, unless we get tremendous help from experts so that we can hopefully narrow it down and actually make good policy solutions.

I have a question. My understanding is since the '80s—they may have called it something differently—since the '80s or so, there have been this surprise billing issue facing American families.

This isn't just five and ten years old. Is that correct? I think, Ms. McAndrew, can you shed some light on that?

Ms. MCANDREW. That is correct. Networks, from our perspective, are a necessary function because they are—they have an ability to rein in costs for consumers.

But, of course, if you have a network, which was part of the managed care revolution that we saw begin in the '80s and increase in the '90s, you can get either in-network care or you can get out-of-network care.

So if you end up inadvertently going to an out-of-network provider you will get a surprise bill. And I mentioned that this issue is something that our organization, Families USA, has been working on for over 20 years.

We've published on it in the early '90s. So this is absolutely not a new problem.

Mr. CÁRDENAS.T1 OK. SO THIS HAS BEEN DOING ON FOR DECADES?

Ms. MCANDREW. Absolutely.

Mr. CÁRDENAS.T1 AND HAS ANYBODY HERE BEEN AT THE TABLE BEFORE CONGRESS TO TALK SPECIFICALLY ABOUT THIS ISSUE OVER THE LAST, YOU KNOW, 40 OR 50 YEARS? OH, YOU HAVE, DR. ZAAFRAN?

Dr. ZAAFRAN. Well, not for 50 years. But since 2009 actually we have been addressing it in Texas and it's been a progression. Of course, we addressed it in New York. But——

Mr. CÁRDENAS.T1 SO AT THE STATE LEVEL. BUT AT THE FEDERAL LEVEL?

Dr. ZAAFRAN. Not at the Federal level. Correct. Well, there's the greater of three standards that the Federal level has—actually had and has been in place since then and it's probably——

Mr. CÁRDENAS.T1 SINCE WHEN? SINCE, ROUGHLY, WHEN? DECADES?

Dr. ZAAFRAN. It has been—it has been at least a decade. Mr. CA´RDENAS.T1 OK. GOT IT.

Dr. ZAAFRAN. I wouldn't say decades. But at least about a decade.

Mr. CÁRDENAS.T1 OK. RIGHT. OK.

The reason why I want to point that out is because I hope that the dialogue doesn't get mired into, you know, what caused this. It's been going on long enough.

We got to figure out how to remedy it, and I think that if we keep clear heads and we are able to focus on the common denominator—to me, the common denominator is the patient. That's the common denominator, and then try to figure out how do systems fulfil their obligation to stay afloat and provide services out there in the communities.

I am sorry I overstepped my time. Sorry about that, Madam Chair. I yield back.

Ms. ESHOO. Always nice to listen to you, Mr. Cárdenas. You're wonderful.

The gentleman——

Mr. BURGESS. Reserving the right to object. Ms. ESHOO. Now—the gentleman yields back.

We have a vote on the floor, and I don't know if there will be any subsequent votes to the one that's on the floor. If there aren't, I think that we all have a 20-minute break at least and I hope we can just—that that's what the case will be. So we'll recess now. We'll go to the floor, take our vote, hoping, again, that it is one— to return. And but if it is longer you just have to be flexible. I ask you to be flexible. So the subcommittee will recess.

[Recess.]

Ms. ESHOO. All right. The subcommittee will come back to order. I would like to—the chair would like to now recognize the gentleman from California, Dr. Ruiz, for his five minutes of testimony, and one of our members that has worked very hard to come up with a solution to what we are grappling with.

It's so ludicrous that this could ever be called balanced. It's not balanced. It's totally out of whack billing. But I want to attach that compliment to Dr. Ruiz's name because he's worked very hard since the beginning of this year on the subject matter.

You're recognized for five minutes of questioning.

Mr. RUIZ. Thank you, Madam Chair.

And the reason why I worked so hard is because, as a physician, we try to eliminate the pain and suffering and anxiety from our patients, and then you find out that the patients are getting a surprise bill that is adding to the anxiety, which only makes their health worse. It only makes their health worse.

In addition to being concerned, as Ms. Wilkes was about her son, she was also concerned to tears in the anxiety of going bankrupt or what do you do and how do you cut costs. That's an outrage. It's unconscionable that families are going through what they're going through, and that's the number 1, 2, and 3 reasons why I set out to find this solution.

We have to close every loophole imaginable so that patients are not stuck in the middle of this dispute—so that patients don't have to decide between, you know, staying in their house, renting an apartment, paying their bills, versus paying their medical bills because of a life-threatening situation for their child.

We need to keep patients out of the middle and, quite honestly, those State models, even with arbitration, don't do enough. There's always a fine print.

There's always a window that a patient has to go through to mail an envelope back or make a call and if they don't—if they don't understand and they're the ones that are not going to have those protections.

And I am concerned with this current bill that there are—like you, Ms. McAndrew, that there are too many loopholes that still allow providers to find a way to say, no, it is your fault—you didn't see the sign, or it is your fault—you didn't make the effort to look at the online list, or it is your fault because you weren't aware that this hospital or these providers were out of network.

In fact, asking an emergency department patient or an in-hospital patient if they consent to be seen by the on-call physician, if they are out of network doesn't work in the real world and it takes somebody who cares for patients who actually has cared for patients to understand that because those patients will most always choose yes because they're under duress or because their care will be delayed or because they will not understand the implications.

And if they consent to yes in this bill, then yes, I will be seen by the anesthesiologist because I've been in the hospital too long, then that allows the physician to balance bill. It's not good for patients.

And to expect that a physician who's on call that night, who doesn't deal with their bills or doesn't deal with being in-network or out-of-network that's a department—billing department issue and they've got 15 different people—to expect them to then just say, no, let me check right now to see if you're in network or out of network or if I am in network or out of network is not based in reality or in the real world.

So creating a loophole where, quote, "adequate information was provided," right, that somebody would say that gives a way to balance bill. It will put the responsibility on the patient to read the fine print or be aware of all the ways the providers can say they were made aware beforehand and it was patient's fault they didn't read it or understand it, and that needs to end.

In the bill that I propose, Protecting People from Surprise Billing Act, has the most robust patient protections out there from any State model or any proposed bill, because that is my number one, number 2, and number 3 priority as someone who cares deeply, who has devoted my entire life during the arduous training to become a physician, to do everything possible to relieve pain and suffering and promote wellness in everyday Americans.

So the second part is how are we going to solve this dispute, and we need to understand that we need to pick a system that is fair— that we are not picking winners or losers—that we address the underlying problem.

The concern is cost. So, Dr. Zaafran, talk about cost—inflationary rates. What does the evidence show in terms of the models that are out there?

Dr. ZAAFRAN. Thank you, Dr. Ruiz, and thank you again for the effort that you have put into the bill that is out there.

Well, again, if you look at the data that is out there on New York, which has been out there for many, many years, the inflationary costs with that dispute resolution process has simply not been any different than the inflationary cost data in California. I believe the number is somewhere along the lines of 6 to 7 percent, not 67—6 to 7 percent and it has been the same whether you have a benchmark process in California——

Mr. RUIZ. So you're saying that there is absolute data showing that an arbitration does not increase inflationary costs? Because otherwise—if the data were otherwise——

Ms. ESHOO. The gentleman's—excuse me. Excuse me. The gentleman's time has expired.

Mr. RUIZ. Thank you so much for your patience.

Ms. ESHOO. Yes. Thank you.

Now I would like to recognize the gentlewoman from Indiana, Mrs. Brooks, for her five minutes of questioning.

Mrs. BROOKS. Thank you, Madam Chairwoman. I apologize. I've been going back and forth to other things as well, and at this point I yield my time to Dr. Burgess, the ranking member.

Mr. BURGESS. Thank you. We are so glad you came back.

Ms. Wilkes, I would just like to ask you, if I could, there has been State legislation passed in Colorado, correct, dealing with this? How would that have impacted your situation when your son was born?

Ms. WILKES. Thank you. I actually am not aware if there has been legislation passed in Colorado, to be perfectly honest. But depending on what this legislation said, it maybe would have prevented us from having the bad credit rating that we had.

Quite frankly, it is not just surprise billing in my family's case. It's billing overall. I mean, high cost dollars—we have gone to arbitration several times to deal with debt to the hospital. So it is not just this.

Mr. BURGESS. Because of that initial episode or subsequent?

Ms. WILKES. It's a chronic disorder. I mean, you know, we are not going to get rid of it. So there's going to be cost. He's about a million dollar a year kid.

Mr. BURGESS. Which is why the hope for the gene therapy is— and when we talk about how do we price that it does have to be in the context of what is it costing us to do nothing and, clearly, in your case the cost is almost intolerable.

Dr. Zaafran, you were answering a question from Dr. Ruiz a minute ago and the clock ran out on you. While I am very sensitive to that because it runs out on me all the time, but you want to continue your discussion just a little bit?

Dr. ZAAFRAN. Yes. Thank you, Dr. Burgess.

No, I was just reiterating that in New York, where they have had a New York arbitration process and dispute resolution process that is robust and expedited that there has not been any difference in the inflationary costs as compared to other states.

It hasn't increased. It hasn't been any different than it has been before and it has resulted in a decrease in the out-of-network providers.

Mr. BURGESS. Mr. Gelfand, you kind of indicated that that was not an acceptable solution from your perspective—that data that now Dr. Zaafran has shared with us. Does that—is that good news from your perspective or news that is not—doesn't necessarily move the needle one way or the other?

Mr. GELFAND. Dr. Burgess, many of the comments that you have heard today are without context of what the markets looked like before these State proposals were brought forward.

So specifically in Texas and New York the question is could things have possibly gotten any worse. When we look at arbitration models, we know that outside counsel charges us $500 an hour on a good day and we know that the filing fees for many of these arbitration groups are $1,500 per party per claim, right. So we beg you spend healthcare dollars on healthcare, not on attorneys.

Mr. BURGESS. Can I just ask you about that? Because now, I've been told from my counterparts in the State House that the fact that arbitration is available means the parties move to an agreement before, prior to getting to that arbitration phase. Just the fact that it is out there means that they are going to talk. Is that something that you have seen?

Mr. GELFAND. Dr. Burgess, we would defer to the Congressional Budget Office that has looked at several proposals and said that if you change to an arbitration model it increases costs by $5 billion. That money will be paid by patients.

Mr. BURGESS. The Congressional Budget Office isn't always high on my list of my favorite people.

But, Dr. Zaafran, can you comment on that? And Dr. Friedman, I would like you to comment as well.

Dr. ZAAFRAN. Dr. Burgess, the cost of arbitration in New York is $300 for arbitration and it is split evenly between the insurer and the physician so—and it is a 2-week process. That is all entered electronically and it is adjudicated right away.

So this cost of arbitration being excessive, again, the data in New York and the way it is going to be in Texas it is a very low cost. It's split between the insurer and the provider with very specific guardrails.

And, again, in Texas what we did is we referenced the previous contracted rates, which is basically saying that you don't have to have just charges out there.

There's a teleconference that happens before arbitration that allows for both sides to sit down at the table and try to come up with a fair payment that they both agree on.

If they don't, that final offer is what goes to arbitration. That final offer could be your previous contracted rate before the insurance company dropped you out of a contract.

And so that allowed in Texas the fiscal note, the score, to come down significantly.

Mr. BURGESS. I see.

And Dr. Friedman, do you have a thought on that?

Dr. FRIEDMAN. Yes. I just want to point out that in New York in seven million emergency department visits in the year 849 cases went to this dispute resolution process, which is about .01 percent. So the process in New York, at least, has worked in that people are—the parties are resolving their dispute before they even utilize the dispute resolution process.

Mr. BURGESS. All right. Thank you. I yield back.

Ms. ESHOO. The gentleman yields back.

Now I would like to recognize the gentleman from Vermont, Mr. Welch, for his five minutes.

Mr. WELCH. Thank you, Madam Chair. Vermont does have a law. Since 1987 it has banned balance billing in the emergency department settings only. And while that addresses a major issue it still had a number of holes. It doesn't do anything to prevent surprise bills from anesthesiologists, pathologists, or radiologists.

It doesn't protect Vermonters who seek care in other states, and many of our Vermonters get care at Dartmouth Hitchcock right across the Connecticut River, which is in New Hampshire.

And finally, the bill doesn't set a rate of reimbursement. I want to ask a few questions, but first this whole surprise billing situation—I think of Dr. Bucshon—is reflective of how it is so opaque what the billing mechanisms are in the healthcare industry, and consumers have no power.

And what it feels like on the outside is that all of the providers who are seeking to get reimbursement of the maximum rate and make their claim as to why they need that, the lack of transparency in fact works to their advantage, and this is just one manifestation of it.

And the challenge for consumers they are totally powerless—totally powerless. So the question I have fundamentally is should the burden to bear the cost of this lack of transparency and opaque billing system be on the consumer, who shows up sick and powerless to affect anything, or should it be on, collectively, the delivery system?

And that would take a lot of cooperation and probably a lot of legislation. But I don't believe it should fairly fall on the shoulders of a consumer who shows up and is absolutely powerless and had nothing to do with creating the mess in the first place.

So just a few questions. I will start with you, Mr. Nickels. How do you see the proposed legislation—the Pallone-Walden bill—affecting our situation in Vermont?

Mr. NICKELS. Well, I think it would actually address one of the problems that you currently have in Vermont. It does address, of course, the emergency situation, which you have protection for.

That bill also reaches into situations where a consumer goes into a facility that's in-network and they knew it was in-network and they did it all in good faith and they got a bill from an out-of-network physician.

That situation which, apparently, is not taken care of in your State law, would be taken care of by the Pallone bill.

Mr. WELCH. OK.

Mr. NICKELS. That would be an improvement. Now, we have some concerns about the Pallone-Walden bill but on that case it would be better for consumers than what you have in Vermont.

Mr. WELCH. OK.

Ms. McAndrew, what about the situation for Vermonters who get their care across the river in New Hampshire? And that's about 40 percent of people in the region of Vermont that I live in.

Ms. MCANDREW. Thank you for that question. One of the reasons we think a Federal solution is ideal is that we believe wherever you live, wherever you receive care, you should be fully protected. We shouldn't be relying on a patchwork state-by-state system for protection.

Mr. WELCH. OK. And while consumers are seeking specialized care, they're bombarded with an enormous amount of information dealing with being sick or injured, and how do we ensure that patients are informed in a clear and meaningful way but one that doesn't put an undue burden on providers? Do you have any thoughts on that, Ms. McAndrew?

Ms. MCANDREW. Yes. Well, I think one of the ways the legislation recognizes that consumers shouldn't be bearing this burden is that in facility-based provider situations the legislation actually doesn't rely on notice requirements. If you are getting care from a facility-based provider like an anesthesiologist or emergency provider, my understanding in the legislation that the protection actually is automatic.

Mr. WELCH. OK. Thank you.

Ms. MCANDREW. The 24-hour notice requirements, as I understand them, although I do believe longer notice should be required, are applying in nonemergency situations or nonfacility-based providers.

Mr. WELCH. Thank you.

Ms. MCANDREW. But I think that can be done to make it even more automatic, so we are getting rid of any phone calls, any emails, any going back and forth between insurers and providers is the ideal solution.

Mr. WELCH. Thank you for that. I want to yield my last minute to Dr. Ruiz, who's been a leader on this for us.

Thank you.

Mr. RUIZ. I appreciate it. Oftentimes, during negotiations insurance companies have a take-it-or-leave-it approach with no communication in any of—and no negotiation.

Why, Dr. Zaafran—what makes baseball-style arbitration so appealing to states that want to impact a fair system?

Dr. ZAAFRAN. Thank you, Dr. Ruiz. Because in that baseball-style arbitration where you have a final offer you have some specific guardrails or specific criteria that the arbitrator is referencing, which is acuity, complexity, quality, previous contract rates, et cetera.

But the key thing is that you have got two numbers. Those two numbers are one—you only have to choose one of them. You're not trying to pick a number somewhere in between, and it forces both sides to be fair.

Mr. RUIZ. Another question, Dr. Friedman. When New York implemented their solution, many feared that it would allow providers to drive up prices exponentially. Has that been the case?

Dr. FRIEDMAN. No, it has not. What we have seen in New York is that providers are charging reasonable rates when they go to arbitration or they go to negotiation and insurers in fact are paying at reasonable rates when those bills come in, for the most part.

What's happened is, is that it has taken care of outliers—the extraordinary cases that where people—and there are folks on both sides abusing the system. It has taken care of those.

Ms. ESHOO. The gentleman's time has expired.

The gentleman from Virginia, Mr. Griffith, is recognized for five minutes for his questions.

Mr. GRIFFITH. Thank you very much, Madam Chair, and I apologize to the members of the committee. I've been bouncing between this one and the others.

You have heard several other people say, and the other one is now over—but I did want to ask some questions and I have—during the time I have been in the room I have learned a tremendous amount. Appreciate you all being here.

Mr. Sherlock, I want to ask you some questions about air transport, and it comes up and I don't know whether the person that told me this is accurate or not, but I had a child in my district recently that was hit and I know that they were airlifted to a hospital.

About a week later, a constituent comes in with a whole laundry list of things and one of them was he says the family was charged $40,000. So that's where I start my questions with that just as a backdrop.

But you opened your written testimony by referencing the Association of Air Medical Services support for the Air Ambulance Patient Billing Advisory Committee in the 2018 FAA reauthorization.

Now, we don't have jurisdiction over that. But that means that a lot of our members of this committee may be less familiar with how that consensus language became law.

Can you share with us the background of what led to the establishment of the advisory committee and while you're at it also tell us has it actually been established—because sometimes we put it into law and it doesn't happen—and have they started meeting?

Mr. SHERLOCK. Thank you for the questions.

First, the Air Ambulance Patient Advisory Committee was put into effect because there are—currently the Department of Transportation has a consumer protection division that has the ability to investigate and look at how charges were determined and hold patients harmless.

We agree with Ms. Wilkes that the medical needs of a patient should be first and no patient should be in the middle of a discussion between payers and providers.

That committee also includes a representative of Health and Human Services and so it is a joint committee. We would encourage Congress to urge them to get that committee seated and started. They have a requirement to investigate and recommend solutions to hold patients harmless as well as to look at the economics of the ambulance industry, and we think Congress would be well served by that.

We also don't believe that—our industry doesn't believe that any patient should be caught in the middle. We have supported legislation that would increase 100 percent transparency of the industry by mandating 100 percent industry reporting of comprehensive cost data that would then be turned over to the Centers for Medicare and Medicaid, which would then be used and analyzed to actually rebase the Medicare rates for air ambulances at the cost of providing the services.

That Medicare gap is the single largest driver in raising costs in the air ambulance industry and in balance bills. When you get those comprehensive data reported and they get analyzed and they become public data, then everybody will see where everybody falls out on the cost curve, and in addition to that quality of care where everybody will see where programs fall out on the quality of care curve.

So when those become public data, that will increase both the transparency and the accountability of the industry, and we support—we support that legislation that was introduced and sponsored by Mr. Ruiz and Mr. Johnson and actually cosponsored by Chairwoman Eshoo in the previous Congress.

Mr. GRIFFITH. And my understanding is currently the Medicare and Medicare reimbursement is somewhere between $3,000 and $6,000 but the average for somebody that's paying without that coverage is about $26,000. Is that accurate?

Mr. SHERLOCK. The median cost of a helicopter air transport is $10,199 according to a study conducted in 2017. If you look at the cost of uncompensated care because Medicare pays less than $0.60 on the dollar of that $10,199—about $5,998. Medicaid pays significantly less than that, less than $3,500 on average, and the uninsured pay about $350. Those make up—those three groups make up 70 percent of air medical transports.

So when you take that cost of uncompensated care and you add it to the median cost of $10,200, that's the average charge of $36,000 that the—that the representative from New Mexico referenced earlier.

When you—when those kinds of situations happen, no one in our industry wants to see a patient or their family placed in jeopardy because they've just had a health emergency.

Our members will sit down with each individual and their families and work out a solution tailored for them, and a comment that was made earlier today about a snake bite victim that was transported across State lines, in fact, that was resolved and that patient and their family received no balance billing in that because our programs will work with each patient to develop a solution tailored for them.

Mr. GRIFFITH. All right. I appreciate it and I yield back.

Ms. ESHOO. The gentleman yields back.

Now I would like to recognize the gentlewoman from Delaware, Ms. Blunt Rochester, five minutes of questioning.

Ms. BLUNT ROCHESTER. Thank you. Thank you, Madam Chairwoman.

And I think you have coined a new term—shock billing. I wrote that one down. I want to also thank the witnesses especially for your flexibility and your patience with all that we have—many of us have been through today. But thank you for your time.

Investigative reporting by journalists like Sarah Kliff for Vox and Kaiser Health News and NPR's Bill of the Month series have really shed a light on how patients, often at their sickest and most vulnerable, get stuck in the middle of payment disputes between providers and insurers.

We've heard countless times today that patients shouldn't serve as an intermediary between these two entities.

Holding the patients harmless should be the crux of any legislative solution that Congress puts forward, and I was really encouraged today by the discussion, the fact that there seems to be bipartisan and across the panel support that something needs to be done and it needs to be done now, and this No Surprises Act also maintains that standard.

In a May 2018 article by Sarah Kliff, a 34-year-old man received a surprise $7,924 medical bill from an emergency oral procedure after a violent attack the night before. Kliff noted that this bill was a case she saw regularly—patients who had large medical bills because they went to an in-network hospital but were seen by out-of-network doctors.

The good news is that the entire bill was reversed. The bad news is that it was after the news article.

So, Ms. McAndrew, I am sure I know the answer to this question, but should patients have to rely on news coverage of their surprise medical bill in order for them to negotiate a lower bill?

Ms. MCANDREW. Thank you very much for that question and, of course, the answer is absolutely not, and we, you know, indicated in our testimony that this problem has been going on for a very long time.

But, unfortunately, before consumers had advocates like reporters or their members of Congress to reach out to, a lot of consumers don't know to take that recourse or are too sick to take that line of recourse and are sometimes paying these bills, going into bankruptcy, going into debt.

And so there should be policy in place that automatically protects consumers, so they don't have to take these great lengths to get protection.

Ms. BLUNT ROCHESTER. Thank you.

I've also heard stories from emergency care physicians in my State where patients delay their care because of their concerns about surprise medical bills.

Ms. McAndrew or any other member of the panel, have you seen this where people are afraid to get care because they're afraid that they might be—receive a shock bill?

Ms. WILKES. I would like to respond to that because it just happened within the last couple of months for my family.

Thomas fell at school and broke his arm, and I legitimately did not know where to go. I didn't know whether to go to the urgent care or to the ER.

So, ultimately, we went to urgent care, got an x-ray. Sure enough, the arm was broken, and ended up in the ER because of his chronic illness.

That delayed his care. He was in pain for a number of hours while we were making that transfer.

Ms. BLUNT ROCHESTER. Thank you.

I want to transition to the question of transparency. Even when patients are diligent about making sure that they're receiving in-network care they can still end up with a surprise medical bill.

Often, this is because they're unable to ultimately know if every physician involved in their episode of care is in-network, and I am going to ask—direct this to Dr. Zaafran.

How can we increase transparency for consumers and make sure that they're able to easily find out what providers are in-network?

Dr. ZAAFRAN. Thank you.

So the short answer to that is that the insurance industry has to have directories that are updated in a real-time fashion. Again, there is no such thing as an out-of-network provider. There is a provider who may happen to be out of network with that specific product.

So the only one who knows what that product is is, of course, the patient and the insurance carrier and they're the only ones who really have the information as to whether they're in network or out of network.

Ms. BLUNT ROCHESTER. I just want to close by saying I commend the committee and everybody who are involved with this. I recall when my husband passed away unexpectedly to receive bills not when I was living in Delaware. You're already going through a tough time, and then to be surprised with these kind of unexpected costs are unacceptable, and I am glad to see in this committee that we are looking at this, we are taking leadership and that there is a sense of urgency because people are counting on us.

Thank you, and I yield back.

Ms. ESHOO. The gentlewoman yields back.

I now would like to recognize the gentleman from Georgia, Mr. Carter.

Mr. CARTER. Thank you, Madam Chair, and thank all of you for being here. I know it has been a long day. So you're almost home. Just hang in there.

You know, this is a very complex issue. We all understand that. But it is a very important issue, and Ms. Wilkes, I want to thank you for being here today and for your testimony. It's certainly compelling and certainly something we have to work with.

Full disclosure—currently, I am the only pharmacist serving in Congress and I have experienced the wrath, if you will, of the insurance companies.

At the same time, I understand where they're coming from, too, and that's what makes it such a complex issue. One of the things that we deal with, and Dr. Zaafran and Dr. Friedman, I will tell you that we use the old adage that misery loves company. I am in misery with you.

So, you know, it is tough. I deal with PBMs and, oh by the way, what we have in common with PBMs is that they're owned by the insurance companies.

So, nevertheless, one of the things that we have in pharmacy, though, is, you know, we have any willing provider and that is if we're—you know, quite often we are shut out. Patients don't have a choice. If they come to me and I am out of network or I am not a member of that network, they can't get their prescription filled under their insurance. They'd have to pay for it out of pocket. But some states have laws that say if you're willing to accept what the insurance company is willing to pay, then you can participate.

Well, the insurance companies don't want to do that because then they can't go out and build networks, is what they're telling me, because if anybody's going to accept it then the companies— the pharmacies that are agreeing to be in that network and bidding to be in that network—aren't going to get the volume that they are anticipating.

It seems to me like this is just the opposite of what the economics are on why you would not want to be a part of that. Can you help me out, Dr. Zaafran, as far as the economics of how that works when you have—when you have the insurance company paying you out of network like that?

Dr. ZAAFRAN. So what I would first say is, again, in our organization, Physicians for Fair Coverage, 90 to 95 percent of us are in network.

We want to be in network. We strive to be in network. We negotiate with insurance companies to be in network. In many instances the times we are out of network is when it is a patient coming from another State or, in some instances, we are in network with everybody but there may be one specific plan or one carrier that is not really negotiating with us in good faith.

Typically, most of them are and we are in network with all of them. It is in our interest to be in network. The volume, the cost of providing that service, the cost of billing, the timeliness of payment from the insurance carrier—these are all factors that actually strive to make all of us as physicians want to be in network because it is so much easier.

Mr. CARTER. OK.

Well, let me ask you, Dr. Friedman, and by the way, yours is somewhat of an unusual circumstance. Yours is kind of an outlier, if you will, because, as you say, you're in Orlando and you got a lot of people coming but, even more so, why we should be addressing it. Can you speak to the economics of it?

Dr. FRIEDMAN. Well, I think for all emergency providers, whether you work in Orlando where I work or anywhere else in the country, we want, as Dr. Zaafran has mentioned and I have as well, we want to be in network. It is—we want to take care of patients.

I became an emergency physician to take care of patients. I didn't take care of—go to medical school to do billing. I, frankly, didn't think I would ever be in Congress talking about anything like this. We want to take care of the patients and——

Mr. CARTER. Right.

Dr. FRIEDMAN [continuing]. We want the—we would like the back end, the business side, to take care of it as well. In emergency medicine, we have a unique circumstance in that I can't tell the patient what the cost is going to be.

I don't even know if they have insurance when I take care of them. So everything happens afterwards. I can't identify the insurance product.

Sometimes my billing company doesn't know if they're out of network for a couple of weeks because it is so difficult. I have a United Healthcare card. Nothing against United Healthcare, but all it says on there is what my co-pay is. That's it.

Mr. CARTER. Right. Right. And, oh by the way, United Healthcare owns their own PBM and they also own their own mail order pharmacy.

Dr. FRIEDMAN. Right. But I don't know where I am in network with that card.

Mr. CARTER. Right.

Dr. FRIEDMAN. And, you know, if I am in DC. if I try to find a doctor——

Mr. CARTER. Sure.

Dr. FRIEDMAN [continuing]. I have no idea.

Mr. CARTER. Well, and thank you for that. Now, before—my time is about up, but Mr. Nickels, I have to tell you, out of all due respect, sir, the chairlady asked you a question at the first of this hearing that I thought you tried to dodge; and I will tell you that whereas I respect the Hospital Association I do think you have more of a responsibility to be a mediator, if you will, between the insurance companies and the providing physicians to try to help them to avoid the surprise billing that we are seeing.

So I think that is a responsibility that I hope that you will take—that you all take seriously, and I hope that we can count on you to do just that.

Mr. NICKELS. Definitely. I know the time has expired but I totally agree with that. We do our best to work the insurers and the physicians——

Mr. CARTER. Well, as I say, I thought you avoided her question. But nevertheless——

Mr. NICKELS. Well, I could—I could try——

Mr. CARTER [continue]. And the last thing is one thing about the Pallone bill that I do like is that they would let states decide, because we do know that there are states where it's working what they're trying to do. I hear New York is working with arbitration, and I hope that we don't precede that with any legislation that we pass.

And I yield back.

Ms. ESHOO. I thank the gentleman and he yields back.

I just would like to add something to Mr. Nickels. This business of anti-trust and what the hospital association keeps referring to it, I think that when you answer members' written questions that you take another look at this.

I don't understand how anti-trust can be thrown around in this. But maybe it's because I don't know enough about it.

Mr. NICKELS. Be glad to answer that.

Ms. ESHOO. We have—thank you.

Mr. NICKELS. I would be glad to answer it. Thank you.

Ms. ESHOO. Is Mr. Sarbanes still here? No? He left? Anyone else?

Mr. BURGESS. Why don't we let Mr. Nickels—are you willing to speak to that now—the anti-trust issue?

Ms. ESHOO. If he can in a succinct way.

Mr. NICKELS. I will do my best. The anti-trust concerns we raised goes along with so-called network matching where requirements which is not in the Pallone-Walden bill but I wanted to mention it because it's in other bills—where there's an attempt to put a requirement on hospitals to get—to make the doctors be in network with them, with us, and we believe that that would raise—I think a physician would be forced to adhere to a third party contract. Could very easily come after us on anti-trust grounds. We are more than willing to work with them to——

Ms. ESHOO. I don't get that. I don't get that. I mean, I chaired a hospital board of directors. We had—it was our own county hospital. It was a public hospital. We had docs from the community that worked there and the contract that we had was for the ER and those docs. And so I don't know what you mean by you can't do this, you can't do that. You already have all these different groups that you contract with.

Mr. NICKELS. Right.

Ms. ESHOO. I mean, the out-of-network starts when they're in your network.

Mr. NICKELS. If we employ the docs then that's not a problem. There is no anti-trust concern of any kind. The concern is, and again——

Ms. ESHOO. What's the difference between employee and contract?

Mr. NICKELS. Well, if it's contracted then if they work for us one of the things we do is if we are in a network, you're in a network. That's required. The issue is we can persuade. We can try to work with the physicians to get them to do what I just described. But the issue that concerns us is what if we try to——

Ms. ESHOO. When was the last time you tried really hard and it failed?

Mr. NICKELS. Say that again. I am sorry.

Ms. ESHOO. When was the last time you tried really hard and it failed?

Mr. NICKELS. I could get you examples of people—my members who have tried to do that. Again, my view is—our view is we want those docs——

Ms. ESHOO. And then was there—were there—was there the threat of anti-trust as a result of trying to work it out?

Mr. NICKELS. There have been—I can give you examples where there has been threatened litigation if you tried to do that. I can also give you examples of where it worked—where we were able to persuade the doctors——

Ms. ESHOO. All right. Well, I am going to have several questions for you. I appreciate it, and now I would like to recognize the gentleman from Maryland, Mr. Sarbanes, for his five minutes of questioning.

Mr. SARBANES. Thank you very much, Madam Chair. Thank you all for being here much of the day.

Your perspectives, obviously, on this issue are very valuable. You have got a lot of expertise you have brought to bear with respect to this issue of surprise billing, and it's incredible, I guess, but not totally surprising that it's affecting as many as 1 in 7 patients in America. We all hear stories from family members and friends of this kind of gotcha moment that they face.

And the thing is even when patients are trying to anticipate a situation and do their homework to make sure they're getting the services in network and so forth, they can still get caught short and be surprised with medical bills and, you know, these can total tens of thousands of dollars and it can wipe somebody out, again, even though they're taking every precaution that they can—they can manage to do.

And as we heard from Ms. Wilkes, the impact of those bills, the examples of how devastating it can be to patients and their families is very sobering.

I am glad we are here talking about different kinds of responses to this problem and solutions. I am sort to attracted to the No Surprises Act right now because I think it achieves that balance in a way that works best for patients, which is the perspective I am bringing to bear for the most part here, and it would take them out of the middle of these out-of-network payment processes, set that benchmark rate for out-of-network payments, as you know, to resolve payment disputes between providers and insurers.

Maryland, the State I represent, has chosen to address the surprise billing through this benchmark approach and in 2011 implemented that system which requires out-of-network bills to be sent to insurers and not to patients and define a formula that could be used for those out-of-network payments.

The goal was to reduce patients' financial burden while still paying providers at an adequate rate and maintaining network adequacy.

To monitor the success of the benchmark plan, the Maryland Health Care Commission was looking at out-of-pocket costs, reimbursement rates before and after the implementation of the law to see what the effect would be.

Ms. McAndrew, would you agree that the rates agreed to between providers and insurers for medical services are in fact a consumer issue and would setting a benchmark rate for out-of-pocket costs go a good way towards protecting patients from unexpected and exorbitant medical bills?

Ms. MCANDREW. Thank you very much for question. We absolutely do believe the rate between insurers and providers is a consumer issue. Consumers, of course, ultimately do bear the costs of healthcare and they bear them both out of pocket, which has been the crux of our discussion today, but they also bear them in their premiums.

And so if the legislation to affect surprise bills ultimately inflates healthcare costs in the system, that will affect consumers' premiums.

And so we do prefer a benchmark methodology. We believe that is what will ultimately lower costs the most for consumers. Other methods can be better than the status quo but they can have less of an effect on lowering costs for consumers, and costs are rising and rising. We see that voters care about that more than anything else about healthcare, and so it's important to us as patient advocates.

Mr. SARBANES. Well, that's certainly my perspective. As a matter of fact, the Maryland Health Care Commission from its study found that in three years after implementation of the benchmark system the total amount of out-of-network payments decreased from 20 percent to 11 percent, and those patients that had still had out-of-network charges saw their total spending decrease as well. So I think it shows the benefits of that.

Some groups have expressed concerns that setting a benchmark rate could lead to providers leaving networks and the networks shrinking over time. Have you seen evidence of like a dramatic negative effect that way or not really?

Ms. MCANDREW. We have absolutely not seen evidence that benchmark rates will cause problems in networks. Our colleagues in California who have worked very deeply on the implementation of this law have not reported any such effects.

I would caution making any conclusions about the California law since it's so early. But I think you have also presented very strong evidence from the State of Maryland, and I would also, you know, acknowledge that the reason this law is being implemented is because right now people can make very large amounts of money by going out of network through balance billing. And so once that's no longer possible that is a very big deterrent for remaining out of network. And so I think that will have a very positive effect on networks.

Mr. SARBANES. Well, I appreciate that and what you just said certainly aligns well with the experience in Maryland because, again, from the study that was done and the monitoring the Maryland Health Care Commission found that although out-of-network payments decreased, as you would expect, in the three years after a benchmark was set, overall provider participation in those networks did now show a decline. So I think there's a lot of promise there in terms of the response we need to see to this surprise billing issue.

With that, I yield back my time. I thank the panel.

Ms. ESHOO. The gentleman yields back, and I think that is it. I don't see any other members on either side.

On behalf of all the members of the subcommittee, I want to thank the witnesses. You have been patient. You have been here since before 10:00. It is now—well, you have been here for four hours, and we are very grateful to you.

You have had to field some tough questions but that makes for a good hearing. None of it is personal and we have to—I always first try to remind myself that there has to be a great deal of friction wave action to—for the sand in the shell to produce a pearl.

Now, the pearl we are looking for is good solid legislation for consumers in the country. So that friction in terms of tough questions and testing each case the best we know how, the best we can, is to benefit the American people. So we all thank you.

I want to remind members, whoever is left in the room, that pursuant to committee rules they have 10 business days to submit additional questions for the record to be answered by the witnesses who have appeared.

I ask each witness to respond promptly—we need that in terms of our considerations here—to any such questions that you may receive. So I don't think any of you are going to purposely drag your feet, but I think it's worth underscoring that we would like a timely response.

Now, I would like to ask unanimous consent to enter into the record the following: a statement from the National Observation Stays Coalition, statement from the American Medical Association, a statement from the College of American Pathologists, a statement from the Association of American Medical Colleges, a statement from the American College of Radiology, a statement from Blue Cross Blue Shield Association, from the Partnership for Employer-Sponsored Coverage, from the American Federation of State, County, and Municipal Employees, a statement from AARP, and from Business Group on Health, SEIU, United Healthcare Workers West, and Blue Shield of California.

So I ask unanimous consent to enter this into the record. I hear no objections.

Ms. ESHOO. And at this time, with your—with all of our thanks, the subcommittee is adjourned.

[Whereupon, at 2:00 p.m., the committee was adjourned.] [Material submitted for inclusion in the record follows:]

H.R. 3630, the No Surprise Act

Mr. PALLONE (for himself and Mr. WALDEN) introduced the following bill; which was referred to the Committee on Energy and Commerce.

A Bill

To amend the Public Health Service Act and title XI of the Social Security Act to protect health care consumers from surprise billing practices, and for other purposes.

Be it enacted by the Senate and House of Representatives of the United States of America in Congress assembled,

SECTION 1. SHORT TITLE.

This Act may be cited as the "No Surprises Act."

SECTION 2. PREVENTING SURPRISE MEDICAL BILLS.

(a) EMERGENCY SERVICES PERFORMED BY NON-PARTICIPATING PROVIDERS.—Section 2719A of the Public Health Service Act (42 U.S.C. 300gg–19a) is amended—

(1) in subsection (b)—

(A) in paragraph (1)—

(i) in the matter preceding subparagraph (A)—

(I) by striking "offering group or individual health insurance issuer" and inserting "offering group or individual health insurance coverage"; and

(II) by inserting "or, for plan year 2021 or a subsequent plan year, with respect to services in an independent freestanding emergency department (as defined in paragraph (2)(C))" after "emergency department of a hospital"; and

(III) by striking "paragraph (2)(B)" and inserting "paragraph (2)";

(ii) in subparagraph (B), by inserting "or a participating emergency facility, as applicable," after "participating provider"; and

(iii) in subparagraph (C)—

(I) in the matter preceding clause (i), by inserting "by a nonparticipating provider or a nonparticipating emergency facility" after "enrollee";

(II) by striking clause (i);

(III) by striking "(ii)(I) such services" and inserting "(i) such services";

(IV) by striking "where the provider of services does not have a contractual relationship with the plan for the providing of services";

(V) by striking "emergency department services received from providers who do have such a contractual relationship with the plan; and" and inserting "emergency services received from participating providers and participating emergency facilities with respect to such plan;"

(VI) by striking "(II) if such services" and all that follows through "were provided in-network" and inserting the following:

"(ii) the cost-sharing requirement (expressed as a copayment amount or coinsurance rate) is not greater than the requirement that would apply if such services were provided by a participating provider or a participating emergency facility;"; and

(VII) by adding at the end the following new clauses:

"(iii) the group health plan or health insurance issuer offering group or individual health insurance coverage pays to such provider or facility, respectively, the amount by which the recognized amount (as defined in paragraph (2)(H)) for such services exceeds the cost-sharing amount for such services (as determined in accordance with clause (ii)); and

"(iv) there shall be counted toward any deductible or out-of-pocket maximums applied under the plan any cost-sharing payments made by the participant, beneficiary, or enrollee with respect to such emergency services so furnished in the same manner as if such cost-sharing payments were with respect to emergency services furnished by a participating provider and a participating emergency facility." and

(B) in paragraph (2)—

(i) in the matter preceding subparagraph (A), by inserting "and subsection (e)" after "this subsection";

(ii) by redesignating subparagraphs (A) through (C) as subparagraphs (B) through (D), respectively;

(iii) by inserting before subparagraph (B), as redesignated by clause (ii), the following new subparagraph:

"(A) EMERGENCY DEPARTMENT OF A HOSPITAL.—The term 'emergency department of a hospital' includes a hospital outpatient department that provides emergency services."

(iv) in subparagraph (C), as redesignated by clause (ii)—

(I) in clause (i)—

(aa) by inserting ", or as would be required under such section if such section applied to an independent freestanding emergency department" after "section 1867 of the Social Security Act"; and

(bb) by inserting "or of the independent freestanding emergency department, as applicable" after "of a hospital"; and (II) in clause (ii)—

(aa) by inserting "or the independent freestanding emergency department, as applicable" after "at the hospital"; and

(bb) by inserting ", or as would be required under such section if such section applied to an independent freestanding emergency department," after "section 1867 of such Act";

(v) by redesignating subparagraph (D), as redesignated by clause (ii), as subparagraph (I); and

(vi) by inserting after subparagraph (C), as redesignated by clause (ii), the following subparagraphs:

"(D) INDEPENDENT FREESTANDING EMERGENCY DEPARTMENT. —The term 'independent freestanding emergency department' means a facility that provides emergency or unscheduled outpatient services to patients whose conditions require immediate care in a setting that is geographically separate and distinct from a hospital and independently licensed.

"(E) MEDIAN CONTRACTED RATE.—

"(i) IN GENERAL.—The term 'median contracted rate' means, with respect to an item or service and a group health plan or health insurance coverage offered by a health insurance issuer, the median of the negotiated rates recognized by the plan or issuer as the total maximum payment (including the cost-sharing amount imposed for such services (as determined in accordance with paragraph (1)(C)(ii) or subsection (e)(1)(A), as applicable) and the amount to be paid by the plan or issuer) for the same or a similar item or service that is provided by a provider in the same or similar specialty and provided in the geographic region in which the item or service is furnished.

"(ii) RULEMAKING. — Not later than 2 July 1, 2020, the Secretary shall through rulemaking determine the methodology the plan or issuer shall use to determine the median contracted rate, the information the plan or issuer shall share with the non-participating provider involved when making such a determination, and the geographic regions applied for purposes of this subparagraph.

"(F) NONPARTICIPATING EMERGENCY FACILITY; PARTICIPATING EMERGENCY FACILITY.—

"(i) NONPARTICIPATING EMERGENCY FACILITY. — The term 'nonparticipating emergency facility' means, with respect to an item or service and a group health plan or health insurance coverage offered by a health insurance issuer, an emergency department of a hospital or an independent freestanding emergency department, that does not have a contractual relationship with the plan or coverage for furnishing such item or service.

"(ii) PARTICIPATING EMERGENCY FACILITY. — The term 'participating emergency facility' means, with respect to an item or service and a group health plan or health insurance coverage offered by a health insurance issuer, an emergency department of a hospital or an independent freestanding emergency department, that has a contractual relationship with the plan or coverage for furnishing such item or service.

"(G) NONPARTICIPATING PROVIDERS; PARTICIPATING PROVIDERS. —

"(i) NONPARTICIPATING PROVIDER.— The term 'nonparticipating provider' means, with respect to an item or service and a group health plan or health insurance coverage offered by a health insurance issuer, a physician or other health professional who is licensed by the State involved to furnish such item or service and who does not have a contractual relationship with the plan or coverage for furnishing such item or service.

"(ii) PARTICIPATING PROVIDER.—The term 'participating provider' means, with respect to an item or service and a group health plan or health insurance coverage offered by a health insurance issuer, a physician or other health professional who is licensed by the State involved to furnish such item or service and who has a contractual relationship with the plan or coverage for furnishing such item or service.

"(H) RECOGNIZED AMOUNT.—The term 'recognized amount' means, with respect to an item or service—

"(i) in the case of such item or service furnished in a State that has in effect a State law that provides for a method for determining the amount of payment that is required to be covered by a health plan or health insurance issuer offering group or individual health insurance coverage regulated by such State in the case of a participant, beneficiary, or enrollee covered under such plan or coverage and receiving such item or service from a nonparticipating provider, not more than the amount determined in accordance with such law plus the cost-sharing amount imposed for such item or service (as determined in accordance with paragraph (1)(C)(ii) or subsection (e)(1)(A), as applicable); or

"(ii) in the case of such item or service furnished in a State that does not have in effect such a law, an amount that is at least the median contracted rate (as defined in subparagraph (E)(i) and determined in accordance with the regulations promulgated pursuant to subparagraph (E)(ii)) for such item or service."

(b) NON-EMERGENCY SERVICES PERFORMED BY NONPARTICIPATING PROV-IDERS AT CERTAIN PARTICIPATING FACILITIES.—

(1) IN GENERAL.—Section 2719A of the Public Health Service Act (42 U.S.C. 300gg–19a) is amended by adding at the end the following new subsection:

"(e) NON-EMERGENCY SERVICES PERFORMED BY NONPARTICIPATING PROVIDERS AT CERTAIN PARTICIPATING FACILITIES.—

"(1) IN GENERAL.—In the case of items or services (other than emergency services to which subsection (b) applies) furnished to a participant, beneficiary, or enrollee of a health plan (as defined in paragraph (2)(A)) by a nonparticipating provider (as defined in subsection (b)(2)(G)) during a visit at a participating health care facility (as defined in paragraph (2)(B)), with respect to such plan, the plan—

"(A) shall not impose on such participant, beneficiary, or enrollee a cost-sharing amount (expressed as a copayment amount or coinsurance rate) for such items and services so furnished that is greater than the cost-sharing amount that would apply under such plan had such items or services been furnished by a participating provider;

"(B) shall pay to such provider furnishing such items and services to such participant, beneficiary, or enrollee the amount by which the recognized amount (as defined in subsection (b)(2)(H)) for such services exceeds the cost-sharing amount imposed for such services (as determined in accordance with subparagraph (A)); and

"(C) shall count toward any deductible or out-of-pocket maximums applied under the plan any cost-sharing payments made by the participant, beneficiary, or enrollee with respect to such items and services so furnished in the same manner as if such cost-sharing payments were with respect to items and services furnished by a participating provider.

"(2) DEFINITIONS.—In this subsection:

"(A) HEALTH PLAN.—The term 'health plan' means a group health plan and health insurance coverage offered by a heath insurance issuer in the group or individual market.

"(B) PARTICIPATING HEALTH CARE FACILITY.—

"(i) IN GENERAL.—The term 'participating health care facility' means, with respect to an item or service and a group health plan or health insurance coverage offered by a health insurance issuer, a health care facility described in clause (ii) that has a contractual relationship with the plan or coverage for furnishing such item or service.

"(ii) HEALTH CARE FACILITY DESCRIBED.—A health care facility described in this clause is each of the following:

"(I) A hospital (as defined in 1861(e) of the Social Security Act).

"(II) A critical access hospital (as defined in section 1861(mm) of such Act).

"(III) An ambulatory surgical center (as defined in section 8 1833(i)(1)(A) of such Act).

"(IV) A laboratory.

"(V) A radiology or imaging cen11 ter."

(2) EFFECTIVE DATE.—The amendments made by this subsection shall apply with respect to plan years beginning on or after January 1, 2021.

(c) PREVENTING CERTAIN CASES OF BALANCE BILLING.—Section 1128A of the Social Security Act (42 U.S.C. 1320a–7a) is amended by adding at the end the following new subsections:

"(t)(1) In the case of an individual with benefits under a health plan or health insurance coverage offered in the group or individual market who is furnished on or after January 1, 2021, emergency services with respect to an emergency medical condition during a visit at an emergency department of a hospital or an independent freestanding emergency department (as defined in section 2719A(b)(2) of the Public Health Service Act)—

"(A) if the emergency department of a hospital or independent freestanding emergency department holds the individual liable for a payment amount for such emergency services so furnished that is more than the cost-sharing amount for such services (as determined in accordance with section 2719A(b)(1)(C)(ii) of the Public Health Service Act); or

"(B) if any health care provider holds such individual liable for a payment amount for an emergency service furnished to such individual by such provider with respect to such emergency medical condition and visit for which the individual receives emergency services at the hospital or emergency department that is more than the cost-sharing amount for such services furnished by the provider (as determined in accordance with section 2719A(b)(1)(C)(ii) of the Public Health Service Act); the hospital, emergency department, independent freestanding emergency department, or health care provider, respectively, shall be subject, in addition to any other penalties that may be prescribed by law, to a civil money penalty of not more than $ [___] for each specified claim.

"(2) The provisions of subsections (c), (d), (e), (g), (h), (k), and (l) shall apply to a civil money penalty or assessment under paragraph (1) or subsection (u) in the same manner as such provisions apply to a penalty, assessment, or proceeding under subsection (a).

"(3) In this subsection and subsection (u):

"(A) The terms 'emergency medical condition' and 'emergency services' have the meanings given such terms, respectively, in section 2719A(b)(2) of the Public Health Service Act.

"(B) The terms 'group health plan', 'health insurance issuer', and 'health insurance coverage' have the meanings given such terms, respectively, in section 2791 of the Public Health Service Act.

"(u)(1) Subject to paragraph (2), in the case of an individual with benefits under a health plan or health insurance coverage offered in the group or individual market who is furnished on or after January 1, 2021, items or services (other than emergency services to which subsection (t) applies) at a participating health care facility by a nonparticipating provider, if such provider holds such individual liable for a payment amount for such an item or service furnished by such provider during a visit at such facility that is more than the cost-sharing amount for such item or service (as determined in accordance with section 2719A(e)(1)(A) of the Public Health Service Act), such provider shall be subject, in addition to any other penalties that may be prescribed by law, to a civil money penalty of not more than $ [___] for each specified claim.

"(2) Paragraph (1) shall not apply to a nonparticipating provider (other than a facility-based provider), with respect to items or services furnished by the provider at a participating health care facility to a participant, beneficiary, or enrollee of a health plan or health insurance coverage offered by a health insurance issuer, if the provider is in compliance with the requirement of paragraph (3). For purposes of the previous sentence, the term 'facility-based provider' means emergency medicine providers, anesthesiologists, pathologists, radiologists, neonatologists, assistant surgeons, hospitalists, intensivists, or other providers as determined by the Secretary.

"(3) (A) For purposes of paragraph (2) a nonparticipating provider is in compliance with this paragraph, with respect to items or services furnished by the provider at a participating health care facility to a participant, beneficiary, or enrollee of a health plan or health insurance coverage offered by a health insurance issuer, if the provider—

"(i)(I) provides to the participant, beneficiary, or enrollee (or to a representative of the participant, beneficiary, or enrollee), on the date on which the participant, beneficiary, or enrollee makes an appointment to be furnished such items or services, if applicable, and on the date on which the individual is furnished such items and services—

"(aa) an oral explanation of the written notice described in item (bb) and such documentation of the provision of such explanation, as the Secretary determines appropriate; and

"(bb) a written notice specified, not later than July 1, 2020, by the Secretary through rulemaking that—

"(AA) contains the information required under subparagraph (B); and

"(BB) is signed and dated by the participant, beneficiary, or enrollee; and

"(II) retain, for a period specified through rulemaking by the Secretary, a copy of the documentation described in subclause (I)(aa) and the written notice described in subclause (I)(bb); and

"(ii) obtains from the participant, beneficiary, or enrollee (or representative) the consent described in subparagraph (C).

"(B) For purposes of subparagraph (A)(i), the information described in this subparagraph, with respect to a nonparticipating provider and a participant, beneficiary, or enrollee of a health plan or health insurance coverage offered by a health insurance issuer, is a notification of each of the following:

"(i) That the health care provider is a non-participating provider with respect to the group health plan or health insurance coverage.

"(ii) The estimated amount that such provider will charge the participant, beneficiary, or enrollee for such items and services involved.

"(C) For purposes of subparagraph (A)(ii), the consent described in this subparagraph, with respect to a participant, beneficiary, or enrollee of a group health plan or health insurance coverage offered by a health insurance issuer, who is to be furnished items or services by a non-participating provider, is a document specified by the Secretary through rulemaking that—

"(i) is signed by the participant, beneficiary, or enrollee (or by a representative of the participant, beneficiary, or enrollee) not less than 24 hours prior to the participant, beneficiary, or enrollee being furnished such items or services by such provider;

"(ii) acknowledges that the participant, beneficiary, or enrollee has been—

"(I) provided with a written estimate and an oral explanation of the charge that the participant, beneficiary, or enrollee will be assessed for the items or services anticipated to be furnished to the participant, beneficiary, or enrollee by such nonparticipating provider; and

"(II) informed that the payment of such charge by the participant, beneficiary, or enrollee will not accrue toward meeting any limitation that the group health plan or health insurance coverage places on cost-sharing; and

"(iii) documents the consent of the participant, beneficiary, or enrollee to—

"(I) be furnished with such items or services by such nonparticipating provider; and

"(II) in the case that the individual is so furnished such items or services, be charged an amount that may be greater than the amount that would otherwise be changed the individual if furnished by a participating provider with respect to such items or services and plan or coverage.

"(4) For purposes of this subsection, the terms 'non-participating provider' and 'participating health care facility' have such meanings given such terms under subsections (b)(2) and (e)(2), respectively, of section 2719A of the Public Health Service Act."

(d) STATE ALL PAYER CLAIMS DATABASES.—

(1) IN GENERAL.—The Secretary of Health and Human Services shall make one-time grants to eligible States for the purposes described in paragraph 14 (2).

(2) USES.—A State may use a grant received under paragraph (1) for one of the following purposes:

(A) To establish an All Payer Claims Database for the State.

(B) To maintain an existing All Payer Claims Databases for the State.

(3) ELIGIBILITY.—To be eligible to receive a grant under paragraph (1) a State shall submit to the Secretary an application at such time, in such manner, and containing such information as the Secretary specifies. Such information shall include, with respect to an All Payer Claims Database for the State, at least specifics on how the State will ensure uniform data collection through the database and the security of such data submitted to and maintained in the database.

(4) ALL PAYER CLAIMS DATABASE.—For purposes of this subsection, the term "All Payer Claims Database" means, with respect to a State, a State database that may include medical claims, pharmacy claims, dental claims, and eligibility and provider files, which are collected from private and public payers.

(5) AUTHORIZATION OF APPROPRIATIONS.—To carry out this subsection, there are appropriated $50,000,000, to remain available until expended.

Letter by A.J. Wilhelmi, President and CEO, Illinois Health and Hospital Association, to Mr. Shimkus, June 10, 2019

IHA Illinois Health and Hospital Association

June 10, 2019

The Honorable John Shimkus
United States House of Representatives
2217 Rayburn House Office Building
Washington, DC 20515

Dear Congressman Shimkus:

On behalf of the Illinois Health and Hospital Association's (IHA) more than 200 hospitals and nearly 50 health systems, we applaud your work to protect patients from surprise medical bills. Illinois is one of only nine states with comprehensive laws that ensure patients are not burdened by unanticipated medical bills after receiving emergency care or treatment in an in-network hospital. These successful state-level approaches should be considered as a model for federal legislation. We also appreciate the opportunity to share our concerns about some of the alternative approaches being considered.

Illinois Laws as a Model for Federal Legislation

Illinois laws protect patients from surprise medical bills by banning the practice of balance billing and removing the patient from disputes between providers and insurance plans. Importantly, all of the legislative proposals introduced in Congress to date also include this IHA-supported patient protection.

Specifically, Illinois *Public Act 96-1523* holds insured patients harmless for any increased out-of-pocket obligations from certain facility-based out-of-network practitioners who provide services at an in-network hospital. The law explicitly defines an "out-of-network practitioner" as one who provides radiology, anesthesiology, pathology, neonatology or emergency department services in a participating hospital or ambulatory surgical treatment center.

Illinois *Public Act 94-0885* requires insured patients to be provided with advance notice that healthcare professionals affiliated with the hospital may not be participating within the same insurance plans and networks as the hospital.

In the event a dispute arises between providers and health plans, Illinois uses "baseball-style" arbitration as the binding dispute resolution process. In this process, each party must submit a proposed best and final offer to the arbitrator, who chooses one of the two, without modification. In addition to expediting dispute resolution, this approach has proven to be significantly less costly than traditional arbitration or litigation

Several of the proposals introduced in Congress would establish arbitration as the dispute resolution mechanism; however, other proposals being considered use government rate setting to determine the amount paid to providers. **IHA strongly opposes setting rates for physicians and hospitals in federal statute and requests that you protect the role of private contract negotiation in healthcare.**

Rate-setting Proposals Would Threaten Access to Care

Over half of the reimbursement rates paid to Illinois hospitals are set in law by the Medicare and Medicaid programs, and fall short of covering the cost of care. Medicare reimburses Illinois hospitals 11 percent below the cost of providing care, and Medicaid reimburses 25 percent below the cost of providing care. Currently, 42 percent of Illinois hospitals are operating on negative or extremely thin margins.

IHA is concerned that expanding government rate-setting to the private sector could lead to an immediate, harmful reduction in hospital resources, which would threaten access to care. Additionally, health insurance companies would have no incentive to negotiate with providers or establish adequate coverage networks, which could especially harm patients living in rural areas. If insurers are allowed to pay out-of-network providers less than they would pay if those providers were in their network, these insurers will have little incentive to contract with these providers and pay them an appropriate rate.

Again, we appreciate the opportunity to highlight Illinois' successful solutions to protect patients from surprise medical bills and to express our support for preserving private contract negotiation for providers, thereby promoting adequate coverage networks for patients.

We look forward to working with you to enact meaningful legislation.

Sincerely,

A.J. Wilhelmi
President & CEO
Illinois Health and Hospital Association

New Mexico, Office of Superintendent of Insurance, Air Ambulance Memorial, Study Report, January 2017

Introduction

New Mexico's Legislature, under House Memorial 78 and Senate Memorial 62, directed the New Mexico Office of Superintendent of Insurance (OSI) in consultation with the Department of Health, the Risk Management Division of the General Services Department, and the Workers' Compensation Administration to study the impacts and cost of air ambulance transports and related insurance policies and payments on consumers, beneficiaries, and payers in New Mexico.

Executive Summary

Data collected by OSI for workers' compensation and health insurance carriers between the years of 2005 and 2016 shows that [next page]:

- Air ambulance providers have increased in numbers since 2009, from approximately 13 in-state aircraft operating that year to 21 aircraft in 2016.
- The average charge per claim for air ambulance services increased 229% between 2006 and 2015.
- The average claim paid by health and workers' compensation insurance for air ambulance charges increased 50% from 2006 to 2015.
- The average portion of the claim unpaid by insurance carriers as of 2015 is $26,829. In some circumstances, providers may balance bill insureds for this unpaid balance.
- Prior to 2015, four air ambulance providers conducted approximately 55% of transports in the state. Three of these companies have recently been purchased by the largest air ambulance provider in the nation, Air Methods.

State regulation of the air ambulance industry has, historically, been limited. Courts have repeatedly ruled that the federal Airline Deregulation Act preempts state regulation of air ambulance industry practices. Recent legal developments, however, may provide a road to challenge this presumption of preemption. Texas recently had success arguing that the McCarran-Ferguson Act grants states sole, reverse-preemptory authority to regulate the business of insurance, including regulation of the rates paid by insurance companies to reimburse air ambulance providers.

Air Ambulance Industry Changes Overview

Until the late 199o's, Helicopter Emergency Medical Services (HEMS) programs in the United States were largely not-for-profit hospital or public safety operations. These programs were generally well integrated with state and local EMS systems.[107] However, as a result of the Balanced Budget Act of 1997, the federal Centers for Medicare and Medicaid Services changed the way they paid for air ambulance services for Medicare recipients. To effect this change, they implemented a fee schedule that provided more favorable reimbursement for air ambulance services. The national fee schedule redistributed, on a budget-neutral basis, payments among various types of ambulance services. Prior to 2002, Medicare reimbursement differed depending on the air ambulance provider's business model: Medicare reimbursed hospital-based providers based on reasonable costs, while it reimbursed independent providers based on reasonable charges. This policy contributed to wide variation in the reimbursement rates for the same service, with hospital based providers generally receiving higher reimbursement than independent providers for similar services. The new national fee schedule established one payment rate for fixed-wing transports and another rate for helicopter transports. The fee schedule also provides higher reimbursement rates for transports in rural areas, but does not differentiate payments according to the business model followed, the size of the aircraft used, or level of medical or safety equipment on board.[108]

---

[107] National Association of State EMS Officials - Air Medical Services Committee, *Brief Outline of the Federal Pre-Emption Issues in Regulating Air Medical Services* (October, 2011) (available at https://www.nasemso.org/projects/airmedical/documents/HelicopterEMS.pdf).

[108] United States Government Accountability Office, *Air Ambulance: Effects of Industry Changes on Services Are Unclear*, 6 (September 2010) (available at http://www.gao.gov/assets/320/310527.pdf).

The effects of this change in the reimbursement landscape was almost immediate. From 1999 through 2008, the number of patients transported nationally by air ambulance helicopters increased from just over 200,000 to over 270,000, or by about 35%. The data also shows that the number of air ambulance helicopters operating nationwide increased from 360 to 677, or by about 88%.[109]

With the change in the reimbursement structure for air ambulance procedures came a change in the make-up of the air ambulance industry. Prior to 1999, most air ambulance providers were hospital-based, whereas today, about half of the providers are private, independent companies with no support from hospitals in terms of ownership, risk, and financial support. Stakeholders interviewed by the federal Government Accountability Office attributed these changes to downsizing or closing of some community hospitals, leading to increased need for air transportation services in emergency situations, especially in rural areas. Additionally, the Government Accountability Office attributed some of these changes to the establishment of regional medical facilities, such as cardiac and stroke centers that provide highly specialized care for critically ill patients, which encouraged the use of air ambulances, again, because they could transport patients more quickly from outlying areas. Finally, and most importantly, implementation of the Medicare fee schedule provided those wishing to provide air ambulance services a degree of predictability for Medicare reimbursement, which stakeholders noted enabled air ambulance providers to develop more accurate financial plans.[110] Nationwide data suggests that this increased stability in funding for air ambulance providers contributed significantly in the number of providers competing to serve this market. These trends may hold true in New Mexico, but, as noted below, the data is unclear.

Air Ambulance Claims Data

Process for Gathering Data

For purposes of this study, OSI requested air ambulance claims data from the four largest and longest operating major medical carriers providing fully-insured individual and small group plans. For the two youngest carriers, this data reached back to the beginning of Affordable Care Act coverage in 2014. For the two oldest carriers, this data reached back to 2005 and 2009, respectively. OSI was also able to longitudinally track data from workers' compensation claims information voluntarily provided by select employers. Additional data for the study came from the New Mexico Public Schools Insurance Authority, which provided air ambulance claims for its self-funded plans from 2011 to 2015.

OSI also sought information from the New Mexico Department of Health on state operations of air ambulance providers. The Department of Health provided the names of the companies operating in the state, as well as their base locations. This information, along with trends observed in air ambulance claims data, is outlined below.

---

109 Ibid.

110 Ibid. at 7-8.

Air Ambulance Providers

According to a federal Government Accountability Office report, as of 2009, New Mexico had 13 air ambulance helicopters operating in the state.[111] The New Mexico Department of Health reports that there are currently 25 air ambulance agencies registered in the state, operating 35 rotary aircraft and 67 fixed-wing aircraft as a part of their multi-state operations. While these aircraft are registered in New Mexico, only eight of these air ambulance providers have home bases in New Mexico. The rest of these providers have a home base in other states, with locations throughout New Mexico and bordering states as extended base sites. The Department of Health estimates that each provider registered with the state operates at least one air ambulance for an estimated total of 21 aircraft operating in New Mexico at any given time.

Air ambulances that transport New Mexico residents also may be registered in other states. As a result, it is difficult to pinpoint the exact number of air ambulance providers serving New Mexico residents. However, it generally appears that there has been an increase of approximately 8 providers operating in the state at any given time since 2009. As noted above, this is a trend observed nationwide as Medicare reimbursement rates for air ambulance providers stabilized.

Claims Payment

When an air ambulance provider charges for its service, it typically charges a base rate for liftoff and a separate rate for mileage. For example, an air ambulance company may charge $10,000 as a base liftoff charge, and then $100 per mile traveled. As a result, in its analysis of air ambulance claims data, OSI conducted a separate analysis of trends in base liftoff charges and mileage charges. Additionally, due to operational differences between rotary (helicopter) and fixed-wing (airplane) providers, where noted, OSI tracked payments to these types of providers separately.

Trends in Base and Mileage Paid by Carrier

In 2006, the first full year for which OSI has significant data on air ambulance charges, the average amount paid by insurance carriers for the base fee was $6,423. Fluctuations likely caused by changes in the amount of data we received for each year aside, the sum paid by insurance carriers for these base charges has steadily increased in the intervening years. As of 2015, the last year for which OSI has complete data, the average base charge amount paid by insurance carriers was $8,943, a 40% increase over the span of nine years. Likewise, for mileage charges, data shows that insurance carriers paid claims averaging $6,356 in 2006. By 2015, insurance carriers paid an average of $11,843 per flight. The average increase in mileage charges paid between 2006 and 2015 was $5,487, reflecting an 86% increase.

In total, insurance carriers in 2006 paid an average of $12,779 for base and mileage charges per flight. As of 2015, this amount had risen to an average of $19,194 paid per claim, for an average difference of $6,415 or a 50% increase in total paid charges for air ambulance services. These payments, however, may not include any amounts recouped from patients for air ambulance services. If the air ambulance provider has a contract with the health insurance carrier to provide services, the patient may pay an additional amount for the service via their deductible or other contractual cost-sharing obligations, such as a co- insurance or co-pay. If the insurance company does not have a contract with the air ambulance provider, the air

[111] Ibid. at 8.

ambulance provider may balance bill the patient, seeking additional payment for the charged services. OSI was not able to obtain direct information about average amounts charged directly to consumers in balance billing. However, we have collected the information below about insurance carriers' unpaid charges.

Charges Unpaid by Insurance Carrier

In 2009, the first year for which the most complete data is available, the average difference between the amount charged by air ambulance providers and the amount paid by health insurers was $13,518 per flight. As of 2015, this amount had risen an additional $26,829 per flight. This amount represents a 98% increase in the amount charged by air ambulance providers but unpaid by insurance carriers between 2009 and 2015. As noted above, whether and how air ambulance companies pass these charges along to patients depends on whether the health insurance carrier has a contractual relationship with the air ambulance provider.

Another way to look at the issue of charged amounts versus paid amounts is to analyze the amounts billed per mile versus the amounts paid per mile. Taken as a whole, for all claims between 2005 and 2016, the most frequent amount air ambulance providers billed per mile was between $274 and $294-Providers billed between $274 and $294 per mile for 1,224 claims out of the 6,825 claims OSI evaluated for this report. Conversely, health insurance carriers paid between $1 and $21 per mile for 2,959 claims out of 6,510 paid claims within the relevant data obtained by OSI. As a result, there is an average $273 difference in the most predominant billed charge per mile versus paid charge. Again, it is unclear from the data obtained by OSI how much of these costs are shifted onto consumers by air ambulance providers.

Total Average Charge by Provider

In 2006, the first year for which OSI has significant data, the average total charge billed by air ambulance providers for their services was $13,984. In 2015, the last year for which OSI has significant data, these charges amounted to an average of $45,937 per flight. This represents an average growth of $31,953 per flight, or 229% increase over a nine-year period.

In a meeting with OSI, Air Methods, the largest air ambulance service provider in the country, stated that this increase in charges is due to an upsurge in flights by patients covered by public programs that do not sufficiently reimburse for their services. Specifically, Air Methods cited that 78% of its flights in the State of New Mexico were transports of patients with Medicaid, Medicare or the uninsured. Air Methods estimated that the break- even cost of the average air ambulance transport, including medical services and maintenance costs, was about $10,000. Medicaid reimburses at a rate of $1,500 to $3,000 per flight. Medicare reimburses at a rate of $5,000 to $6,500 per flight. As a result, Air Methods argued, the air ambulance industry is forced to shift costs to the privately insured and workers' compensation insureds.

However, the figures provided by Air Methods do not support the costs currently charged per air ambulance flight. As an example scenario, using the percentages and costs provided by the air ambulance industry, we will assume that an air ambulance provider provides 100 flights per year. Additionally, we will assume that approximately 80 of these flights are for patients with public insurance, such as Medicaid or Medicare. At an even split of Medicaid and Medicare patients, with Medicaid reimbursing approximately $2,000 per flight and Medicare reimbursing approximately $6,000 per flight, this pool of flights generates $320,000 in reimbursements. If the air ambulance industry's costs are currently an average of $10,000 per flight, this business leaves a $680,000 shortfall. The air ambulance industry admits that it shifts this shortfall to its privately insured payers, including workers' compensation payers. Assuming that the privately insured payers make up approximately 20% of flights, and that the air ambulance industry must generate at least $1 Million to break even on costs (100 flights x $10,000 in operating costs), an air ambulance provider must charge approximately $34,000 per flight to break even. This is approximately $12,000 short of the current $46,000 average charge per flight.

These figures, again, assume that the air ambulance industry has provided OSI with accurate data about their operations costs. As described by the air ambulance industry, operations costs include purchase and maintenance of aircraft, air ambulance staffing, including medical technicians, and medical equipment. It is worthwhile noting that as late as 2010, air ambulance providers were accepting an average of $10,500 per flight for payment of services, including operations costs and any profit expected to be made on flights. In contrast, as of 2015, air ambulance providers billed an average of $45,937 per flight and accepting an average of $19,194 from carriers for payment of services (this figure does not include amounts recouped from privately insured payments). While the issue of disparities in payment between public and private payers certainly contributes to the amount charged to break even, it does not explain why the break-even amount has increased in just six years to be an amount previously accepted as profitable. Air ambulance industry watchdogs have pointed out that this increase in operations costs may be due to a glut of providers in the market resulting in fewer flights per vehicle, which means fewer opportunities to recoup operational expenses.

Rotary versus Fixed Wing

Air ambulance providers can be broken into two groups, providers that offer helicopter, or rotary services and providers that offer services via fixed-wing airplanes. While some air ambulance providers have both rotary and fixed-wing ambulances in their fleets, many concentrate on providing services via only one type of aircraft. Accordingly, OSI examined the billed and paid charges for these two types of providers to determine if there is any meaningful difference between these types of aircraft.

For the years for which data was collected, rotary wing aircraft provided more services to patients than fixed wing aircraft. Between 2005 and 2016, rotary wing providers flew 6,836 flights as opposed to fixed wing providers' 4,723 flights. The average paid claim for rotary flights per patient for the period of time covered in OSI's claims survey is $16,465 for base charges combined with mileage charges. The average paid claim for fixed wing flights during that same timeframe is $15,582. This accounts for an average difference of $883 between rotary flights and fixed wing flights. Accordingly, the data presented to OSI shows no meaningful difference between the charges for these flights.

Between 2006 and2015, the amounts insurance carriers paid for rotary wing flights increased an average of 54.7%. In contrast, the percent increase for fixed wing flights was slightly less at 43%. The difference between the increases in paid claims for these two types of services may be related to operating costs for the various types of fleets, differences in ownership and management practices of rotary and fixed wing fleets, or other factors such as flight distances and fuel costs.

Insurer Networks

In October of 2016, OSI surveyed the six major medical carriers offering coverage in the fully-insured and small group markets in the state about their contracted air ambulance providers. Of these carriers, two do not have any preferred provider agreements with air ambulance providers. These carriers have stated that they pay claims for air ambulance services as incurred by enrollees. The remaining carriers do have contracts with air ambulance providers, however, these contracts are constantly evolving due to company buy-outs, mergers or movement from state to state. Other states' efforts to control the impact of air ambulance charges on insureds have been largely focused on educating hospitalists on how to ensure that air transport of patients is in-network for their insurance.

While OSI agreed not to share carriers' specific negotiated payment for services, it can report generally that there is no clear pattern linking patient volume to payments. As a result, the payers surveyed do not appear to necessarily be paying less for air ambulance services based on patient load. Additionally, there does not necessarily appear to be a distinguishable trend in the amount paid for services based on number of provider contracts. Unusually, the carriers reporting higher numbers of contracts with air ambulance providers do not necessarily see a lower price paid for their enrollees' care.

Air Ambulance Provider Market Share

As a part of its data request, OSI asked insurers to supply the names of the air ambulance Providers serving their patiens. This information allowed OSI to evaluate the market share of each provider and see if market share in any way correlates to average paid charges. However, it is important to note that there has been significant consolidation within the air ambulance provider industry. Namely, many of the top air ambulance providers in the state have been bought out or merged. For instance, Air Methods, the largest air ambulance provider in the nation, recently acquired Tri-State Care Flight, Rocky Mountain Holdings, LifeNet, and Native American Air, several of the major air ambulance providers in the state.

In total, prior to acquisition, Tri-State Care provided the most patient transports, with 1,969 flights provided in the survey period for the claims data received. The second largest air ambulance provider was Rocky Mountain Holdings/LifeNet at 1,881 transports. The third largest air ambulance provider is the nation's second largest air ambulance company, PHI Air, with 1,287 flights. PHI Air largely operates out ofTexas. The fourth largest air ambulance provider, Native American Air, at 915 transports, was also acquired by Air Methods. These four providers, prior to acquisition, made up approximately 55% of the air ambulance transports in the state.

Interestingly, the claims data shows that the four air ambulance providers with the largest market share also had amongst the highest billed charges for services. With the exception of two other transport companies, these companies charged more for their services than the 20 other named companies surveyed. Consequently, the conglomeration of three out of four of these companies and resulting decline in competition may have led to an increase in charges for air ambulance services for New Mexico residents.

Regulatory Authority

Airline Deregulation Act Preemption Overview

Few states have attempted regulation of the air ambulance industry due to federal court interpretations of the preemption language in the Airline Deregulation Act (ADA) of 1978. This federal statute was designed to remove government control over air fares and routes and increase efficiency of airline operating costs. The ADA was passed after Congressional investigators compared fares of regulated airlines flying between states with fares of unregulated airlines within states. Investigators found that unregulated airlines charged lower fares. The Act was passed with bipartisan support, but was strongly opposed by the airline industry itself.[112] The Act states that through deregulation, the air transport industry should rely on "competitive market forces" to further "efficiency, innovation, and low prices" as well as "variety and qualify...of air transportation services."[113] To ensure that states would not undo federal deregulation with regulation of their own, the ADA included a preemption provision, prohibiting states from enforcing any law "relating to rates, routes, or services of any air carrier."[114]

This prohibition was interpreted extremely broadly by the U.S. Supreme Court in *Morales v. Trans World Airlines, Inc.,* 504 U.S. 374 (1992). In this case, airlines sued to enjoin Texas from enforcing state deceptive marketing practice laws against airlines' advertising. The U.S. Supreme Court ruled that state regulation of air fare advertising was expressly preempted by the ADA. Over the years, various courts have further interpreted the ADA to directly preempt state regulation related to rates, advertising, scheduling, insurance coverage, routing, accounting and reporting systems, and air ambulance subscription programs.

States are still able to require an air ambulance operator to be licensed as a medical services provider, but licensing requirements can apply only to the quality of medical services and equipment required for an ambulance service. However, the patchwork of federal Department of Transportation (DOT) and court opinions does not provide a clear picture of what state regulations of air ambulances are permissible. Although the DOT has indicated that state regulations serving primarily a patient care objective are properly within the states' regulatory authority, it has also indicated that a state medical program, ostensibly dealing with only medical equipment and supplies aboard the aircraft, could be so pervasive or so constructed as to be indirect regulation of prices, routes, or services, which is preempted. As a result, the line delineating where state regulation of public health constitutes impermissible economic regulation is not so bright.

The DOT, however, recently issued a document outlining the "Guidelines for the Use and Availability of Helicopter Emergency Medical Transport (HEMS)" which outlines opportunities for permissible state regulation on the:

- Quality of emergency medical care provided to patients
- Requirements related to the qualification and training of air ambulance medical personnel

---

[112] Smithsonian National Air and Space Museum, *America By Air: Deregulation: A Watershed Event,* https://airand space.si.edu/exhibitions/america-by- air/online/jetage/jetageo8.cfm (last accessed October 26, 2016).

[113] *Morales v. Trans World Airlines, Inc.* et al. 504 U.S. 374 (1992).

[114] Ibid.

- Scope of practice and credentialing
- Maintenance of medical records, data collection, and reporting
- Medically related equipment standards
- Patient care environments
- EMS radio communications
- Medically related dispatch requirements
- Medical transport plans including transport to appropriate facilities
- Other medical licensing requirements[115]

Few states have attempted to enact laws, regulations, or policies regarding air ambulance safety for fear that it would conflict with ADA's preemptive powers. For example, states have tried to ensure that the number and location of air ambulance providers corresponds with patient need. However, in 1987, the Attorney General of Arizona concluded that the ADA precluded the state from asserting Certificate of Need (CON) regulation of the number and location of air ambulance services within its boundaries. Similarly, in 2006, the Attorney General of Hawaii also issued an opinion to the Hawaii State Health Planning and Development Agency and the Department of Health advising that the state cannot require a CON for air ambulances to operate in Hawaii. Hawaii's ruling resulted from a Federal Aviation Administration (FAA) advisory to the state declaring that it could not regulate air carriers; even those involved in a specialized service that otherwise would be regulated at the state level.[116]

Most recently, in 2015, the North Dakota legislature passed a law requiring air ambulance operators to become participating providers with certain North Dakota health insurance companies to be listed on a "primary call list" for air ambulance services. The legislation assigned the state's Department of Health the task of housing this "primary call list." Specifically, North Dakota House Bill 1255 provided that:

1. The department shall create and maintain a primary call list and a secondary call list of air ambulance service providers operating in this state.
2. To qualify to be listed on the primary call list, an air ambulance service provider shall submit to the department attested documentation indicating the air ambulance service provider is a participating provider of the health insurance carriers in the state which collectively hold at least seventy-five percent of the health insurance coverage in the state as determined by annual market share reports.
3. The department shall provide the primary call list and the secondary call list for air ambulance service providers operating in this state to all emergency medical services personnel, each hospital licensed under chapter 23-16, each 911 coordinator in this state, and each public safety answering point operating in this state.
4. The department shall establish air ambulance service response zones for rotary wing aircraft which are based on response times and patient health and safety.
   a. Upon receipt of a request for air ambulance services, emergency medical services personnel, a hospital licensed under chapter 23-16, or a public safety answering

[115] National Association of State EMS Officials, *State Model Rules for the Regulation of Air Medical Services*, 4 (September 2016).

[116] Maryland Health Care Commission, *Air Ambulance Study Required Under Senate Bill* 770, 11 (December 2006) (available at http://dlslibrary.state.md.us/publications/EXEC/DHMH/MHCC/ AirAmbulance_2006.pdf).

point operating in this state, shall make a reasonable effort to inform the requesting party of the estimated response time for the requested air transport versus the ground transport for that designated response zone. If at any point during the request for air ambulance services the requester withdraws the request, the receiving party is not required to complete that call for air ambulance services.

b. If emergency medical services personnel, a hospital licensed under chapter 23-16, or a public safety answering point operating in this state receives a request from emergency medical services personnel for air ambulance services, the recipient of the request shall comply with the call priority under this subdivision in responding to the request.
   - First, the recipient of the request shall call an air ambulance service provider listed on the primary call list which is within the designated response zone.
   - Second, if each of the air ambulance service providers listed on the primary list is not available or is not able and willing to respond to the call, the recipient of the request shall notify the requester of this fact and shall call an air ambulance provider listed on the secondary call list within the designated response zone.
   - Third, if each of the air ambulance service providers listed on the secondary list is not available or is not able and willing to respond to the call, the recipient of the request shall notify the requester of this fact and shall inform the requester of primary and secondary air ambulance service provider options outside the designated response zone.

5. Upon request of the department, a potential patient, or a potential patient's legal guardian, an air ambulance service provider shall provide that provider's fee schedule, including the base rate, per loaded mile rate, and any usual and customary charges.
   a. The department shall compile and distribute this fee information to each hospital licensed under chapter 23-16, each hospital emergency department in the state, each physician the department determines is likely to generate an air ambulance transport, each emergency medical services operation, each emergency medical services professional, emergency medical services personnel, each public safety answering point in this state, and each 911 coordinator in this state.
   b. Before a hospital refers a patient to an air ambulance service provider, the hospital shall make a reasonable effort to inform the patient or the patient's legal guardian of the fees for the air ambulance service providers licensed under this chapter, for the purpose of allowing the patient or legal guardian to make an informed decision on choosing an air ambulance service provider. A hospital is exempt from complying with this subdivision if the hospital determines compliance might jeopardize the health or safety of the patient.
6. The state health council shall adopt rules establishing air ambulance service provider requirements that must address transport plans, including auto launch protocol and auto launch cancellation protocol; transporting to the nearest appropriate medical facility; medical necessity; and informed consent. As necessary, the state health council shall adopt rules relating to quality of care standards and other appropriate requirements regarding air ambulance service providers.[117]

[117] N.D.C.C. § 23-27-04.10.

The intention of North Dakota's legislation was to curb the billing of consumers for out-of-network air ambulance charges. Air ambulance industry practices often result in "out-of-network," surprise medical bills for patients needing emergency air transportation. The air ambulance industry, however, promptly sued the state for running afoul of the Airline Deregulation Act. Valley Med, the air ambulance carrier suing North Dakota, asserted that because the law in question has a significant impact on the prices, routes, and services of air ambulance service providers, the law was preempted. In March of 2016, the U.S. District Court for the District of North Dakota sided with Valley Med and applied a broad reading of the ADA's preemption authority. The court reasoned that because an air ambulance provider must accept the reimbursement rates offered by the predominant insurance carriers of the state in order to be placed on the "primary call list," the state was essentially forcing air ambulance providers to accept an insurer's rates or discontinue operating in the state. Accordingly, the law impacted the air fare rates and services deregulated under the ADA, and thus was preem pted.[118]

North Dakota's governing body is not alone in its concerns with the practices of the air ambulance industry. Growing concerns about the impact of air ambulance billing on patients has led to the introduction of federal legislation to limit the ADA's preemption authority. Spring of 2016 saw the introduction of federal legislation allowing state insurance regulators the flexibility to protect consumers from excessive out-of-network charges by regulating how air ambulance carriers are reimbursed. Specifically, members of Congress attempted to introduce an amendment to Federal Aviation Authority reauthorization legislation that would remove federal preemption of state regulation of air ambulances. This legislation would allow states to regulate air ambulance participation in health insurance networks, balance billing of patients, and allow states to require increased transparency for consumers. The legislation stated that:

Nothing in this subsection shall be construed as affecting or in any way interfering with the ability of any State or Territory to enact or enforce a law, regulation, or other provision having the force and effect of law related to network participation, reimbursement, and balance billing, or transparency for an air carrier that provides air ambulance service.

Diverse groups such as the National Association of Insurance Commissioners (NAIC) and the Association of Health Insurance Plans lobbied for the change. However, the Senate Commerce Committee Chair blocked the amendment, and it did not advance to the Senate floor. Legislation to remove federal preemption of states regulation of air ambulance services has not been reintroduced.[119]

Reverse Preemption Overview

Recent litigation between the state of Texas and the air ambulance industry has shed light on another potential path for legal regulation of air ambulance services. Texas's Department of Insurance, Division of Workers' Compensation, set guidelines regarding what insurers must pay for air ambulance transport of injured workers. These guidelines then required insurers to pay the full, billed charges of these set payments. Texas' Workers' Compensation Division set these charges at 125% of the Medicare-approved fee for air ambulance services.

The air ambulance industry promptly sued the state of Texas and its Workers' Compensation Division, claiming that the state had violated the ADA The Workers'

[118] *Valley Med Flight, Inc. v. Dwelle,* 171 F.Supp.3d 930 (2016).

[119] National Association of Insurance Commissioners, *Air Ambulance Regulation Issue Brief* (April 2016) (available at http://www.naic.org/documents/government relations air ambulance regulation issue brief.pd£).

Compensation Division, however, made the relatively novel legal argument that the state had the authority to regulate air ambulance reimbursement, as it related to insurance, under states' authority to regulate the business of insurance via the federal McCarran-Ferguson Act. The McCarran-FergusonAct, which was passed by Congress in 1945, provides that,

> No Act of Congress shall be construed to invalidate, impair, or supersede any law enacted by any State for the purpose ofregulating the business of insurance...unless such Act specifically relates to the business ofinsurance: Provided, [federal antitrust statutes]...shall be applicable to the business of insurance to the extent that such business is not regulated by State Law.[120]

The legal concept for the effect of the McCarran-Ferguson Act is called "reverse preemption." Reverse preemption occurs when states are given the exclusive or near exclusive authority to pass laws and regulate an issue area. Its practical effect is to bar federal action on issues given solely over to states for regulation.

Courts have interpreted the McCarran-Ferguson Act's grant of reverse preemption to states broadly. In a 1993 case, *U.S. Treasury v. Fabe,* the U.S. Supreme Court defined the concept of the "business of insurance" as "The relationship between insurer and insured, the type of policy which could be issued, its reliability, interpretation, and enforcement - these were the core of the 'business of insurande." The Court then went on to clarify that a state directly regulates the "business of insurance" if it "prescribes the terms of the insurance contract." The Court also stated that there can "also be no doubt that the actual performance of an insurance contract falls within the business of insurance."[121]

In support of its regulation of air ambulance reimbursement fees, Texas' Workers' Compensation Division argued that setting the fee schedule was legally within its authority to regulate the business of insurance. As a result, its actions were protected under the McCarran-Ferguson Act's reverse preemptory authority given to states. Texas argued that since the ADA did not explicitly remove states' reverse preemptory authority to regulate the business of insurance, its authority to regulate insurers' payments for air ambulance services were intact and not preempted. In December 2016, a Texas district court judge agreed with the Texas Department of Insurance, Workers' Compensation Division, and upheld the state's authority to set air ambulance fees. Appeals are expected in the case.

Other Federal Preemption

In addition to the ADA, other federal laws may impact state action on air ambulance regulation. The first, the Emergency Medical Treatment and Active Labor Act (EMTALA), applies to all hospitals receiving Medicare payments. This law states that hospitals must not transfer an individual with an emergency medical condition that has not been stabilized unless several conditions are met, including arranging appropriate transfer. This requirement directly impacts air ambulance transport from the sending hospital, and creates liabilities for the sending hospital to ensure appropriate care.[122]

Secondly, the Federal Employee Retirement Income Security Act (ERISA), exempts self-insured companies or entities from state insurance laws. This statute hasa preemptive effect similar to the ADA in that self-insured entities may ignore any state-imposed insurance

---

[120] 15 U.S.C. § 1012(b).

[121] Id. at 502-503.

[122] 42 U.S.C. § 1395dd.

coverage mandates, required reimbursement floors for specific services, e.g., coverage for out-of-network service providers, as well as any other insurance requirement that a state enacts. Employers that self-insure their employees' health cannot be compelled to offer a benefit (i.e., air ambulance service) under state law. The preemption applies regardless of whether an employer self-administers the insurance benefits or pays an insurance company "administrative services only" to administer the benefit on behalf of the employer.[123] Notably, more than half of New Mexico's employers who provide health insurance are self-insured.

Lastly, as mentioned elsewhere in this report, federal Medicare and Medicaid provisions have definite implications for the provision of air ambulance services for patients covered by these program. Significantly, Medicare has developed extensive rules for appropriate use of ambulance services, including air ambulance services. Medicare pays for use of air ambulance services when medically necessary, time is essential, and/or other modes of transport are not available or not appropriate. Transport is only provided to the nearest hospital offering the treatment needed by the patient.[124] Medicare, as a major payer for air ambulance services, can and has shaped many of the operations of the air ambulance industry. Accordingly, while Medicare provisions may not have preemptive authority, their impact cannot be understated.

Current State Regulation

Department of Health Regulation

Current New Mexico state regulation of air ambulance providers was enacted in 2006, pursuant to the state's Emergency Medical Services Act, N.M.S.A. 1978, § 24-10B-4-H. The regulations, which can be found at 7.27.5 NMAC, were drafted to achieve compliance with federal guidance on ADA preemption. New Mexico's Department of Health has noted that these regulations will likely be updated to incorporate additional federal Department of Transportation guidance issued in 2015, and model law developed by the National Association of State EMS Officials.

New Mexico Department of Health air ambulance regulations delineate processes for state certification of air ambulance services, fees for operation in New Mexico, medical standards, radio communications operations, and complaint procedures. Notably, these regulations avoid topic areas preempted by federal law, per DOT guidance. Current recommendations for regulation by the National Association of State EMS Officials expand upon some areas currently not covered by the Department of Health's regulation. As a result, the Department of Health has indicated that it is considering revising its current state regulation of air ambulance services.

Superintendent of Insurance Regulation

Currently, there are no laws or regulations flowing from New Mexico's Insurance Code that directly regulate air ambulance providers. However, the Insurance Code does require coverage for emergency services. More specifically, the Patient Protection Act requires insurance companies to pay for emergency services for health insurance policy holders, including emergency services provided outside the network, at no additional cost to consum ers.[125] OSI has interpreted this provision to include coverage for air ambulance services and has required

---

[123] 29 U.S.C. § 1001 et seq.

[124] Medicare.gov, *Ambulance Services* (available at https://www.medicare.gov/coverage/ambulance-services.html) (last accessed October 2016).

[125] N.M.S.A. 1978 § 59A-57-4.

carriers to pay air ambulance charges, even when they are out of network. However, OSI does not have control over whether air ambulance providers accept payments by the carriers, or the amount.

Moreover, air ambulances are not just used for emergency services. These companies also transport medically fragile patients from one critical care unit to another. These circumstances are not typically considered an emergency as there is time to receive authorization for transport from the insurance company. Nonetheless, while the flight may be authorized by the insurance company, this authorization does not necessarily preclude an outcome resulting in balance billing. If the only available air ambulance provider is one that is out-of-network, this out-of-network provider may balance bill a patient where the provider deems the insurer's reimbursement for its services insufficient. Currently, New Mexico's Insurance Code does not preclude out-of-network providers from balance billing patients in non-emergency circumstances.

Workers' Compensation Regulation

Like many other states, New Mexico sets a maximum amount workers' compensation insurers can pay health care providers to care for injured employees.[126] These compensation amounts are called a fee schedule, and are established by the Workers' Compensation Administration. This fee schedule does not set an absolute reimbursement amount, *but* an acceptable range for payment of services, and providers and insurers are permitted to negotiate for payment of services within that range.[127] This range is set based on an evaluation of health care providers' usual and customary charges for services typically provided to injured workers.[128] Unfortunately, however, air ambulance services are excluded from this fee schedule.

Under Workers' Compensation regulations, services that are not on the fee schedule are "billable and payable on a by-report (BR) basis," meaning that the fee for these services is subject to negotiation between the provider and the payer. Current Workers' Compensation regulations dictate that this negotiation process is triggered by the filing of a report that describes why an established fee schedule code was not used to bill for the services.[129] The provider and workers' compensation carrier then negotiate payment for the services rendered outside the fee schedule, including, as relevant here, air ambulance services. Should there be a dispute as to the reasonableness of the fee charged for the BR service, Workers' Compensation regulations provide for a dispute resolution process.[130] In the event of a billing or payment dispute, any party may submit a request to the Workers' Compensation Cost Containment Bureau for a director's determination of reasonable charges for the service. The Bureau director's determination of reasonable payment for the service is deemed final, but subject to appeal under workers' compensation law procedures.[131] Regardless of the outcome of fee negotiations or any resulting dispute resolution process for BR services, New Mexico law prevents balance billing of injured workers for any claims charges unpaid by workers' compensation insurers.[132]

---

[126] N.M.S.A. 1978, § 52-4-5.
[127] NMAC 11.4.7.
[128] N.M.S.A. 1978, § 52-4-5.
[129] NMAC 11.4-7.8(B).
[130] NMAC 11.4.7.11 (A).
[131] N.M.S.A. 1978, § 52-5-8.
[132] NMAC 11.4.7.8(B)(13).

Air ambulance companies providing services in New Mexico have begun to challenge the authority of the state's Workers' Compensation Administration to resolve fee disputes and prohibit balance billing of injured workers under state law. Air ambulance providers are arguing that the ADA preempts the state from deciding these disputes. As a result, it has been reported to OSI that New Mexico's Workers' Compensation Administration is dismissing these cases due to lack of jurisdiction.[133] Furthermore, New Mexico's workers' compensation insurers and self-funding groups are reporting an uptick in litigation on this issue, with at least two claims reported as having been filed in state district court on this issue.

Recommendations

Based on the data collected, feedback provided by stakeholders, and legal research, OSI makes the following recommendations to policymakers and officials to protect New Mexico consumers and businesses against unfair practices and billing by the air ambulance industry:

- Consider intervention in lawsuits challenging the Workers' Compensation Administration's jurisdiction to settle air ambulance fee disputes under the Airline Deregulation Act
- Consider proactive legislation/regulation under the states' McCarran-Ferguson authority to regulate the business of insurance. Proactive legislation or regulation may include, like Texas, setting a fee schedule for workers' compensation claims or dictating health insurer policy language governing fees paid by health insurers for these claims.
- Enact surprise or balance billing legislation that prohibits balance billing of insureds by health care providers, including air ambulance companies.
- Educate health care providers, including emergency doctors and hospitalists, on the impact of air ambulance charges on consumers. Provide training on the selection of in-network providers for patients needing transport.
- Evaluate the impact of any legislative or regulatory action on the provision of air ambulance services provided in the state.
- Centralize and continue communications with other states about litigation related to unfair practices by the air ambulance industry and monitor opportunities for federal class action suits."

"Taken for a Ride: Your Medical Emergency Could End in Bankruptcy" by Larry Barker, KRQE News, February 21, 2019

ALBUQUERQUE, N.M. (KRQE) - Former New Mexico Insurance Superintendent Chris Krahling calls an obscure insurance practice, "Cold. Unethical. Wrong."

We buy health insurance for protection from unforeseen medical emergencies. That's the way it's supposed to work. However, a four-month News 13 investigation has uncovered a cruel and heartless tactic that's leaving some families on the brink of bankruptcy.

[133] *See Gallup Med Flight* v. *Builders Trust of New Mexico,* D-m;-CV-2016-00394.

Melvin and Tricia Banister know the issue first hand. While working on a piece of machinery in Carlsbad last year, Melvin fell and fractured his hip.

"It's the worst pain I've ever had in my life," Melvin Banister said. "Anytime they moved me I would just start screaming and hollering because it hurt so bad."

Melvin required emergency surgery. However, the Carlsbad hospital where he was being treated did not have an on-call orthopedic surgeon.

"The E.R. doctor said that he needed to be airlifted out," Tricia Banister said. "I said, 'Can I take him by car?' And she said no. And I said, 'By ambulance?' And she said no, he needs to be airlifted."

Melvin was flown by air ambulance 160 miles to a hospital in Lubbock. He underwent surgery the next day and made a full recovery. However, the Carlsbad retiree would soon learn this ordeal was just beginning. It was triggered by an invoice that came in the mail a few weeks after Melvin's accident: a $64,999 bill for that 75-minute medical helicopter transport.

"I thought it was a crazy amount. That's just ridiculously high, and I thought the insurance would pay for it," Tricia Banister said.

The Banisters submitted the bill to their insurance company, Blue Cross Blue Shield, for payment. However, BCBS rejected the claim, sticking the Banisters with the $64,999 obligation.

In an appeal, Melvin's doctors in Carlsbad and Lubbock asked BCBS to reconsider. The doctors said Melvin needed an air ambulance because of his severe pain and need for emergency surgery.

But just because your doctor said you need a medical airlift doesn't mean the insurance company will pay for it. In this case, Blue Cross Blue Shield refused to pay the Banister's helicopter bill because, in the insurance company's opinion, an air ambulance was "not medically necessary."

It's all right there in the BCBS Benefit Book, "...Because a health care Provider prescribes, orders, recommends, or approves a service does not make it Medically Necessary... BCBSNM will determine Medical Necessity based on (stated) criteria."

According to a staff attorney in the New Mexico Insurance Superintendent's Office, Blue Cross Blue Shield is the only New Mexico insurance carrier with language in its benefit booklets giving the insurance company authority to deny coverage based on 'medical necessity.'

"It just really chaps me that with the premiums we paid, and they come up and say it's not medically necessary," Melvin Banister said. "They're not there. They're not in the emergency room. They're not the ones that see you there in pain and...they're basically second-guessing the doctors."

Former New Mexico Insurance Superintendent Chris Krahling reviewed the Banister file. Krahling is critical of Blue Cross Blue Shield for denying to pay Melvin Banister's air ambulance bill.

"The one and only person in the whole world that has the authority to determine what is medically necessary in an emergency room situation is the attending physician," Krahling said. "The insurance company doesn't have any authority to override the decision of the attending physician."

"It is not right. It's not correct. It's not fair," said John Franchini, New Mexico's current Insurance Superintendent. "My message to the insurance companies is quit deciding what is medically necessary. Let the doctors and the hospitals decide what is medically necessary."

Melvin Banister is not the only victim.

"It's devastating. I mean you end up losing sleep at night because you're wondering how in the heck am I going to be able to pay this bill," said Southeast New Mexico cotton grower Travis Ludwig.

Last summer while burning weeds at his Anthony, New Mexico farm, Travis suffered first and second degree burns over 7 percent of his body.

"I was in a lot of pain," Ludwig said. "We went to the closest hospital … on the west side of El Paso. The surgeon stated that I needed to go to a burn unit."

The nearest Burn Unit to El Paso is 300 miles.

"They put me on (an air ambulance) plane and transported me…to Lubbock, Texas," Ludwig said. "I was thinking this is probably going to be a very expensive situation. But I didn't think I had any sort of worry given the fact that I had insurance."

Little did Travis Ludwig know that one year later his insurance company, Molina Healthcare, would flat out refuse to pay the air ambulance bill leaving Travis with a $65,000 debt.

"I was flabbergasted. I just was completely floored," Ludwig said.

On appeal, Molina Healthcare reconsidered and agreed to pay a small portion of the air ambulance bill. However, Travis Ludwig was stuck with paying the balance, $55,243, out of his pocket.

It's so exorbitant, it's so unreasonable and unconscionable. How can anybody pay that? Nobody," Ludwig said.

A spokesperson for Molina Healthcare said the insurance company could not discuss its handling of the Ludwig claim.

What's going on here? Well, if you thought health insurance covers big-ticket expenses like an air ambulance, think again. In fact, in New Mexico, if you have a medical emergency and need to be transported by air, you could be stuck with the bill, and it might set you back as much as $60,000-$70,000.

"It's a huge issue in the state of New Mexico. It's at a crisis level," said Insurance Superintendent John Franchini. Franchini calls air ambulance billing practices outrageous.

"The bills are not justified. They're highway robbery. They are charging excessive amounts of money," Franchini said.

However, Air Methods, one of the largest air ambulance companies in the country, said it is not gouging consumers. Air Methods executive Doug Flanders said it costs the medical airlift firm millions of dollars to run a 24/7 New Mexico operation staffed by teams of medical and flight professionals.

"We are basically a flying ICU," Doug Flanders said. "We can do things that you can't do by ground, and we can get there quicker, thus making sure that these patients have a greater degree of success from a health care recovery."

Flanders said Air Methods loses money on 80 percent of its New Mexico transports which are primarily Medicaid, Medicare or uninsured patients. In order to stay in business, he said the unreimbursed costs are shifted to private insurance companies.

"We have to then work with the health insurance company to try to get as much reimbursement on behalf of that patient," Flanders said. "We work very hard to try to do that on a regular basis. Sometimes we're successful. Other times we're not."

In Melvin Banister's case, the air ambulance didn't actually cost $65,000. His bill was inflated to make up for all the other transports that weren't paid. When Melvin's insurance company refused to pay the bill, then Banister was on the hook for the full amount.

"When we pick (a patient) up we're hoping that the insurance is going to be able to cover their medical emergencies. If you're looking at, why do you have insurance? It's for medical emergencies," Doug Flanders said.

"We've seen an increase of 336 percent over the last four years where the insurance company will receive the claim and then say, 'this was not medically necessary, the doctor who deemed this medically necessary was incorrect,' and they would deny the claim," Flanders said.

"What that means to the patient is then they are now stuck in the middle because the insurance company has said 'sorry, but the care you received is not medically necessary, so therefore, you now have to pick up the bill,'" Flanders said.

A spokesperson for Blue Cross Blue Shield of New Mexico said some 'out of market' air ambulance bills are unreasonably high. BCBSNM said it is in negotiations with Air Methods to arrive at a negotiated rate so that policyholders are not stuck with huge bills.

Despite the excessive charges and insurance company fine print, you can fight back. Melvin Banister and Travis Ludwig challenged their air ambulance bills and appealed their cases to New Mexico's Insurance Superintendent. Ultimately, Banister and Ludwig won their cases and got their air ambulance charges reversed.

"A lot of people just give up and pay it," Melvin Banister said. "I've made up my mind that I wouldn't just give up and pay it. I was going to fight them to the bitter end," the retired Carlsbad businessman said.

Travis Ludwig wonders, which was worse, the accident or the bill? "I would say they were pretty neck and neck because it only took me a month to get over the physical pain, but the mental anguish created many a sleepless night for me."

Statement from Blue Cross and Blue Shield of New Mexico

As it relates to air ambulance companies, noncontracted rates are generally much higher when compared to Commercial contracted rates and Medicaid and Medicare rates.

As an example, a noncontracted air ambulance company liftoff rate can be $30,000 or higher. When mileage rates of $250 per mile for noncontracted air ambulance companies are added to the liftoff rate, we have seen total charges up to $65,000 for relatively short flights.

That is compared to liftoff rates for Medicaid and Medicare that range from about $1,800 to $4,000. When mileage rates ranging from $7 to $35 per mile are added in, total charges for a similar flight would more likely be in the range of $6,500.

Contracted air ambulance companies include San Juan Regional Medical Center AirCare, CSI Aviation Inc., Med Flight Air Ambulance, University of New Mexico Hospital's Lifeguard Air Emergency Services, Critical Air Response Enterprises, PHI Air Medical, and Southwest Med. Evac. Inc.

List of Air Ambulance Cases in the Office of the New Mexico Superintendent of Insurance as of August 2018

TH New Mexico Health Connections NMHC,
Air Ambulance Provider: Mercy Air Service

Grievant TH filed a complaint against NMHC. TH is being balance billed for $37,579.77. NMHC paid Mercy Air Service $15,920.45. Total bill for the services provided by Mercy Air Service is $53,500.22. Grievant was transported from Pahrump, Nevada to University Medical Center, Las Vegas, NV for treatment of a gunshot wound to the right knee (traumatic injury).

This appeal was for two fixed wing air ambulance transports. In May, JG was transported due to altered mental status after being found unresponsive in his home. In June, JG was reported to have epilepticus with seizures for two hours or more and needed large doses of benzodiazepines. Dr. H ordered air transport from Silver City to the Tucson AZ Medical Center for neurology specialty services, as the specialty services were unavailable at the sending facility. JG was transported 166 miles.

Total Bill: $82,645.00

As of September 11, 2018, a Post Service Internal Review of Adverse Determination approved the reprocessing of these claims.

TL Molina,
Air Ambulance Provider: Rocky Mountain Holdings, LLC

The total initial bill is $64,999.00. Molina is paying $8,755.86 and the grievant has a co-insurance responsibility of $2,188.96, with an unpaid balance of $54,054.18. TL was transported by ground ambulance from The Hospitals of Providence Transmountain Campus to El Paso International Airport El Paso, TX, then transported by air to Lubbock Preston Smith International Airport Lubbock, TX, then transported by ground to University Medical Center (UMC) of Lubbock: TL was transported from El Paso due to 1st degree burns to his cheek and 2nd degree burns to right hand and upper leg. Airtime is 70 minutes and ground is 360 minutes. Molina stated that they reached out to their UM Department to review the claim submission.

YS New Mexico Health Connections
Air Ambulance Provider: PHI Air Medical

YS was transported by ground to the Presbyterian Emergency Room in Socorro where she was diagnosed with a brain aneurysm and then air lifted to UNMH, Albuquerque due to the severity of the bleeding in the brain. YS remained in Neuro ICU for thirteen days.

Dr. TB ordered the air transport and YS was transported 76 miles. YS filed a complaint against NMHC. YS is being balance billed $30,526.56. NMHC paid PHI Air Medical $16,559.44. Total bill for the services provided by PHI Air Medical $47,186.00.

PA New Mexico Health Connections,
Air Ambulance Provider: Rocky Mountain Holdings, LLC

PA transported by air from Roswell, NM to Albuquerque, NM for treatment of a wrist fracture (Subdural hernatoma-HCC); comminuted intra-articular minimally displaced fracture involving the distal radius, with accompanying fracture fragment of the ulnar styloid. There were degenerative changes at the base of the thumb. The amount of the total bill is $64,999.00. NMHC paid $20,113.63 and the unpaid balance is $44,785.37.

KS BCBSNM,
Air Ambulance Provider: PHI Air Medical, LLC

KS was seen in the ER and had obstructed right pyelonephritis associated with right ureteral stone, along with ESBL bacteremia and Nephrolithiasis. Dr. B ordered air transport from Gallup, NM to UNMH in Albuquerque, NM. The total balance of the bill is $62,363.05, Discounts, reductions and payments applied $1,593.05, and the amount not covered $60,770.00.

Statement for the Record of the National Observation Stays Coalition to the U.S. House of Representatives, Committee on Energy and Commerce, Subcommittee on Health Hearing, "No More Surprises: Protecting Patients from Surprise Medical Bills," June 12, 2019

Chairwoman Eshoo, Representative Burgess, and distinguished Members of the Health Subcommittee, thank you for the opportunity to share the perspectives of the Observation Stays Coalition as the Subcommittee examines protecting patients from surprise medical bills.

The undersigned organizations of the Observation Stays Coalition have come together to address a surprise medical billing issue that affects Medicare patients in hospitals who are called observation status patients or outpatients, although the medically necessary care they need and receive is no different from the medically necessary care provided to formally admitted inpatients. The classification as observation or outpatient is significant, however, because the Medicare statute covers a post-hospital stay in a skilled nursing facility only if the patient was hospitalized for three consecutive days as an *inpatient*.

Recent efforts have focused on eliminating burden and unanticipated/surprise medical bills that are having a significant negative impact on out-of-pocket-costs and patient-provider relationship. The observation stays matter is one such area that should be addressed as part of comprehensive efforts to eliminate surprise medical bills. Counting observation status toward the 3-day inpatient requirement in the Medicare program is a common-sense policy that does not affect hospital care – but does protect the ability of beneficiaries to receive needed postacute nursing home care.

Earlier this Congress, the bipartisan legislation *Improving Access to Medicare Coverage Act* (H.R. 1682/S. 753), sponsored by Representatives Courtney and 'GT' Thompson and Senators Brown, Collins, Whitehouse, and Capito, was re-introduced to update a current loophole in Medicare policy that would help protect seniors from high – and often – surprise medical costs for the skilled nursing facility care they require after hospitalization. The *Improving Access to Medicare Coverage Act* would allow for the time patients spend in the hospital under "observation status" to count toward the requisite three-day hospital stay for coverage of skilled nursing care. This legislative fix is important for several reasons, including the fact that our nation's most vulnerable seniors could be surprised with high out-of-pocket costs due to being admitted to the hospital under observation status.

There are currently 33 national beneficiary and provider organizations that support this legislation, and it is our hope that this issue gets addressed in this Congress. Unfortunately, there have been countless heart-wrenching stories from older people and their families who have had to pay high out-of-pocket charges since they were deemed to be on observation status, and Medicare did not cover their necessary skilled nursing facility care. Often, these individuals didn't even know they were on observation status – or know to ask. But even if they received and understood the Medicare Outpatient Observation Notice (MOON), required by the Notice of Observation Treatment and Implication for Care Eligibility Act (NOTICE Act) and advising them of their outpatient status, they have no right to appeal and to request that their status be changed to inpatient.

It is simply not right to limit access to quality care for those most in need. Now is the time for Congress to pass legislation that addresses this issue once and for all. Thank you again for the opportunity to weigh in on this important matter. The Coalition looks forward to working with Members of Congress in both chambers on the observation stays issue.

Sincerely,
American Association of Healthcare Administrative Management (AAHAM)
American Association of Post-Acute Care Nursing (AAPACN)
American Case Management Association (ACMA)
Aging Life Care Association®
American Geriatrics Society (AGS) American Health Care
Association (AHCA) Association of Jewish Aging Services (AJAS)
Alliance for Retired Americans
AMDA - The Society for Post-Acute and Long-Term Care Medicine
American Physical Therapy Association (APTA)
Center for Medicare Advocacy
The Jewish Federations of North America Justice in Aging
LeadingAge
National Academy of Elder Law Attorneys, Inc. (NAELA)
National Association of Area Agencies on Aging (n4a)
National Association of Health Care Assistants (NAHCA)
National Association of State Long-Term Care Ombudsman Programs (NASOP)
National Association for the Support of Long Term Care (NASL)
National Center for Assisted Living (NCAL)
National Committee to Preserve Social Security & Medicare
The National Consumer Voice for Quality Long-Term Care
Society of Hospital Medicine (SHM)
Special Needs Alliance

Statement for the Record of the American Medical Association, to the U.S. House of Representatives, Committee on Energy and Commerce, Subcommittee on Health, Re: Protecting Patients from Surprise Medical Bills, June 11, 2019

The American Medical Association (AMA) appreciates the opportunity to provide testimony to the U.S. House of Representatives Committee on Ways and Means Health Subcommittee as part of the hearing titled, "Protecting Patients from Surprise Medical Bills," and to offer our perspective on the important issue of unanticipated out-of-network care and solutions to protect patients from the financial impact of "surprise" coverage gaps.

The focus of most congressional discussions and state legislative efforts has been on the specific coverage gap that occurs when a patient unexpectedly receives out-of-network care during a scheduled procedure at an in-network hospital or receives out-of-network care in an emergency situation. As such, our testimony offers solutions that address those narrow situations.

It is important, however, to view this issue as a subset of the coverage gaps and unanticipated medical bills that are plaguing patients and families. Recent efforts to lower health care premiums have induced the rise of high deductible, narrow network, and other limited plan options that may increasingly leave patients with health care bills their insurer will not pay. Moreover, patients are increasingly coming face-to-face with payer policies that attempt to inappropriately narrow the scope of the coverage they purchased. For example, a major health insurer implemented a policy in several states last year that forced patients to pay out-of-pocket for emergency care if the insurer retroactively determined that the patient was not, in fact, experiencing an emergency based on the final diagnosis.

The problem of unanticipated out-of-network bills is complex and requires a balanced approach to resolve. The AMA agrees that any solution must keep patients out of the middle of payment rate negotiations and ensure that when patients seek emergency care or otherwise do not have the opportunity to select their provider, they should not be responsible for cost sharing beyond what they would face if they had seen an in-network provider. Any proposed solutions should also require both providers and insurers to be transparent about anticipated charges and the amount of those charges that insurance will cover. We also agree that in these cases balance billing the patient should be banned if there is a process in place to ensure that providers receive fair reimbursement for their services.

Specific to the issue of surprise billing, the AMA has long been working with our colleagues in the states, calling for patient-centered solutions that prevent patients from receiving unanticipated out-of-network care and balance bills associated with that care. The AMA encourages Congress to look to states that have already acted to address unanticipated medical bills, specifically those state laws that are functioning well such as those in New York and Connecticut. The AMA is committed to working with Congress to find a fair solution for all stakeholders that protects patients from unanticipated out-of-network bills.

Key Principles in Addressing Unanticipated Out-of-Network Medical Bills

Fair and workable solutions to unanticipated out-of-network care can come in many forms. The AMA believes that the best solutions have several common principles at their cores.

- *Protect patients.* The AMA supports solutions that keep patients out of the middle of payment rate negotiations. In situations where patients do not have the opportunity to select an in-network provider, they should not be charged any more than the in-network amount. Moreover, payments should count toward their deductibles and out-of-pocket maximums.
- *Network regulation.* Critical to any solution is a focus on increasing the adequacy of provider networks, especially when it comes to hospital-based providers. Network adequacy standards should require, at a minimum, an adequate ratio of physicians, including hospital-based physicians and on-call specialists and subspecialists, to patients, as well as geographic and driving distance standards and maximum wait times. Regulation should also include the active evaluation of networks to determine access to in-network, hospital-based care at participating hospitals.
- *Fair payment to providers.* To ensure that appropriate market incentives remain in place, any solution must incorporate a mechanism to ensure fair payment to providers. Such mechanisms could include a minimum payment standard based on physicians' rates and/or a binding arbitration process that requires the consideration of a number of market-related factors.
- *Transparency.* Any solution to address unanticipated medical bills must also require transparency so that all patients who choose in advance to obtain scheduled care from out-of-network physicians, hospitals, or other providers are informed prior to receiving care about their anticipated out-of-pocket costs, scope of their coverage, and breadth of their provider network. When scheduling services for patients, providers should be transparent about their own anticipated charges.

Nearly all stakeholders agree that patients should be financially protected from these specific out-of-network bills and that transparency is an important component of a solution, though not a solution in-and-of-itself. However, disagreement among stakeholders has most heavily surrounded the two middle principles we identify above. As such, we would like to provide additional detail as to the importance of addressing these issues in any federal legislation.

Facilitating In-Network Contracting

It is important to recognize that most physicians want to be included in payers' networks, if fair contracts are offered; however, many physicians are in a weak bargaining position relative to commercial health insurers. The majority of health insurance markets are highly concentrated and characterized by insurers with high market shares of patients.[134] This increases the risk of those insurers exercising monopsony power and paying physicians below competitive levels. Moreover, given that 56.5 percent of physicians providing patient care are in practices with 10 or fewer physicians, physicians are regularly in a weak bargaining position relative to

---

[134] American Medical Association. *Competition in Health Insurance, A Comprehensive Study of U.S. Markets, 2018* Update. https://www.ama-assn.org/system/files/2018-11/competition-health-insurance-us-markets_1.pdf. Publish ed 2018.

commercial health insurers.[135] We therefore urge Congress to incentivize insurers to come to the negotiating table with physicians and offer fair contracts. The most promising way for policymakers to facilitate contracting between providers and health plans is to ensure regulation of provider networks. Strong network adequacy requirements create a more balanced environment for all stakeholders where: insurers are incented to maintain meaningful access to in-network providers by offering providers competitive contracts; providers are incented to come to the table knowing that it will be a fairer process; and patients will have access to in-network care and get greater value for their premiums paid.

While there has been a great deal of discussion about the growth of narrower provider networks, relatively little has been done to create or enforce network adequacy requirements, especially as they relate to hospital-based providers. Moreover, ensuring that patients have appropriate access to primary and specialty care will go a long way in preventing emergency department visits and other hospitalizations that may lead to unanticipated, out-of-network bills.

The basis of network adequacy standards should be quantitative, measurable requirements on the front-end, before insurance products are brought to market. The quantitative standards should include minimum time and distance requirements, maximum patients-to-provider ratios, and maximum wait times. In addition, and specific for hospital-based specialties, it is critical that standards also measure access to in-network physicians at in-network hospitals.

Meaningful regulation of provider networks must also be ongoing. Consistent monitoring of the network's ability to provide in-network, hospital-based care is particularly important, given that patients may not evaluate access to these providers simply through a directory or other tool, as is normally the case when choosing a provider.

Finally, it is important to recognize the connection between accurate provider directories and meaningful access to in-network providers for patients. The AMA encourages greater oversight of provider directories and stronger requirements that they be transparent and up-to-date. Patients need access to robust, up-to-date provider directories to enable them to determine which providers are in-network as they purchase their plans, and which providers continue to be in-network as their medical needs change.

Additionally, providers need accurate information from health plans to allow for in-network referrals when further treatment is needed.

Some have recently attempted to separate the issue of network adequacy with that of surprise billing, suggesting that surprise billing solutions should solely be stopgap measures, retroactively addressing the network failure. However, we believe this is an oversimplified view and devalues the goal of reducing the frequency of surprise bills. Our views are shared by the nation's insurance regulators, who prominently addressed the issue of unanticipated out-of-network care in the National Association of Insurance Commissioners' (NAICs) recently revised model legislation on network adequacy regulation.[136] The NAIC noted that the revised model legislation "establishes strong standards for network adequacy, while balancing the need for states to establish specific standards that are effective for their markets and geography."[137]

[135] Kane C. Updated Data on Physician Practice Arrangements: For the First Time, Fewer Physicians are Owners Than Employees. *Policy Research Perspectives*, 2019. https://www.ama-assn.org/system/files/2019-05/prp-fewer-owners-benchmark-survey-2018.pdf. Published May 2019.

[136] https://www.naic.org/store/free/MDL-74.pdf.

[137] https://www.naic.org/cipr_topics/topic_network_adequacy.htm.

Payment for Out-of-Network Providers

In general, the AMA urges Congress to avoid any solutions that set minimum payment standards for out-of-network care at noncompetitive rates. Any guidelines on out-of-network provider payment should reflect actual charge data for the same service in the same geographic area and should not be based on a percentage of Medicare rates, which have become increasingly inadequate in covering overhead costs, or be based on in-network rates, as such a standard would eliminate the incentive for insurers to create adequate networks and negotiate contracts in good faith.

Negotiated Rates

Some proposals to establish a payment standard point to in-network rates as a benchmark for provider payment. Such rates are negotiated by physicians and insurance plans during the contracting process and physicians agree to significantly discount their fees in exchange for contracted benefits, such as increased patient volume, being listed in the plan's provider directory, and prompt payment of claims.

Setting out-of-network payments at those discounted rates would place physicians at a competitive disadvantage when the attempt to negotiate a fair contract, especially when the repercussions of limited networks on plans have been removed. It also further disrupts the increasing market imbalance favoring health insurers. Moreover, proposals often use the "average" in-network rate or a percentage of the in-network rate. This is incredibly problematic for those physicians who have negotiated contracts for amounts above the mean, as a health plan would have an incentive to quickly drop a physician from the plan's network knowing they could use the physician's services for less when the physician is outside their network.

Medicare Rates

Medicare payment rates should not be considered as a benchmark standard. Medicare payment rates would be even more problematic than using in-network rates in terms of incenting insurers to fairly contract—they simply do not reflect the costs of providing care, especially in the commercial market where the population varies greatly.

Medicare uses the resource-based relative value scale system to establish physician payments, determined by the resource costs associated with the total amount of physician resources required to provide a specific service. However, before Medicare rates are finalized, they go through adjustment and conversion processes to meet federal budgetary requirements. Adjustments are done in a budget neutral manner, meaning that if an adjustment increases the payment for one service, it must account for this increase by decreasing payment for another service. This establishes artificial decreases in payment for many physician services ever year. And before the final Medicare payment is set, geographically adjusted values are multiplied by a conversion factor—a monetary payment determined by Medicare each year that changes based on the Medicare economic index, adjustments pertaining to budget neutrality, and other adjustments stipulated by legislation. After everything is complete, the resulting payment rates are not reflective of markets rates for physician services.

As illustrated by the chart below, Medicare physician payments have not kept up with inflation over the past decade. According to data from the Medicare Trustees, Medicare physician pay has barely changed over the last decade and a half, increasing just six percent from 2001 to 2018, or just 0.4 percent per year on average. And, under the Medicare Access and CHIP Reauthorization Act (MACRA), physician payment rates will be frozen for calendars years 2020 through 2025.

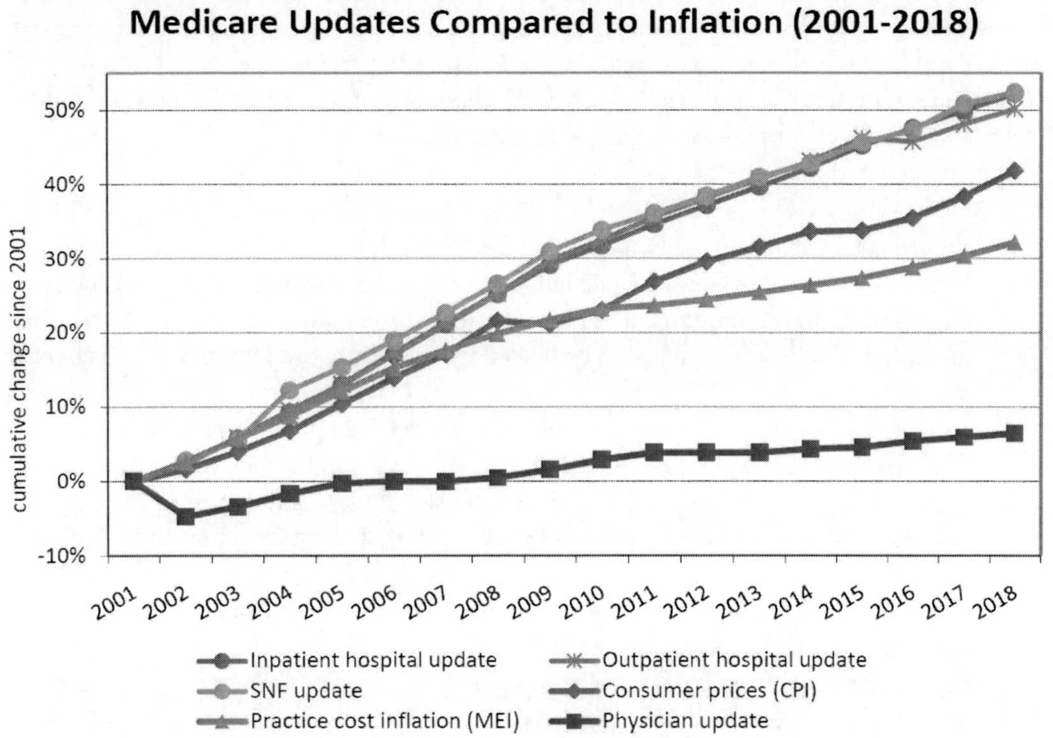

In comparison, the cost of running a medical practice increased 32 percent between 2001 and 2018, or 1.7 percent per year.[138] In addition economy-wide inflation, as measured the Consumer Price Index, increased 42 percent over this time period (or 2.1 percent per year, on average). Over time, the adequacy of Medicare physician payment rates has eroded significantly. Adjusted for inflation in practice costs, Medicare physician pay declined 19 percent from 2001 to 2018, or by 1.3 percent per year on average. As such, the AMA opposes efforts to cap or benchmark out-of-network physician payments on a percentage of Medicare. Linking out-of-network rates to Medicare would eliminate any incentive for insurers to build adequate networks or offer physicians fair contracts.

Arbitration

The AMA urges consideration of structured binding arbitration to help determine a fair payment, either as a backstop when a set payment standard is inappropriate for a particular case, or potentially as a way to achieve fair payment when informal negotiations between insurers and providers fail. Successful implementation of this approach would require an

[138] Inflation in the cost of running a medical practice, including increases in physician office rent, employee wages, and professional liability insurance premiums, is measured by the Medicare Economic Index or MEI.

arbitrator to have expertise in medical billing and the health care system, as well as guidelines that includes reference to a percentile of charges for the particular service in the same geographic area as reported by an independent database. A solution that incorporates arbitration, including so-call "baseball style" arbitration, also has the potential to encourage parties to reach agreement outside of and before the arbitration process if structured appropriately. We encourage the Committee to work with providers on an arbitration model that considers a number of market-related factors, such as the complexity of the patient's medical condition, the special expertise required, comorbidities, and other extraordinary factors. Perhaps the most successful state law addressing surprise billing, New York's 2014 law, uses an arbitration-based model, and has an impressive track record in protecting both patients and incentives for physicians and plans to negotiate.

Specifically the law:

- Protects patients from unanticipated out-of-network bills.
- Emphasizes the role of network adequacy in solving the "surprise" billing problem and puts in place new requirements to regulate networks and affords patients the right to an independent external appeal to be treated by a non-network provider if the network is inadequate.
- Establishes a strong independent dispute resolution (IDR) process made by a reviewer with training and experience in health care billing, reimbursement, and usual and customary charges in consultation with a licensed physician in active practice in the same or similar specialty as the physician providing the service that is the subject of the dispute.
- Requires that the IDR process incorporate the consideration of factors, including the rate that non-participating physicians charge for the service in the area based on independent data, usual and customary charge for the service based on independent data, the complexity of the case, and the physician's experience, training and education.

A study released last week by Georgetown University Health Policy Institute and the Robert Wood John Foundation,[139] reports that New York state officials have seen a dramatic decline in consumer complaints about balance billing since enactment, with one regulator stating to researchers that the law has "downgraded the issue from one of the biggest [consumer concerns out call center receives] to barely an issue."

Meanwhile, the study points to nearly evenly split numbers in IDR decisions among physicians and insurers and reports among stakeholders that physicians and insurance are incented to work out their payment disputes before filing with IDR. And, importantly, the study notes that regulators report there has not been any indication of an inflationary effect in insurers' annual premium rate filings.

[139] https://georgetown.app.box.com/s/6onkj1jaiy3f1618iy7j0gpzdoew2zu9.

Independent Data

The AMA is concerned with proposals that allow insurers to develop benchmarks using internal data or data controlled by health insurance plans. Such proposals represent a significant step backwards in efforts to promote fairness and transparency in the health care system, especially with health care costs.

Moreover, using insurer-controlled data to determine out-of-network benchmarks opens the door for manipulation and consumer harm. For example, in 2009 a report from the New York Attorney General and a preceding settlement between United Health Group and the AMA, the Medical Society of the State of New York, and the Missouri State Medical Association, illustrated the dangers of using data controlled by insurers to set benchmarks for reimbursement rates. The New York Attorney General concluded that, because United Health Group owned Ingenix (the database used nationwide by health plans to set out-of-network benchmarks), there was an inherent conflict of interest. By using a flawed and conflicted database to determine reimbursement rates for out-of-network care, insurers were increasing profits at the expense of patients and physicians. In order to avoid this conflict, the report stated that "market rates for health care charges should be determined by an independent third party free of conflicts of interest, using a fair, objective, and reliable database."[140] Given this history of data manipulation, the AMA urges Congress to require that an independent data source be used for any benchmarking that is including in a surprise billing solution.

The AMA was pleased to see funding in the Chairman and Ranking Member's draft legislation for state all payer claims databases (APCDs). The AMA believes that APCDs have the potential to play an important role in establishing out-of-network payment benchmarks and advancing price transparency, as well as assisting policymakers in understanding price variation, trends in costs and gaps in coverage. Beyond the scope of this legislation, APCDs' data can also be excellent tools for studying utilization trends, health care disparities, alternative payment models and population health. As such, we would encourage your committee to allow states to mandate submission of data from federally-regulated health plans to APCDs. We believe that states' ability to create complete datasets that include data from federally regulated plans is critical to the viability of these databases.

Conclusion

The AMA thanks the Subcommittee for this hearing and for your commitment to addressing the problems associated with unanticipated out-of-network care. We welcome the opportunity to work with the Subcommittee and Congress to draft legislation that will both protect patients and promote greater access to in-network care.

---

[140] https://ag.ny.gov/sites/default/files/pdfs/bureaus/health_care/FINALHITIngenixReportJan.13,%202009.pdf.

Statement for the Record of the College of American Pathologists to the U.S. House of Representatives, Committee on Energy and Commerce, Subcommittee on Health Hearing, "No More Surprises: Protecting Patients from Surprise Medical Bills," June 12, 2019

COLLEGE of AMERICAN PATHOLOGISTS

Statement for the Record
United States House Committee on Energy and Commerce
Subcommittee on Health
No More Surprises: Protecting Patients from Surprise Medical Bills

June 12, 2019

Statement by
College of American Pathologists

The College of American Pathologists (CAP) appreciates the opportunity to share our comments in response to the committee's hearing on surprise out-of-network medical bills. We appreciate the discussion of this important issue so that all stakeholders can work together to protect patients and ensure continued access to high-quality health care. The CAP has been constructively engaged on this issue for many years. It has always been our position that patients should not be financially penalized for the failure of health insurance plans to provide in-network access to hospital-based physician specialties.

As the world's largest organization of board-certified pathologists and leading provider of laboratory accreditation and proficiency testing programs, the CAP serves patients, pathologists, and the public by fostering and advocating excellence in the practice of pathology and laboratory medicine worldwide. The CAP believes that to protect patients from gaps in their health insurance coverage, insurers and providers should settle all payments without the patient's involvement, even if an independent arbitrator settles disputes. Network adequacy standards for health plans should be set, and at a minimum, there should be network standards for ensuring that an appropriate number of specialty physicians are available to provide medically necessary services at "in-network" facilities. Additionally, it is critically important that out-of-network payment mechanisms not in any way deter, displace, or discourage equitable contracting for physician services, as we believe such contracting is critical to maintaining the private commercial marketplace that consumers wish to avail. Finally, any reimbursement for out-of-network services should be based on the market value of physician services according to commercial data compiled by independent, non-affiliated organizations, like FAIR Health Inc. or a state's all-payor claims database (APCD). For these reasons, we urge a fully deliberative and engaged physician specialty stakeholder process, as has occurred to date in multiple states, to produce an optimal legislative outcome that protects patients and preserves the non-governmental health care marketplace.

College of American Pathologists
1001 G Street, NW, Suite 425W
Washington, DC 20001
202-354-7100

COLLEGE of AMERICAN PATHOLOGISTS

Remove burden of surprise bills from patients

Limiting unexpected patient cost sharing is an essential part of any congressional action. Through no fault of their own, patients are caught off guard when an insurer doesn't cover certain physician services. Patients do not need additional financial stress when they are at their most vulnerable. Congress should create a system whereby insurers and providers can come to agreement independent of the patient, who should only pay for care at an in-network rate.

Alternative dispute resolution (ADR) can help address this problem when set up appropriately. If there is a dispute over payment between an insurer and provider, an independent arbitrator can step in and consider several factors pertaining to the case. An arbitrator should be able to consider things like complexity and duration, but also other factors that either the insurer or provider may submit. Parameters that include geographically-based charges by providers and payments from insurers should be used in order to determine the fair market value of the physician service. It is imperative that in-network rates not be an exclusive factor in determining a starting point or an outcome for any arbitrator, as this would immediately bias the process and defeat the goal of the ADR option.

Several states have policies that protect patients from out-of-network bills resulting from gaps in health insurance plan contracting. States with laws that are reasonable and that appropriately protect patients include: Arizona, New Jersey, Maryland, Massachusetts, Illinois, Minnesota, Florida, Washington, and New Hampshire.

In particular, the law enacted by New York State is the optimal approach to protect patients from surprise medical billing. In New York, patients are financially held harmless and there is an effective method for resolving disputes between providers and insurance plan payers. Further, not only is there mediation/arbitration between insurers and providers, but the payment methodology upon which the "usual and customary rate" (UCR) is calculated is based upon the 80th percentile of FAIR health database charges to reflect the market value of physician services. Most importantly, it is clear this approach is working. Researchers at Georgetown University recently determined that "insurer, provider, and consumer stakeholders generally agree that the implementation of New York's Surprise Billing law went smoothly, was relatively fair to all parties, and is working as intended to protect consumers from a significant source of financial hardship."[1] The Georgetown study also notes that state officials have reported a dramatic decline in consumer complaints about balance billing and physicians are largely satisfied with the process and its results. Finally, concerns about inflated charges are thus far proven unfounded, as the Georgetown researchers cited a study that found

[1] https://georgetown.app.box.com/s/6onkj1jaiy3f1618iy7j0gpzdoew2zu9

College of American Pathologists
1001 G Street, NW, Suite 425W
Washington, DC 20001
202-354-7100

COLLEGE of AMERICAN PATHOLOGISTS

a 13 percent average reduction in physician payments since the law was enacted in New York.

Enact network adequacy standards

The CAP strongly believes inadequate networks are the root cause of surprise bills. Unfortunately, many of the legislative proposals released do nothing to address the issue. Without adequate networks of contracted physicians, a patient cannot be properly guarded from out-of-network health care at an in-network facility. If there are fewer out-of-network providers to begin with, there will be fewer patients receiving their bills.

It is important to recognize that the vast majority of providers, including pathologists, wish to contract with health plans. Health plans have deliberately and systematically denied network participation to, or ejected pathologists and clinical laboratories from network participation, and states are starting to take notice. In December of 2017, the Washington State insurance commissioner fined a health insurer $1.5 million and detailed steps it must take to fix its provider networks. Most recently, in Texas, the Center for Public Policy Priorities reported in 2014 that one health plan in the state had no pathologist providers at 20 percent of their in-network hospitals. Then, in October 2018, this health plan was fined $700,000 by the Texas Department of Insurance for failure to contract with a hospital-based physician specialty in multiple counties.

The CAP supports federal enactment of network adequacy requirements similar to the law of Louisiana (Network Adequacy Act 22§1019.1 et seq,) that expressly require health insurance plans to "maintain a network of providers that includes but is not limited to providers that specialize in mental health and substance abuse services, facility-based physicians, and providers that are essential community providers." Facility-based physicians are defined in the Louisiana Act to include: "anesthesiologist, hospitalist, intensivist, neonatologist, pathologist, radiologist, emergency room physician, or other on-call physician, who is required by the base health care facility to provide covered health care." Such requirements should be subject to regulatory oversight and enforcement to ensure that patients have reasonable and timely access to in-network physician specialists at in-network hospitals and facilities. California (Code of Regulations (CCR) Title 10, Section 2240.5 (d) (14)) and New Hampshire (RSA 420.J:7 II(e)) are two other states with specific hospital-based physician network adequacy requirements. However, at present, the vast majority of states have no such hospital-based physician network adequacy requirement and thus should be compelled under federal law to adopt such requirements.

Of note, transparency alone cannot solve the surprise bill problem for patients, as many physician services are unexpected and cannot be anticipated by the patient. For example, the type of specimen or complexity of the analysis done by the pathologist is often not known in advance of the initial microscopic analysis, making it impossible to provide a reliable estimate of charges or costs. Moreover, patients under anesthesia during a procedure cannot exercise choice or control over pathology or laboratory

College of American Pathologists
1001 G Street, NW, Suite 425W
Washington, DC 20001
202-354-7100

COLLEGE of AMERICAN PATHOLOGISTS

referrals. Thus, creating regulatory standards that require health insurance plans to contract with the requisite number of providers covering the full array of physician care at an in-network facility, including pathology and laboratory services, is a more appropriate component of the solution to reduce surprise bills.

Fair reimbursement for out-of-network services

In order to encourage health plans to contract for physician services, and to ensure that the health care delivery system is financially viable, a fair market rate should be paid for physician services. In general, caps on payment for physicians treating out-of-network patients should be avoided. If pursued, guidelines or limits on what out-of-network providers are paid should reflect actual charge data for the same service in the same geographic area from a statistically significant and wholly independent database.

Further, if in-network rates are used as a benchmark for payment, insurers have a clear economic incentive to lower rates without any constraint and have the unilateral ability to do so.

Several proposals from Congress rely on a median in-network rate to determine payment to providers delivering care to out-of-network patients. **The CAP opposes the use of a rate that can be wholly controlled by the health insurance industry**. In the end, it is important to remember that it is doctors who care for patients, not insurance companies. Any prohibition, whether state or federal, on out-of-network billing should be paired with a corresponding payment process that is keyed to the market value of physician services.

A caution regarding price transparency

A lack of information about the cost of health care services can be an impediment to transparency and patient empowerment, but the CAP generally opposes adding additional administrative requirements on physicians that interfere with or impair the patient's medical diagnosis and care. Transparency alone cannot solve the surprise bill problem for patients, as many physician services are unexpected and cannot be anticipated by the patient.

Specifically, we wish to emphasize the unique difficulty that pathologists have in providing patients with information about out-of-pocket costs in advance of services. For instance, a surgical or invasive diagnostic procedure performed by a dermatologist, surgeon, gastroenterologist, urologist, or other clinician may result in no specimens obtained or it may result in multiple specimens requiring anatomic evaluation. Additionally, anatomic pathology services typically involve a pathologist performing microscopic analysis of tissue or body fluids to determine whether cancer or other disease is present and, if so, its characteristics. The type of specimen or complexity of the analysis is often unknown in advance of the initial microscopic analysis conducted by the pathologist, making it impossible to provide a reliable estimate of charges or costs.

College of American Pathologists
1001 G Street, NW, Suite 425W
Washington, DC 20001
202-354-7100

COLLEGE of AMERICAN PATHOLOGISTS

Providers should be transparent about their own anticipated charges at the time of scheduling, and insurers should be transparent about the amount of those charges they will cover. However, in going any further, the difficulty of price transparency poses administrative hurdles and significant risk for patient harm from any delays.

Summary

As the committee moves to address the issue of surprise billing, it is of paramount importance to strike a compromise that holds patients harmless but also allows providers and insurers to come to agreement on outstanding bills. The CAP would be supportive of a legislative proposal that includes:

1.) Language that holds patients harmless and enacts a process, like ADR, that allows insurers and providers to settle any billing disputes without involving the patient;
2.) Network adequacy standards that ensure a proper number of physicians can provide services at in-network facilities; and
3.) If necessary, a payment benchmark that precludes the unilateral ability of health insurance plan to determine payment as would be the case with in-network rates. Instead, there must be a balance of geographic rates from an independent database to either inform an arbitrator in an ADR process or to ensure that the commercial value of the service is considered in determining payment.

Specifically, the CAP is supportive of the direction of the section-by-section legislative proposal released by Representatives Raul Ruiz, M.D., and Phil Roe, M.D., that addresses surprise billing. The solutions as proposed would take necessary steps to accomplish the goals of holding patients financially harmless from surprise medical bills while creating a fair reimbursement system that keeps patients out of the middle of billing disputes. The CAP is pleased to see inclusion of a baseball-style arbitration process that allows consideration for a range of factors, including the usual and customary rate that reflects the market value of physician services. Although the proposal does not address network adequacy, we appreciate that the proposal's goal of avoiding the use of a rate that could be wholly controlled by insurers.

Thank you for your consideration of this important issue and we look forward to working with your committee to come up with the best solution for ensuring patients have in-network access to physician services or are otherwise protected from out-of-network charges that result from health plan inadequacies. The CAP urges the committee to work with Representatives Ruiz and Roe on their proposal to address surprise billing. If you would like to meet, or have any questions, please contact Sarah Bogdan, Assistant Director, Legislation and Political Action, at Sbogdan@cap.org or 202-354-7106.

The College of American Pathologists

College of American Pathologists
1001 G Street, NW, Suite 425W
Washington, DC 20001
202-354-7100

Statement for the Record of the Association of American Medical Colleges, et al., to the U.S. House of Representatives, Committee on Energy and Commerce, Subcommittee on Health Hearing, "No More Surprises: Protecting Patients from Surprise Medical Bills," June 12, 2019

AAMC

Association of
American Medical Colleges
655 K Street, NW, Suite 100, Washington, DC 20001-2399
T 202 828 0400
aamc.org

Statement for the Record
of the
Association of American Medical Colleges
for the
Committee on Energy and Commerce
Subcommittee on Health
of the
U.S. House of Representatives
"No More Surprises: Protecting Patients from Surprise Medical Bills."
June 12, 2019

The Association of American Medical Colleges (AAMC) appreciates the opportunity to provide testimony and the perspective of academic medicine for this hearing on protecting patients from surprise medical bills.

The AAMC is a not-for-profit association dedicated to transforming health care through innovative medical education, cutting-edge patient care, and groundbreaking medical research. Its members are all 154 accredited U.S. medical schools; nearly 400 major teaching hospitals and health systems, including 51 Department of Veterans Affairs medical centers; and more than 80 academic societies. Through these institutions and organizations, the AAMC serves the leaders of America's medical schools and teaching hospitals and their more than 173,000 full-time faculty members, 89,000 medical students, 129,000 resident physicians, and more than 60,000 graduate students and postdoctoral researchers in the biomedical sciences.

A surprise medical bill can occur when a patient receives out-of-network emergency care, or when they receive an unexpected bill for care that they thought was covered by their health plan. These surprise bills can deeply financially impact patients, and ultimately undermine academic medicine's core mission of providing outstanding patient care, by introducing an element of uncertainty into the provider-patient relationship.

Thus, the AAMC firmly believes that patients should be protected from surprise medical bills, and that they should be removed from surprise billing disputes. Teaching hospitals often are where individuals present when experiencing an emergency and these patients are at their most vulnerable while seeking and receiving emergency medical services. They should not incur the additional stress of being balance billed when they were unable to choose a provider that would have been in network. Additionally, the AAMC does not believe that patients should be balance billed for services that they could not have reasonably known would be out-of-network, particularly when they took appropriate steps to ensure that their care would be in-network.

The AAMC shares the Committee's approach that patient cost-sharing for emergency health care services should be based on the in-network amount. We are pleased that the proposal would prohibit balance billing and hold patients harmless by only requiring them to pay the in-network cost-sharing amount for out-of-network emergency care and for care in which the patient could not reasonably choose their provider. However, the AAMC has serious concerns with the Committee's proposal to base the provider's reimbursement on a statutory benchmark rate.

As you know, the AAMC joined several hospital association stakeholders in proposing the attached set of guiding principles addressing surprise medical bills. We have used these principles to evaluate several surprise billing legislative proposals, including that of the "No Surprises Act," which has been proposed by the Energy and Commerce Committee ("the Committee"). Additionally, the AAMC has joined with these hospital groups to urge the Committee to re-evaluate several of the proposals in this draft legislation, particularly in regard to benchmark rate-setting. That letter is also attached to this testimony.

The AAMC provides the following comments on the discussion draft:

Prohibiting balance bills and holding patients harmless

The AAMC is pleased that the discussion draft would take patients out of the middle of surprise medical bill situations; however, we are concerned that the draft legislation does not appear to actually prohibit balance billing, but rather, imposes a penalty on providers who issue a surprise bill. The AAMC urges the Committee to specifically include a prohibition on balance billing in order to provide patients with the most protection.

Increasing transparency though notice and consent

The discussion draft requires that, at the time of scheduling, patients receiving scheduled care be given written and oral notice about the provider's network status and any potential charges they could be liable for if treated by an out-of-network provider. Though we support transparency, we believe the patient's health plan is the primary and best source of this information, and they are best positioned to discuss confidential, plan-specific information with the patient, including their cost-sharing. Detailing and communicating a patient's coverage should remain the primary responsibility of the insurer.

With regard to emergency situations, imposing an additional notice requirement on hospitals, and teaching hospitals in particular, would be overly burdensome and also could be detrimental to patients. Major teaching hospitals are common sites for emergency treatment due to their "stand-by capacity" and 24/7 readiness – trauma centers, burn units, psychiatric services, and more. We believe that the notice requirements in the discussion draft could slow emergency care and run counter to the expediency required in emergency situations. Additionally, in an emergency situation, a patient's primary concern should not be with the network status of their providers, but rather, with receiving the treatment that they need.

Energy and Commerce Subcommittee on Health
June 12, 2019
Page 3

Resolving billing disputes

The AAMC opposes statutory rate setting and urges the committee to reconsider this proposal. Statutory rate setting will disincentivize insurers to negotiate with providers, and instead allow them to leverage statutory benchmarks to gradually negotiate lower overall rates with providers. Not only does this undermine the fundamental practice of private negotiation, but it will lead to narrow networks – which oftentimes limit patient access to needed health care services and providers – as health plans will lose the incentive to offer competitive rates and fair business practices to encourage providers to enter into contracts.

The AAMC is specifically concerned that statutory rate setting stands to potentially limit beneficiary access to academic medical centers and their affiliated physicians due to the perceived higher costs of care at our facilities. Major teaching hospitals, medical schools, and their clinical faculty are a critical component of the US health care system because their joint missions of patient care, medical research, and education benefit the health care of all. While only 5% of all hospitals, AAMC's member major teaching hospitals account nationwide for 24% of all Medicare inpatient days, 25% of all Medicaid inpatient days, 31% of all hospital charity care costs, 21% of all psychiatric beds, 61% of all pediatric intensive care beds, 71% of all Level 1 trauma centers, and 96% of all NCI registered cancer treatment centers. We believe it is important that as many patients as possible have access to teaching hospitals, their physician faculty, and the critical services they provide.

Therefore, the AAMC strongly urges the Committee to reconsider this proposal, as it would destabilize academic medicine and workforce training by allowing insurers to use benchmark payments as leverage to pay academic medical centers less, or to justify cutting them out of networks completely. The Committee should preserve the process of rate negotiation between providers and insurers.

The AAMC suggests that the Committee explore other options for resolving disputes between payers and providers. Given the successes of state laws, particularly in New York, the AAMC believes that the Committee should consider an Independent Dispute Resolution (IDR) process. We believe that this may be the most expeditious and fair way to resolve billing disputes, particularly for physicians. The AAMC, however, also urges the Committee to ensure that that any entity certified to complete IDR be informed enough to understand the complexities of the health care system. This entity must ensure that decisions made are fair to both parties, and that the entity has appropriate criteria to make decisions that are standardized and uniform.

American Hospital Association™
Advancing Health in America

AMERICA'S ESSENTIAL HOSPITALS

AAMC
Tomorrow's Doctors, Tomorrow's Cures®

CHA
Catholic Health Association of the United States

CHILDREN'S HOSPITAL ASSOCIATION

Federation of American Hospitals®

May 28, 2019

The Honorable Frank Pallone
Chairman
Committee on Energy and Commerce
U.S. House of Representatives
Washington, DC 20515

The Honorable Greg Walden
Ranking Member
Committee on Energy and Commerce
U.S. House of Representatives
Washington, DC 20515

Dear Chairman Pallone and Ranking Member Walden:

On behalf of our member hospitals, health systems and other health care organizations, we are fully committed to protecting patients from "surprise medical bills" that result from unexpected gaps in coverage or medical emergencies. We agree with the Committee's goal, outlined in its summary of the "No Surprises Act," that America's families need relief from this problem and we welcome the opportunity to share our comments regarding the Committee's discussion draft.

Our organizations have previously outlined to Congress the scenarios in which patients should be protected when they receive a surprise medical bill, as well as the principles that should be used to evaluate legislative proposals. The letter is attached for your reference. For these comments, we would like to focus on one component of the "No Surprises Act:" the establishment of a benchmark payment to resolve out-of-network payment disputes between providers and insurers. Specifically, the discussion draft calls for a median in-network rate to be paid in these instances. We oppose the setting of payment rate in statute and would ask that you instead consider an independent dispute resolution process.

We are concerned that the rate-setting provision of the legislation is a plan-determined, non-transparent process that will upend private payment negotiation. A default rate will become the payment ceiling and remove incentives for insurers to develop comprehensive networks, as there are already increasing numbers of narrow network products offered that exclude certain types of providers. If an insurer can pay the same rate to all out-of-network providers, why would they make the effort to develop robust in-network insurance products for their subscribers? Moreover, setting a payment rate is difficult to do properly in statute, even when a geographic adjustment is provided, given the many factors that are currently used to determine payment. For example, rates usually take into account a provider's volume, services offered and quality improvement efforts.

The Committee should instead consider the establishment of a dispute resolution process, such as arbitration or mediation, as a way to resolve payment issues. Such a process could serve as a backstop after a period of direct negotiation between payers and providers and could, as evidenced by the experience in New York State, both reduce the incidence of out-of-network billing and incentivize network participation.

There are several ways that a dispute resolution process could be structured. We recommend the Committee require the provider or health insurer to initiate the request, rather than the patient, and ensure that the arbiter or mediator is independent and has an understanding of health care and the local market.

A number of states have enacted these dispute resolution processes, ranging from mediation to variations of arbitration. Some have put in place a binding arbitration "baseball style" process that requires both parties to submit a best offer in writing, with the arbiter responsible for choosing from between the two options, without modification. The cost of the arbiter could either be borne by the losing party or could be shared between the negotiating parties. Any dispute resolution process can be implemented quickly and efficiently and allows for similar claims to be batched. Another suggestion would be to follow the National Association of Insurance Commissioners' 2015 Model Act on provider network adequacy standards, which outlined a structured mediation process for disputes between insurers and out-of-network providers for bills of $500 or more. To be useful to all consumers, any dispute resolution process must be applied to those states that have not already enacted surprise medical billing legislation, as well as for self-funded plans regulated by the Employee Retirement Income Security Act of 1974 (ERISA).

We appreciate your consideration of these suggestions and look forward to continuing to work with you on a federal legislative solution to the issue of surprise medical billing.

Sincerely,

American Hospital Association
America's Essential Hospitals
Association of American Medical Colleges
Catholic Health Association of the United States
Children's Hospital Association
Federation of American Hospitals

American Hospital Association
Advancing Health in America

AMERICA'S ESSENTIAL HOSPITALS

AAMC
Tomorrow's Doctors, Tomorrow's Cures®

CHA
Catholic Health Association of the United States

CHILDREN'S HOSPITAL ASSOCIATION

Federation of American Hospitals®

February 20, 2019

Dear Congressional and Committee Leadership:

On behalf of our member hospitals, health systems and other health care organizations, we are fully committed to protecting patients from "surprise bills" that result from unexpected gaps in coverage or medical emergencies. We appreciate your leadership on this issue and look forward to continuing to work with you on a federal legislative solution.

Surprise bills can cause patients stress and financial burden at a time of particular vulnerability: when they are in need of medical care. Patients are at risk of incurring such bills during emergencies, as well as when they schedule care at an in-network facility without knowing the network status of all of the providers who may be involved in their care. **We must work together to protect patients from surprise bills.**

As you debate a legislative solution, we believe it is critical to:

- **Define "surprise bills."** Surprise bills may occur when a patient receives care from an out-of-network provider or when their health plan fails to pay for covered services. The three most typical scenarios are when: (1) a patient accesses emergency services outside of their insurance network, including from providers while they are away from home; (2) a patient receives care from an out-of-network physician providing services in an in-network hospital; or (3) a health plan denies coverage for emergency services saying they were unnecessary.

- **Protect the patient financially.** Patients should have certainty regarding their cost-sharing obligations, which should be based on an in-network amount. Providers should not balance bill, meaning they should not send a patient a bill beyond their cost-sharing obligations.

- **Ensure patient access to emergency care.** Patients should be assured of access to and coverage of emergency care. This requires that health plans adhere to the "prudent layperson standard" and not deny payment for emergency care that, in retrospect, the health plan determined was not an emergency.

- **Preserve the role of private negotiation.** Health plans and providers should retain the ability to negotiate appropriate payment rates. The government should not establish a fixed payment amount or reimbursement methodology for out-of-network services, which could create unintended consequences for patients by disrupting incentives for health plans to create comprehensive networks.

- **Remove the patient from health plan/provider negotiations.** Patients should not be placed in the middle of negotiations between insurers and providers. Health plans must work directly with providers on reimbursement, and the patient should not be responsible for transmitting any payment between the plan and the provider.

- **Educate patients about their health care coverage.** We urge you to include an educational component to help patients understand the scope of their health care coverage and how to access their benefits. All stakeholders – health plans, employers, providers and others – should undertake efforts to improve patients' health care literacy and support them in navigating the health care system and their coverage.

- **Ensure patients have access to comprehensive provider networks and accurate network information.** Patients should have access to a comprehensive network of providers, including in-network physicians and specialists at in-network facilities. Health plans should provide easily-understandable information about their provider network, including accurate listings for hospital-based physicians, so that patients can make informed health care decisions. Federal and state regulators should ensure both the adequacy of health plan provider networks and the accuracy of provider directories.

- **Support state laws that work.** Any public policy should take into account the interaction between federal and state laws. Many states have undertaken efforts to protect patients from surprise billing. Any federal solution should provide a default to state laws that meet the federal minimum for consumer protections.

We look forward to opportunities to discuss these solutions and work together to achieve them.

Sincerely,

American Hospital Association
America's Essential Hospitals
Association of American Medical Colleges
Catholic Health Association of the United States
Children's Hospital Association
Federation of American Hospitals

Statement for the Record of the American College of Radiology to the U.S. House of Representatives, Committee on Energy and Commerce, Subcommittee on Health Hearing, "No More Surprises: Protecting Patients from Surprise Medical Bills," June 12, 2019

On behalf of the more than 38,000 members of the American College of Radiology (ACR), thank you for your leadership in convening a hearing to discuss the Energy and Commerce Committee's bipartisan discussion draft of the "No Surprises Act." Issues surrounding high out-of-pocket costs and shrinking provider networks present real issues for patients in need of life saving diagnostic imaging and other services provided by our members.

Health insurance plans are increasingly relying on narrow and often inadequate networks of contracted physicians, hospitals, pharmacies, and other providers as one mechanism for controlling costs. As a result, even those patients who are diligent about seeking care from in-network physicians and hospitals may find themselves with unanticipated out-of-network bills from providers who are not in their insurance plan's network, simply because they had no way of knowing and researching in advance all the individuals who are ultimately involved in their care. Physicians and other providers are limited in their ability to help patients avoid these unanticipated costs because they, too, may not know in advance the exact plan in which the patient is enrolled and who will be involved in an episode of care, let alone other providers' contract status with all the insurance plans in their communities.

In addition to providing responses to the Committee's specific questions/areas of interest, the College reiterates the importance of the below principles being utilized as a foundation for legislation. We believe legislation based on these principles would provide strong patient protections, while simultaneously improving transparency, promoting access to appropriate medical care, and avoiding the creation of disincentives for insurers and health care providers to negotiate network participation contracts in good faith. As such, we urge the Committee to include provisions in the "No Surprises Act" to:

- **Create a mechanism for insurer accountability.** Since overly narrow provider networks contribute significantly to this problem, strong oversight and enforcement of network adequacy is needed from both federal and state governments.

- **Establish limits on patient responsibility.** Patients should only be responsible for in-network cost-sharing rates when experiencing unanticipated medical bills. However, legislation should also include provisions to ensure the further education of patients about their co-pays and deductibles so they are not "surprised" when they receive a bill based on the contract they have with their plan, un-related to their provider's network status.

- **Avoid benchmarking payments to Medicare or another arbitrarily low-set rate.** Guidelines or limits on what out-of-network providers are paid should reflect actual charge data for the same service in the same geographic area from a statistically significant and wholly independent database. Medicare rates are inadequate for this purpose because they establish artificial rates based on budgetary constraints. Nor should rates be based on negotiated in-network rates, which would have the effect of eliminating the need for insurers to engage in meaningful negotiations.

- **Mirror viable state laws.** Several states have implemented out-of-network billings laws that present tangible templates for a federal solution.
  - New York: The law includes comprehensive patient protections, holds insurers accountable for maintaining adequate networks of physicians and specialists, establishes reasonable patient benchmarks, and a mechanism for effective alternative dispute resolution (ADR).

- **Apply to all plan types.** Any federal legislative solution to address unexpected out-of-network medical bills should apply to all plan types, including ERISA.

As the Committee's efforts on this issue continue to evolve, the ACR strongly urges incorporation of the Protecting People From Surprise Medical Bills Act, a legislative framework recently released by Representatives Raul Ruiz, MD, and Phil Roe, MD. We believe it strikes a necessary balance by providing strong patient protections, while simultaneously improving transparency, promoting access to appropriate medical care, and avoiding the creation of disincentives for insurers and health care providers to negotiate network participation contracts in good faith.

In addition, the College is happy to provide the below detailed comments regarding the Committee's request for feedback on the following topics.

- ***Ensuring Network Adequacy.*** *Consumers deserve adequate networks that offer the right care at the right time. The Committee seeks feedback on ensuring that networks are sufficiently meeting the needs of individuals.*

The College has long viewed "surprise medical bills" as an issue largely stemming from actions of private insurers to shift too much blame to physicians for patients experiencing high bills when treated by out-of-network providers. Instead, the ACR believe a more accurate characterization of these scenarios is of "surprise gaps in insurance coverage." This definition is more reflective of the reality of insurers capitalizing upon consumers' desire for low-cost insurance premiums and failing to disclose potentially costly deficiencies in their plans, resulting in greater responsibility for out-of-pocket costs and the financially burdensome impact of inadequate provider networks. The College appreciates the Committee's acknowledgment that ensuring robust provider networks is a critical aspect of protecting patients from surprise medical bills. To ensure that narrow networks actually provide sufficient patient access to all types of physician specialties, legislation should require an adequate ratio of ancillary physicians, especially radiologists, based on the size of the beneficiary population covered by a given health plan. Furthermore, and with respect to radiologists, any forthcoming legislation should bar insurers from utilizing teleradiology as a primary mechanism to comply with any network adequacy standard, as patients should have access to an adequate number of in-network radiologists at local, in-network facilities. Also, to ensure patients in rural areas have ample access to all types of physicians, network adequacy standards should also take into account geographic and driving distances, as well as potential wait times for appointments. Ideally, patients would not have to travel more than 30 minutes or 30 miles to access in-network ancillary physicians at in-network facilities.

The network adequacy section of any forthcoming legislation should also include provisions requiring the insurance carriers to update their directories of participating providers on a regular basis, preferably via a specific set interval (e.g. every two weeks, last day of each month, etc.). As a byproduct of this requirement, insurance carriers should be held financially responsible for patients who are unable to obtain in-network services due to provider directories deemed out-of-date or not reflective of the total number of physicians participating in a narrow network. Finally, legislation should require insurers to comply with the prudent layperson standard in existing law for determining coverage for emergency care, so that insured patients are not liable for unexpected costs simply because they were unable to accurately self-diagnose ahead of time whether their symptoms were, in fact, due to an emergency medical condition.

The College has also previously voiced concern regarding potential legislative provisions limiting a physician's ability to remain out of network. While the College supports holding beneficiaries financially harmless for bills stemming from surprise gaps in insurance coverage and/or scenarios where the patient was unable to choose their providers, adequately compensating physicians for the care they provide patients is equally important. As such, the College continues to support the inclusion of a mechanism for alternative dispute resolution (ADR), included, but not limited to mediation or arbitration, with the patient's insurance carrier instead of unilateral bans on balance billing in all scenarios. Failure to include such protections will likely result in eliminating the need for insurers to negotiate contracts in good faith.

- ***Encouraging the Development of State All-Payer Claims Databases.*** *All-payer claims databases have the potential to bring greater transparency to health care costs and spur innovative policy solutions. The Committee requests feedback on how to aide states in developing robust all-payer claims databases.*

The College is concerned that the creation of separate state-based claims databases will lead to unnecessary variability in resolving the issue of "surprise" or OON medical bills. Instead, the Secretary of HHS should certify various national independent databases as eligible references for use in arbitration or other processes for determining payment for OON services. For example, the FAIR Health Database, an independent collection of more than 25 billion private healthcare and 20 billion Medicare claims, is typically regarded as the gold standard for analyzing and establishing UCRs for care delivered by OON physicians.

- ***Protecting Consumers from Surprise Bills from Air and Ground Ambulances.*** *While the No Surprises Act does not address the issue of surprise medical bills from ground or air ambulances, the Committee recognizes the need for solutions in these areas and seeks feedback on how to provide relief to consumers burdened with unexpected ambulance bills.*

At this time, the College does not have a formal position relating to the issue of surprise medical bills stemming from ground or air ambulance services.

- ***Establishing a market-based benchmark to resolve out-of-network payment disputes between providers and insurers.*** *Payment disputes between providers and insurers must be resolved in a manner that takes the patient out of the middle, is transparent and does not increase federal healthcare expenditures. The Committee requests feedback on how to adequately provide payment in these situations through a transparent, non-inflationary mechanism.*

The College views average in-network and Medicare fee-for-service payment rates as inadequate payment benchmarks because they are not designed to truly cover the costs of providing care to patients. In-network rates are opaque and easily manipulated by the carrier, and physicians agree to these lower payments in exchange for guaranteed patient populations, prompt payment, etc. Medicare rates simply do not cover the incurred cost of services provided by physicians and can lead to patients being unable to access care. In addition, these rates are inadequate benchmarks because they establish artificial rates based on budgetary constraints and policy agendas rather than market forces. We fear these low potential payment benchmarks will eliminate any financial incentive for the insurer to negotiate meaningful reimbursement rates for all providers, regardless of whether they choose to be in or out-of-network. Instead, the College urges payment to be at least equivalent to the 80th percentile of charges contained in neutral databases unaffiliated with insurers, such as the FAIR Health Database. The FAIR Health database is regarded as the gold standard for analyzing and establishing "usual, customary, and reasonable" rates, and the 80th percentile is a more reasonable mathematical calculation for reimbursement of OON care. In addition, we recommend that any prohibition, whether state or federal, on billing from out-of-network providers not chosen by the patient be paired with a corresponding payment process that is tied to the market value of physician services.

Instead of establishing an arbitrary payment benchmark for OON care, the College urges the Committee to pursue a mechanism for Alternative Dispute Resolution/Independent Dispute Resolution (ADR/IDR). Several states have successfully implemented an ADR process with binding "baseball-style" arbitration and mediation (a negotiated settlement) while patients receive protections from surprise medical bills. For example, New York's statute established a dispute resolution process and enabled the state superintendent of insurance the power to grant and revoke the certifications of independent resolution (IDR) entities. Moreover, the superintendent was charged with promulgating regulations establishing standards for the dispute resolution process. With baseball-style arbitration, the insurer and physician publicly submit unique "final offers" for review by the independent arbiter. The theory behind making the offers public is to encourage the parties to settle outside of the arbitration, as well as to incentivize reasonable bids for review. The ADR/IDR process is particularly important in circumstances where a potential minimum payment standard is insufficient due to factors such as the complexity of the patient's medical condition, the special expertise required, comorbidities, and other extraordinary factors. In addition, the College supports the adoption of the New York statute definition of the usual customary rate:

> "Usual and Customary Cost shall mean the eightieth percentile of all charges for a particular health care service performed by a provider in the same or similar specialty and provided in the same geographical area as reported in a benchmarking database maintained by a nonprofit organization specified by the superintendent. The nonprofit organization shall not be affiliated with any insurer, a corporation, a municipal cooperative health benefit plan, a health maintenance organization, or a student health plan. "

Of note, a May 2019 report from the Georgetown University Health Policy Institute's Center on Health Insurance Reforms concluded that in terms of New York, "...the law has been a success. Consumer complaints have declined dramatically. For the most part, insurers and providers appear to be working out their differences without resorting to arbitration. Further, there is not yet clear evidence that the law's use of UCR as a benchmark price has had broadly inflationary effects." The same report indicated that IDR decisions using the New York model have been relatively even between providers and payers, with 618 disputes decided in favor of the health plan and 561 decided in favor of the provider. Given these compelling results, the College strongly encourages the Committee to include an ADR/IDR process that mirrors the New York model in lieu of establishing an arbitrary payment benchmark.

In fact, the experience of physicians in the state of California reflects the pitfalls of establishing a payment rate tied to Medicare or in-network rates. As was predicted by the California Health Benefits Review Program, "by setting the non-contracted effective rate for potentially surprise professional services, "the new law "put downward pressure on contracted rates among the specialties ...that are most likely to work in non-contracted medical groups within contracted in-network facilities ...". It has also "reduce[d] the negotiated rates for those specialties by setting a ceiling (i.e., based on the Medicare fee schedule) for out-of-network...surprise medical bill payment." According to the California Medical Association, since the passage of the state's surprise medical billing law in late 2016, a substantial number of their member physicians have reported difficulties in renewing contracts with health plans and insurers with which they had longstanding existing contracts for reimbursement greater than 125 percent of the Medicare rate and in obtaining new contracts.

Again, the ACR appreciates the opportunity to provide detailed comments regarding the draft "No Surprises Act," and we look forward collaborating with you to find a federal solution that addresses the issue of surprise medical bills in a comprehensive way that does not compromise access to care through unintended consequences.

If you have any questions and/or would like any additional information regarding the College's comments, please contact Cynthia Moran, ACR's Executive Vice President, Economics, Government Relations and Health Policy, via phone (202-223-1670) or email (cmoran@acr.org).

Sincerely,

William T. Thorwarth, Jr., MD, FACR
Chief Executive Officer

Statement for the Record of the Blue Cross and Blue Shield Association to the U.S. House of Representatives, Committee on Energy and Commerce, Subcommittee on Health Hearing, "No More Surprises: Protecting Patients from Surprise Medical Bills," June 12, 2019

The Blue Cross Blue Shield Association (BCBSA) is pleased to provide a statement in support of the United States House Committee on Energy and Commerce Subcommittee on Health's thoughtful efforts to address surprise medical billing.

BCBSA is a national federation of 36 independent, community-based and locally operated Blue Cross and Blue Shield (BCBS) companies (Plans) that collectively provide healthcare coverage for one in three Americans. For 90 years, BCBS Plans have offered quality healthcare coverage in all markets across America – serving those who purchase coverage on their own as well as those who obtain coverage through an employer, Medicare and Medicaid.

A Kaiser Family Foundation analysis found that 15 percent of patients with large employer coverage who were admitted to an inpatient hospital stay received balance bills from providers, exposing patients to significant and unanticipated costs.[1] We believe that all stakeholders, including issuers, providers and policymakers, have the same goal – to protect consumers from crippling costs when they have a reasonable expectation that they have done everything to seek care at an in-network facility. BCBS companies are invested in this goal, and BCBSA has worked hard to bring forward solutions that offer a meaningful middle ground to protect not only the individuals impacted by the bills, but all consumers. If all stakeholders come to the table ready to give a little, this is a problem that can be solved. To support this goal, we have brought forward a number of common-sense approaches in our discussions with policymakers, including:

- Support for limiting patient responsibility to in-network amounts in these scenarios, understanding that consumers have imperfect information with which to make decisions
- A proposed payment benchmark that ensures out-of-network provider payments are on par with providers who have contracted with payers and agreed to the responsibilities associated with network participation
- A recommendation that the Department of Health and Human Services (HHS) develop the calculation methodology for a reasonable payment benchmark through rulemaking so it is transparent and all stakeholders have the opportunity to inform the approach
- A willingness to consider requiring payers to pay providers directly, a key contracting incentive, in these scenarios so patients are kept out of the middle

We commend the Committee for its thoughtful and bipartisan process in addressing this complicated issue. The Committee's draft legislation will go a long way towards protecting patients from surprise medical bills, will help ensure that patients are informed and engaged and will help protect all consumers from escalating costs. Furthermore, the draft achieves the appropriate balance of incentives that will help ensure that providers are paid fairly while not enabling specific medical specialists to remain out-of-network, which has led to the challenges

[1] Kaiser Family Foundation. "Analysis: For Patients with Large Employer Coverage, About 1 in 6 Hospital Stays Includes an Out-of-Network Bill." Aug. 13, 2018. https://www.kff.org/health-costs/press-release/analysis-for-patients-with-large-employer-coverage-about-1-in-6-hospital-stays-includes-an-out-of-network-bill/

the healthcare system faces today around surprise billing. Below is our specific feedback and recommendations on the Committee's draft.

BCBSA recommendations and feedback on the *No Surprises Act* to address surprise billing

BCBSA strongly supports prohibiting balance billing for all emergency services and by providers that patients cannot reasonably choose, holding patients responsible for only the amount they would have paid in-network.

This is an essential first step to protect consumers by preventing providers from burdening them with additional costs over and above what they owe as part of their cost-sharing obligations and what the providers are already paid by health plans.

The Committee's proposed bill states that the prohibition on balance billing would apply to all out-of-network emergency services and to all out-of-network non-emergency services received at an in-network facility from "facility-based providers," which the bill defines to include anesthesiologists, radiologists, pathologists, neonatologists, assistant surgeons, hospitalists, intensivists, and any additional provider types specified by the Secretary of HHS. We recommend that the Committee also consider including non-physician providers often involved in surprise billing, such as certified nurse anesthetists (CRNAs), in the draft's list of facility-based providers that are subject to the law. Furthermore, understanding that the specific providers most associated with surprise billing may evolve over time, Congress may choose to direct the Secretary of HHS to revisit the specific provider types periodically through rulemaking.

We also support limiting patients' cost-sharing to in-network amounts for surprise bills. The purpose of in-network versus out-of-network cost-sharing is to encourage consumers to seek care with providers who plans have thoroughly vetted and have confidence in. If patients cannot be reasonably expected to know who will be providing them services, then their ability to choose is negated. Patients should not be held responsible for choices they did not actively make by paying out-of-network cost-sharing in these instances.

BCBSA also supports the Committee's proposal that patients receiving scheduled care be given written and oral notice at the time of scheduling about providers' network status and any potential charges they could be liable for if treated by an out-of-network provider.

However, we caution against the use of a consent component as it could be used as a workaround to facilitate balance billing. Furthermore, we believe that the legislation should go further in notifying patients of their rights around surprise billing. To improve transparency, we recommend that facilities be required to make sure patients are informed of their planned providers' network status when scheduling and of their rights regarding balance billing as part of their intake process. Notifying patients of their rights at intake would help inform them of their recourse should they receive a balance bill and where to turn for assistance with interpreting whether it was received in error. To be effective, a notification of rights would need to include information on what qualifies as a surprise out-of-network bill and who to contact (e.g., health plan, hospital, state agency) if the patient is balanced billed in those circumstances. A notification could include a signature of confirmation from a patient to support facilities' and oversight entities' ability to track compliance with the requirement.

BCBSA strongly supports the Committee's proposal to establish a minimum payment standard set at the median contracted (in-network) rate for the service in the geographic area where the service was delivered.

BCBSA commends the Committee's approach to establish a fair payment benchmark for surprise bills that will not increase premiums or impact access for consumers. This approach is superior to other options under consideration in Congress, such as arbitration, that could undermine health plan networks and result in higher costs for consumers over time.

A payment methodology that is simple, transparent and fair to all parties is the most meaningful way to address surprise billing and prevent unintended downstream consequences for consumers when there are disputes between payers and providers. These disputes, in many cases, are driven by forces that distort market dynamics, including inelastic demand for services, lack of transparency in obtaining services and imbalanced negotiating powers that are propelled by limitations on how hospitals contract with certain specialties, and provider consolidation. A benchmark-based payment methodology can rebalance these forces so the environment can function closer to a true market.

We also support the Committee's recommendation to rely on HHS for a determination on how to calculate the median in-network payment rate. We believe this will help address provider concerns with how payers develop contracted rates, while allowing for minimal HHS involvement and resources. The methodology would need to account for provider specialties, lines of business and geographic variation, and HHS should not be permitted to incorporate any rate-setting elements into the methodology (e.g., a calculation plus a specified percent).

Finally, we appreciate the Committee's judiciousness in not tying the payment benchmark to billed charges, relying on a third-party database or defaulting to an arbitration system for settling disputes. These approaches are problematic and will lead to greater costs to the healthcare system in the long-term. The Committee's approach to a clear federal benchmarking methodology brings competition and balance and is a more effective way to support a market-based solution to surprise billing. We urge the Committee to maintain use of the payer's median in-network rate as a fair payment benchmark and to resist using other approaches such as billed charges or arbitration.

- **Currently there is no mechanism to control what providers charge (i.e., billed charges) so charges often increase capriciously and with little transparency.** Any approach that would tie payment to a percentage of billed charges would continue to escalate over time, increasing the impact to premiums exponentially and discouraging network participation by providers. Billed charges are often out-of-sync with costs and can be significantly higher than typical network rates. Setting the benchmark by reference to billed charges creates incentives to artificially inflate billed charges with a so-called "discount" rate that remains well above costs and in-network rates and discourages network participation.
- **Arbitration adds administrative and financial costs to payers and providers, which ultimately leads to higher patient costs. It also increases uncertainty for payers, employers and providers, extends the timelines to resolve claims and adds complexity to the resolution process.** While models focused on arbitration, or dispute resolution, can somewhat rebalance negotiations in a similar way to a benchmark-based

payment, they add new layers of administrative complexity, uncertainty and cost to all entities involved (i.e., payers, providers, employers and the government entity responsible for management of the process) as well as additional complexity to, and prolongation of, the claims resolution process. Arbitration could also have the unintended impact of establishing a baseline for payment as a pattern would likely emerge in how arbiters decide cases. If that amount is too high, it could drive up costs and limit plans' ability to locally manage their networks.

- **Tying a benchmark to a third-party database reduces some of the potential gains of using a defined payment benchmark methodology, particularly around transparency and fairness to all parties.** Payers and other stakeholders have significant concerns regarding the ability and willingness of these databases to be fully transparent with their benchmarking methodologies, the quality of their data and the costs of use. These concerns are compounded by an awareness that with many, if not all, of these databases, their available data remains meaningfully incomplete, creating a potential for bias in their benchmarking.

BCBSA response to common arguments used by physicians and hospitals to turn attention away from their role in surprise billing

Using a payment benchmark to address surprise billing will address current market distortions.

Establishing a payment benchmark replicates the market rate for each individual insurer and does not rely on a government benchmark. Typically, surprise billing happens when patients access care in an emergency or from a provider in an in-network facility that the patient did not know they would need. In these non-elective situations, the patient has limited opportunity to choose his or her providers. Furthermore, due to factors such as market consolidation, these bills occur in situations where the market is not functioning effectively. It is important to correct market imbalances in these instances, and a payment benchmark would be the cleanest, least disruptive solution. However, adoption of a broader payment benchmark in specialties or situations not typically facing surprise billing would be unnecessary, and likely harmful to an already functioning market.

The recommended approach would give authority to HHS to develop the calculation methodology to promote transparency, but would *not* give HHS the authority to determine specific payment amounts. This is not rate setting or "Medicare for all."

Health plans follow state and federal network adequacy laws to ensure consumer have access to the care they need, and current enforcement of network adequacy is robust.

Most, if not all, states have extensive network adequacy laws that require insurers to maintain robust networks based on provider type and/or time and distance standards. Despite these standards and BCBS Plans' compliance with them, consumers have seen a significant uptick in surprise bills in recent years. Surprise bills existed previously, predominately in rural areas, but the number and scale have increased exponentially with little to no change in most network adequacy standards. For example, Texas is a state with some of the strictest network adequacy laws, but is also a state regularly cited for its ongoing issues with excessive surprise billing.

Therefore, arguments that blame surprise billing on network adequacy or narrow networks are unfounded.

When insurers build networks for different products, they focus on which commonly used providers (e.g., primary care, OB-GYNs) and facilities will be in-network rather than the more granular level of which providers within an in-network facility will be in-network. These networks, including narrow networks, are designed to drive consumers to the highest quality, most cost-effective facilities, not to deter access to necessary services. Furthermore, in the narrow network context, products are often designed around the inclusion of particular facilities, and are not aimed at removing specific providers from a network. This is an important distinction for surprise billing purposes, as the goals of current legislative efforts are aimed at surprise bills that are coming from out-of-network providers delivering care at *in-network* facilities. Narrow networks are not relevant to this issue, and are simply an argument made to draw attention away from fair and transparent solutions to solving the problem of surprise billing.

In fact, this point is further confirmed by research from the Commonwealth Fund that indicates that the rate of surprise billing is similar across different types of insurance products.[2] In the case of surprise billing, patients have already used their networks to identify an in-network facility, using the product as designed, regardless of whether the product utilizes a broad or narrow network. The surprise bill comes when an individual provider (or provider group) performing services within an in-network facility refuses to separately contract to be in-network with the insurers with which that hospital contracts.

The Brookings Institution also examined the relationship between network adequacy and surprise billing recently, and noted that "a network adequacy standard for facility-based clinicians would not do anything to address the market failure that leads to surprise out-of-network billing. Network adequacy regulation would strengthen the incentive for insurers to bring these providers into their networks, but surprise bills arise because of the incentives that providers (not insurers) face. Ancillary and emergency providers are guaranteed a flow of patients without regard to their network status and therefore have a lucrative opportunity to remain out-of-network that is not available to their peer physicians in other specialties. Intensifying the pressure on insurers to contract with them would not change their ability to remain out-of-network; it would simply enable them to obtain even higher rates for going in-network – their current in-network rates in relation to Medicare are already extremely high – and would continue to leave consumers exposed."[3]

Both federal and state oversight of insurer networks has been working, and will continue to be robust regardless of what solution is implemented to address surprise billing. At the federal level, the Centers for Medicare & Medicaid Services (CMS) has done nothing to weaken regulatory requirements for qualified health plans. The Affordable Care Act requires plans sold on the Exchanges to maintain a provider network that is "sufficient in numbers and types of providers, including providers that specialize in mental health and substance abuse services, to

---

[2] The Commonwealth Fund. "Rate of "Surprise Medical Bills" Similar for Adults Insured with Employer and Marketplace Coverage." July 6, 2016. https://www.commonwealthfund.org/chart/2016/rate-surprise-medical-bills-similar-adults-insured-employer-and-marketplace-coverage

[3] Young, Christen Linke et al. The Brookings Institution. "The relationship between network adequacy and surprise billing." May 10, 2019. https://www.brookings.edu/blog/usc-brookings-schaeffer-on-health-policy/2019/05/10/the-relationship-between-network-adequacy-and-surprise-billing/

assure that all services will be accessible without unreasonable delay." Recognizing that many states already have strong standards in place and others will consider the best way to improve their oversight based on the updated NAIC Model, the HHS Notice of Benefit and Payment Parameters for 2020 Final Rule indicates that CMS, in its role as Exchange administrator, would defer to state departments of insurance's (DOI) network adequacy evaluations in determining a provider network to be adequate.

While there is considerable variation in state approaches to network adequacy regulation and review, there is good reason to believe that states are, overall, conscientious regulators of provider networks. This is evidenced by:

- Several state-based exchange entities defer to their state's DOI for network adequacy determinations, so the Trump Administration's approach is not unusual.
- As of May 2017, 46 states have enacted some type of provider network adequacy laws.[4]
- States are currently implementing innovative approaches to improve provider network oversight and transparency, including California's provider network utility.
- States conduct robust oversight of their network adequacy provisions. While most health plans are able to demonstrate compliance with the requirements, in instances where a plan does not meet the standard, penalties are assessed. For example, two states assessed fines on insurance carriers for provider network problems in the last two years: Washington fined Coordinated Care (a subsidiary of Centene) $1.5 million and ordered it to stop issuing individual health insurance policies in the state because of inadequate networks; Massachusetts fined Aetna Health Insurance on concerns that their online directories mislead patients and that Aetna has not fully complied with state laws requiring insurers to cover certain substance use disorder treatment without prior authorization.

Our primary recommendation to facilitate network adequacy and encourage provider participation is that Congress include a payment benchmark that is not greater, and is preferably less, than what plans pay to in-network providers. Anything above the median in-network rate will drive providers out-of-network, eroding contracting relationships between insurers and providers, increase costs to consumers and the healthcare system as a whole and undermine efforts to provide care coordination and value-based care programs that ensure patients get the highest quality care in the right setting, at the right time and at the right price. We believe a payment methodology that is simple, transparent and fair to all parties would be the most meaningful way to address this issue given the unique environment where these surprise bills mostly occur.

Networks are core to the business of health plans, and a payment benchmark would support—not hinder—their development.

Creating a benchmark payment will not erode networks. In fact, this argument actually runs counter to a core business proposition for health plans – to develop networks in order to ensure our members have access to high-quality, cost-efficient clinicians and hospitals. Health plans develop different types of network solutions based on client needs, and these range from

[4] America's Health Insurance Plans. "Network Adequacy Requirements: Summary of State Network Adequacy Provisions." May 22, 2017

It also does little to constrain costs. Regarding New York's model, stakeholders (including issuers) raised concerns that the process may incentivize providers to increase their charges.[14] One way this would happen is if a pattern develops where an arbiter considers a percent of charges (e.g., 80 percent) a reasonable concession on the part of providers. This could incent providers to raise their charges since they are not tied to market forces. There is existing evidence to support this possible outcome. When Major League Baseball (MLB) implemented a best-and-final offer arbitration approach to setting players' salaries, which has been the model for the IDR proposals to address surprise billing, the MLB saw players' salaries increase overtime as a result.

This becomes particularly problematic when structured with inherent bias towards providers. For example, requiring the arbiter to have clinical expertise can, on the surface, make sense, but likely translates to the arbiter having a clinical background and an implicit bias in favor of providers' concerns. Given the size of these cases, any escalation over time could have meaningful impacts on premiums for consumers.

The cost of the IDR process itself is also expensive. At least one judge who represents a District Court in Massachusetts has raised concerns on the cost of arbitration generally (i.e., not specific to healthcare), citing a $1,900 filing fee per case, a $750 care management fee and the arbiter's time. One BCBS Plan estimated that the cost of an arbiter would likely be a minimum of $1,000/hr. This would be in addition to the legal costs incurred by both entities to prepare for and be represented in these cases. In many cases, these costs could quickly exceed the cost of the bill itself and will ultimately be passed on to consumers through higher premiums and to taxpayers through federal subsidies and other consumer support mechanisms.

The use of arbitration, and subsequently the burden, will increase over time, especially if the process is extended to employer-sponsored insurance through federal action. The volume of cases going through independent dispute resolution in New York has been increasing since implementation. In 2015, there were 207 emergency service surprise bills and 36 non-emergency surprise bills that went through the process. As of 2017, the use of the process had increased 450 percent (645 and 451 cases, respectively).[15] As another example, when Texas established an arbitration system for surprise medical bills, the number of cases increased significantly - from 43 requests preceding the law to more than 600 a year later. Four years later, there was a backlog of more than 4,000 cases waiting for resolution,[16] and this backlog is expected to be even larger this year.

However, existing state laws only extend to products the states have jurisdiction over, which typically excludes self-insured products used by companies to cover employees. These plans

[14] Corlette, Sabrina and Olivia Hoppe. Center on Health Insurance Reform, Georgetown University Health Policy Center. "New York's 2014 Law to Protect Consumers from Surprise Out-of-Network Bills Mostly Working as Intended: Results of a Case Study." May 2019. https://nationaldisabilitynavigator.org/wp-content/uploads/news-items/GU-CHIR_NY-Surprise-Billing_May-2019.pdf

[15] New York State Health Foundation. "Issue Brief: New York's Efforts to Reform Surprise Medical Billing." February 2019. https://nyshealthfoundation.org/wp-content/uploads/2019/02/new-yorks-efforts-to-reform-surprise-medical-billing.pdf

[16] Root & Najmabadi. Thousands of Texans Were Shocked by Surprise Medical Bills – Their Requests for Help Overwhelmed the State. The Texas Tribune. February 12, 2019. https://www.texastribune.org/2019/02/12/texas-mediation-balance-billing-faces-massive-backlog/

represent over half of all employer-sponsored coverage and a total of 100 million lives.[17] Based on the way self-insured plans are structured between insurance companies and employers, employers would often be the entity responsible for going to arbitration if a provider contests payment. This would be extremely burdensome for many small and mid-sized businesses that would not have the resources to maintain internal staff to resolve these cases but would be forced to either accept provider pricing or hire external legal support, both of which could be extremely costly.

Furthermore, arbitration would not be able to be centralized in a single entity due the nature of existing state laws and legal infrastructure. This will likely result in variation across markets, creating fragmentation and complexity for employers operating in different markets and/or areas of the country.

We believe that use of an arbitration or dispute resolution process should be intended as a *last resort* rather than simply a means to defer decision-making to a third party. A payment benchmark, as referenced above, offers a much simpler, fair, transparent and cost efficient solution.

Conclusion

BCBSA and BCBS Plans believe all patients should be protected from surprise medical bills and remain strongly committed to working with policymakers on solutions to better protect consumers while preventing unintended costs and disruptions to the healthcare system. We strongly support solutions that: protect patients from the significant financial burden tied to surprise medical bills; establish fair and transparent payment for providers that would continue to encourage them to remain in-network; and maintain high-quality networks to ensure consumers have access to high-quality, cost-efficient clinicians and hospitals.

[17] ERISA Industry Committee. "Protecting Patients from Surprise Medical Bills". Testimony before House Ways and Means Health Subcommittee. May, 21, 2019. https://docs.house.gov/meetings/WM/WM02/20190521/109508/HHRG-116-WM02-Wstate-GelfandJ-20190521.pdf

Statement for the Record of the Partnership for Employer-Sponsored Coverage, et al., to the U.S. House of Representatives, Committee on Energy and Commerce, Subcommittee on Health Hearing, "No More Surprises: Protecting Patients from Surprise Medical Bills," June 12, 2019

PARTNERSHIP FOR
EMPLOYER-SPONSORED COVERAGE

STATEMENT FOR
U.S. HOUSE OF REPRESENTATIVES
WAYS AND MEANS COMMITTEE
HEARING ON
NO MORE SURPRISES:
PROTECTING PATIENTS FROM SURPRISE MEDICAL BILLS
JUNE 12, 2019

The Partnership for Employer-Sponsored Coverage is an advocacy alliance of employment-based organizations and trade associations representing businesses of all sizes and the over 181 million American workers and their families who rely on employer-sponsored coverage every day. We are committed to working to ensure that employer-sponsored coverage is strengthened and remains a viable, affordable option for decades to come.

Employer-sponsored coverage has been the backbone of our nation's health system for nearly eight decades. Employers of all sizes contribute vast resources to employees and their families through the employer-sponsored system. Employers have a vested interest in health care quality, value, and system viability. Employers have been on the leading edge of health delivery innovation and modeling for decades.

The Partnership for Employer-Sponsored Coverage applauds the Committee for holding this hearing and working on bipartisan solutions to address surprise medical billing. As the Committee continues its work on *No Surprises Act*, we would like to reiterate our support for protecting patients from surprise billing and enacting a minimum payment standard to resolve out-of-network claims disputes instead of an arbitration system. Attached are our full comments on the draft legislation submitted to the Committee last month.

PARTNERSHIP FOR
EMPLOYER-SPONSORED COVERAGE

May 28, 2019

The Honorable Frank Pallone (NJ)
Chairman
U.S. House Energy & Commerce Committee
2125 Rayburn House Office Building
Washington, D.C. 20515

The Honorable Greg Walden (OR)
Ranking Member
U.S. House Energy & Commerce Committee
2322 Rayburn House Office Building
Washington, D.C. 20515

Dear Chairman Pallone and Ranking Member Walden:

As members of the Partnership for Employer-Sponsored Coverage, we write to commend you on your efforts in drafting the bipartisan *No Surprises Act* to address surprise medical billing in our nation's health care system. We welcome the opportunity to provide you with feedback as you continue your work toward formal introduction of this legislation.

The Partnership for Employer-Sponsored Coverage is an advocacy alliance of employment-based organizations and trade associations representing businesses of all sizes. We are committed to working to ensure that employer-sponsored coverage is strengthened and remains a viable, affordable option for decades to come.

Employer-sponsored coverage has been the backbone of our nation's health system for nearly eight decades. The employer-sponsored coverage system provides health coverage for over 181 million hardworking Americans and their families every day. Employers of all sizes contribute vast resources to employees and their families through the employer-sponsored system. Employers have a vested interest in health care quality, value, and system viability.

As you know, benefits offerings and coverage plans in the employer-sponsored system are as diverse as employers and employees themselves. With self-insured coverage under the Employee Retirement Income Security Act (ERISA), employers tailor coverage to meet their workforce's specific needs across state lines, pay all health claims and bears the financial risk, and utilize a third-party administrator (insurance carrier) for daily plan management. Through the fully insured state-regulated insurance market, employers purchase a prescribed benefit insurance product sold in a state from an insurance carrier and do not bear the full financial risk of claims.

As you work to formally introduce the *No Surprises Act*, we would like to provide you with the following comments for your consideration. The Partnership for Employer-Sponsored Coverage has been working alongside other stakeholders in the employer and plan coverage community on this important issue and our comments below reflect shared policy opinions.

Protecting Patients from Surprise Medical Bills

First and foremost, we strongly agree that patients should be protected when put in a situation in which they lack a choice of providers. We support the draft proposal to prohibit balance billing for all emergency services. We also support the draft proposal to prohibit balance billing from providers that patients cannot reasonable choose in situations in which there was scheduled care with an in-network provider, but associated care was charged at an out-of-network rate.

Increasing Transparency for Consumers

Navigating the health care system for a consumer is most often mindboggling, frustrating and emotionally draining. We support the draft proposal to require providers to give patients receiving scheduled care written and oral notice

www.p4esc.org @P4ESC

PARTNERSHIP FOR
EMPLOYER-SPONSORED COVERAGE

at the time of scheduling about the provider's network status and any potential charges for out-of-network care. Transparency of this information is critical to ensuring patients are better consumers of their health care and protected from surprise medical bills.

Additionally, it is important to note that employer plan sponsors are already required to provide enrollees with benefits guides and materials and devote a lot of time and resources to produce this information in ways that are innovative and interactive such as through web portals and clickable .pdfs. As you continue to identify ways to improve transparency in the system, please call upon employers to provide you with real-world examples about the types of communications they transmit to their employees.

Resolution of Out-Of-Network Payment Disputes

We welcome the draft legislation's recognition that a minimum payment standard should be set to resolve out-of-network claims disputes. We greatly appreciate that the draft legislation does not utilize an arbitration system to settle payment disputes. An arbitration system would be an administrative nightmare to self-insured employers who would have to directly contest claims in court as they are the plan sponsor. For smaller and mid-size employers who self-insure, the legal costs of arbitration could potentially be devastating.

While we do believe that the draft legislation's proposal of a market-based median contracted rate for the geographic area in which the service was delivered is a step in the right direction, we are in support of establishing a federal cap for emergency services at an out-of-network facility at 125 percent of the Medicare rate for the service. Additionally, we support the proposition that all providers in an in-network facility must accept the in-network rate. This will greatly reduce potential consumer confusion as well as the incidence of surprise billing.

Network Adequacy

For talent retention and recruitment reasons, employers are committed to providing robust provider networks that address all of their employees' health care needs. Employers have been at the forefront of developing and implementing high value provider networks at the lowest possible cost, including telehealth, on-site and near-site health centers, utilizing centers of excellence, direct contracting, provider transparency initiatives and wellness programs. Any legislation to address surprise billing should be crafted in a way that ensures these employer innovations and other value-based network initiatives are not hindered. Additionally, we agree that provider directories must be kept up to date. Providers play a key role in keeping these directories current.

All-Payer Claims Database

As you know, current all-payer claims databases in individual states collect data from fully insured products regulated by the state and not from self-insured ERISA plans governed under federal law. While there is understanding that transparency of claims costs and utilization of services through the establishment of all-payer claims databases can help with overall system reforms and plan designs, the administrative details of these databases could have potentially devastating effects on multi-state self-insured employers.

We recommend you proceed cautiously with applying the current fully insured state database model to ERISA self-insured plans. We oppose any effort to preempt ERISA and require self-insured employers to adhere to individual-by-individual state claims databases. Should legislative proposals establish a federal claims database for self-insured ERISA plans, we urge it to 1) include a single federal point-of-entry for uploading this information, and 2) be made available to employer plan sponsors for their utilization of plan development and design.

PARTNERSHIP FOR
EMPLOYER-SPONSORED COVERAGE

Air and Ground Ambulance Services

We are very concerned about the non-participatory status of many air and ground ambulance services. It is unfathomable to think that the travel to a hospital in an air or ground ambulance could impoverish a patient. We believe legislation should prohibit the balance billing of patients for these emergency services and encourage in-network participation by air and ground ambulance providers. We also support applying provider price transparency requirements to air and ground ambulance companies. Further, while we understand there are issues governing air ambulance services under the Federal Aviation Administration (FAA) that complicate the committees of health care jurisdiction from implementing robust policy, we call upon Congress to resolve these issues so patients are no longer subject to exorbitant charges.

Conclusion:

As a coalition representing businesses of all sizes, the Partnership for Employer-Sponsored Coverage has the unique ability to provide operational input across the full spectrum of the employer system – from the smallest family-owned business to the largest corporation. Employers have a great stake in the development and implementation of health care policies, and we look forward to working with you and your colleagues in a bipartisan manner throughout 116th Congress.

PARTNERSHIP FOR EMPLOYER-SPONSORED COVERAGE

American Hotel & Lodging Association
American Rental Association
American Staffing Association
Associated Builders and Contractors, Inc.
Associated General Contractors of America
Auto Care Association
Food Marketing Institute
HR Policy Association
International Franchise Association
National Association of Health Underwriters
National Association of Wholesaler-Distributors
National Restaurant Association
National Retail Federation
Retail Industry Leaders Association
Society of American Florists
Society for Human Resource Management

www.p4esc.org @P4ESC

Statement for the Record of Scott Frey, Director of Federal Government Affairs, American Federation of State, County and Municipal Employees, to the U.S. House of Representatives, Committee on Energy and Commerce, Subcommittee on Health Hearing, "No More Surprises: Protecting Patients from Surprise Medical Bills," June 12, 2019

AFSCME
We Make America Happen

June 12, 2019

The Honorable Anna G. Eshoo
Chairwoman, Subcommittee on Health
Committee on Energy and Commerce
U.S. House of Representatives
Washington, DC 20515

The Honorable Michael C. Burgess
Ranking Member, Subcommittee on Health
Committee on Energy and Commerce
U.S. House of Representatives
Washington, DC 20515

Dear Chairwoman Eshoo and Ranking Member Burgess

On behalf of the members of the American Federation of State, County and Municipal Employees (AFSCME), I ask that this letter be included in the record for the subcommittee's June 12, 2019 legislative hearing on the "No Surprises Act." The health and financial security of working families rests upon solid health care coverage, but coverage alone is not enough when individuals face surprise medical bills. We applaud the subcommittee for working to tackle this problem. The draft "No Surprises Act" is a key step towards protecting patients against punitive balance bills while keeping overall health care costs in check. We appreciate the opportunity to urge further improvements to the bill.

"Surprise medical bills" result from unexpected charges from an out-of-network provider. These bills can be tens of thousands of dollars, leaving working families with huge medical debt and a heavy financial burden. They usually happen with an emergency room visit. In an emergency, patients do not choose the emergency room, treating physicians, or ambulance providers. Surprise medical bills also happen with planned care from an in-network provider (such as a hospital or ambulatory care facility), but other treating providers brought in to care for the patient are not in the network. Typically, anesthesiologists, radiologists, pathologists, surgical assistants, and others may be out-of-network providers at an in-network facility. Like in an emergency, the patient seeking planned care in not in control of who treats at their in-network facility.

Hold Individuals Harmless for a Broad Range of Unexpected Medical Bills

We support that the bill works to hold individuals harmless but urge the subcommittee to expand the scope of services covered to hold individuals harmless against unexpected bills for air and ground ambulances when an individual is not in control of the decision to use the service. In rural areas, geography and hospital closures mean severely injured or ill individuals must rely upon air ambulance services and face surprise bills of $30,000 to $80,000. Air ambulance surprise bills also affect individuals in urban and suburban areas. For example, an individual seriously injured in a highway car crash may need this type of high-cost emergency transportation to be airlifted to a specialized trauma care medical center. The "No Surprises Act" should also cover air and ground emergency medical transportation.

We also urge the subcommittee to clarify in the legislation that hold harmless protections also apply to a patient transitioning from emergency to non-emergency treatment at a non-network facility. The scope of the bill should not leave these patients vulnerable to surprise bills, especially for those admitted to a hospital.

We also encourage the subcommittee to extend surprise billing protections to certain non-emergency services or items originating from the office of an in-network physician or other medical professional, even if that office falls outside the definition of health care facility described in proposed 42 U.S.C. Sec. 300gg–19a(e)(2)(B). For example, we encourage that the subcommittee clarify the bill's identification of health care to ensure hold harmless protections also apply in cases where a physician directs blood or other samples taken in the physician's office to a third-party, non-network laboratory.

Ensure that "No Surprises Act" Protections Wrap Around State Laws

The "No Surprises Act" defers to state surprise billing laws in instances in which a state law provides a method for determining the payment amount. We ask the subcommittee to ensure the "No Surprises Act" protects individuals in cases where the state surprise billing law is less comprehensive and not coextensive with federal law. For example, if a state surprise billing law applies only to specified categories of nonparticipating providers, federal law should still apply with respect to all other nonparticipating providers otherwise covered by the federal requirements.

Base Payment Rates for Out-Of-Network Providers on Medicare Rates

With the patient held harmless for the surprise medical bill, payment for the bill shifts to a resolution between the insurer and the out-of-network providers. Payment rates for out-of-network providers must not lock in soaring prices or increase health care costs. Americans already pay high health care prices even for in-network care. Using median contracted rates, as the "No Surprises Act" proposes, would not correct for the problem of already excessive contracted rates.

The most effective and efficient way to provide for adequate, non-escalating payments would be to link the new payment to Medicare rates plus a percentage for the same or similar services or items provided by a provider in the same or similar specialty in the same geographic region.

A recent analysis found that average contracted rates for emergency physicians and anesthesiologists are 306 percent and 344 percent of Medicare rates, respectively; in comparison, the average contracted rate for all physicians is just 128 percent of Medicare rates. Using Medicare rates as the reference price would correct for the market failures that result in these excessive in-network rates while also addressing surprise medical bills. *See https://www.brookings.edu/research/state-approaches-to-mitigating-surprise-out-of-network-billing/*

We urge the subcommittee to revise the "No Surprises Act" to use reference prices based on Medicare rather than negotiated rates for surprise billing claims because negotiated rates for providers most frequently involved in surprise billing (e.g., emergency room physicians, radiologists and anesthesiologists) are already inflated compared to negotiated rates for other providers.

The minimum rate could be set at Medicare rates plus a percentage, such as Medicare plus 25 percent. Oregon uses this basic method for setting adequate rates in some circumstances. Oregon law sets maximum rates that can be paid by the state's Public Employees' Benefit Board and the Oregon Educators Benefit Board for certain hospital claims as a percent of the amount paid by Medicare, with a lower rate paid to out-of-network hospitals than in-network hospitals and hospitals reimbursed under this method barred from balance billing patients. *See* Or. Rev. Stat. § 243.256 and § 243.879 (as amended in § 31, Ch. 746, Or. Laws 2017) (applies to plan years beginning after July 1, 2019).

Network Adequacy Is Important but Not a Surefire Way to Protect Against Surprise Medical Bills

Some suggest improving network adequacy to protect individuals against surprise medical bills. Surprise billing and network adequacy are different problems. Addressing network adequacy will not solve the surprise billing problem. We note, for example, that individuals already covered by broad networks, including many AFSCME members, are still vulnerable to surprise bills.

Again, we thank the subcommittee for its work in protecting individuals against surprise medical bills.

Sincerely,

Scott Frey
Director of Federal Government Affairs

SF/LB:cg

Statement for the Record of David Certner, Legislative Counsel and Legislative Policy Director, Government Affairs, AARP, to the U.S. House of Representatives, Committee on Energy and Commerce, Subcommittee on Health Hearing, "No More Surprises: Protecting Patients from Surprise Medical Bills," June 12, 2019

AARP
Real Possibilities

601 E Street, NW | Washington, DC 20049
202-434-2277 | 1-888-OUR-AARP | 1-888-687-2277 | TTY: 1-877-434-7598
www.aarp.org | twitter: @aarp | facebook.com/aarp | youtube.com/aarp

June 12, 2019

The Honorable Anna Eshoo
Chairwoman
Subcommittee on Health
Energy and Commerce Committee
House of Representatives
Washington, DC 20515

The Honorable Michael Burgess
Ranking Member
Subcommittee on Health
Energy and Commerce Committee
House of Representatives
Washington, DC 20515

RE: No More Surprises: Protecting Patients from Surprise Medical Bills

Dear Chairwoman Eshoo and Ranking Member Burgess:

AARP, on behalf of our nearly 38 million members and all older Americans nationwide, would like to thank you for holding a hearing on June 12 to examine the issue of surprise medical billing. AARP strongly supports efforts to protect consumers from expensive surprise medical bills when they believe they are appropriately seeking care from in-network providers (facilities or professionals) or during an emergency.

Cost is often a key determinate as consumers decide what care to seek, as well as where to receive it. Unfortunately, there are times when an individual makes every effort to obtain affordable care under their insurance coverage, but is surprised to receive a bill from a non-network provider whom they did not choose or were not given the opportunity to choose. As we noted in our May 28, 2019, letter commenting on the draft *No Surprises Act*, we seek clarification on the following points:

- The draft bill does not appear to apply protections to non-facility based settings, such as physician offices. There are many instances of in-network, office-based providers using non-network labs to process tests, or consulting non-network providers, without the knowledge or permission of the consumer. We urge that the bill be clarified to apply to non-facility based settings as well.

- Allowing exceptions for nonparticipating providers at participating facilities to balance bill if they provide notification may remove the "surprise", but it can still place an undue burden on consumers. Individuals visiting the facility may see multiple providers. Allowing different providers to bill under different rules creates confusion and puts a burden on the consumer. Moreover, consent is not meaningful if there is limited or no choice of provider. Consumers may sign the acknowledgement form because they have no alternative.

Any final legislation must prioritize the consumer experience and follow these three principles:

1. Consumers must be held harmless

Individual out-of-pocket cost-sharing must be limited to the in-network amount when a consumer receives emergency care, chooses to receive care at an in-network facility, or has not elected to receive care from a non-network provider. This applies to any copay, coinsurance, or deductible under the individual's insurance coverage. Disputes about payment, once the in-network coverage obligation has been met, are between the provider and the payer. The consumer has fulfilled their responsibility and should not be subject to further bills or penalties. Furthermore, notifying an individual at an in-network facility that a provider or service is out-of-network does not provide sufficient protection. Notification may remove the "surprise", but it is not a substitute for meaningful choice.

2. Protections must apply to all sites of care and providers of care

An individual seeking care in a medical emergency should not be expected to research provider directories or check network status before calling an ambulance or going to the nearest emergency room. Likewise, we must not penalize consumers for making good choices, or when they are given no choice at all. An individual who does their due diligence, and seeks care from an in-network facility or an in-network provider's office, should not be saddled with a bill from a separate provider or lab for which they had no choice. Once at the facility or doctor's office, the discretion is with the provider – not the consumer – to consult specialists, order tests, and process images.

3. Protections must apply to all payers

Surprise balance billing must be prohibited across all payers – individual/small market, large employer, self-insured, and ERISA plans. This issue impacts all consumers, regardless of their type of coverage. While states should be allowed to have more protective laws, a federal standard or baseline is necessary to prevent loopholes and exceptions.

We also urge you to not overlook the Medicare program as you consider ways to protect consumers from surprise medical bills. There is a glaring absence of consumer protection in Medicare regarding the use of "observation status". Medicare beneficiaries who enter the hospital, spend multiple nights, and receive the same care as *inpatients* are being denied coverage for subsequent skilled nursing facility (SNF) care because they were classified as an *outpatient* under *observation*. We urge you to protect beneficiaries from paying possibly thousands of dollars more in surprise out-of-pocket costs by counting the time a Medicare beneficiary spends in observation toward the three-day stay requirement for Medicare coverage of SNF care.

Thank you again for your bipartisan leadership on this issue. We appreciate the opportunity to provide feedback, and look forward to working with you to protect consumers from surprise medical bills and make health care more affordable. If you have any questions, please contact me, or have your staff contact Andrew Scholnick of our Government Affairs team at ascholnick@aarp.org or 202-434-3770.

Sincerely,

David Certner

David Certner
Legislative Counsel and Legislative Policy Director
Government Affairs

Statement for the Record of Blue Shield of California, Pacific Business Group of Health, SEIU United Healthcare Workers West, to the U.S. House of Representatives, Committee on Energy and Commerce, Subcommittee on Health Hearing, "No More Surprises: Protecting Patients from Surprise Medical Bills," June 12, 2019

June 11, 2019

Dear California Members of the Energy and Commerce Committee:

We are writing to express our support for the Committee's bipartisan work to end the practice of surprise medical bills through the draft No Surprises Act. Our organizations worked together in California to pass an overwhelmingly bipartisan reform, AB 72, which tackled surprise bills in our state. Although we are proud of the work California did to tackle surprise billing, state law cannot protect every consumer. In particular, self-funded plans are exempt from AB 72 because of ERISA preemption. As demonstrated by the recent testimony of Congresswoman Katie Porter to the Ways and Means Committee, enrollees in these ERISA-governed plans can still be balanced billed. Therefore, federal legislation remains critical to close the gaps left for Californians.

We applaud the Energy and Commerce Committee for its work to move the discussion forward with a bipartisan and substantive effort. Most importantly, the discussion draft would protect consumers from surprise bills. As in the California law, the No Surprises Act would provide that, unless the consumer consents to additional charges, they would only be responsible for the amount that they would have paid if the provider had been in network.

Additionally, the draft would help protect the market from price increases that would result from choosing an inflationary and arbitrary benchmark, such as billed charges or arbitration. While many entities, include business groups and insurers, continue to support a benchmark payment set as a percentage of Medicare, we believe the state legislation was the result of a fair and productive compromise. The California law and the Energy and Commerce draft bill rely on the median network rate for each plan in each geography, which is designed to reflect the market rate so as to not inflate commercial or government health expenditures. We agree with a Health Affairs analysis which concluded that the Energy and Commerce draft, "likely would result in lower insurance premiums in most markets and hence reduced federal deficits (from reducing loss of revenue from tax subsidies to health insurance), in addition to eliminating the scourge of surprise bills to patients."

Our experience in California is that AB 72 is working to end surprise billing for health plans regulated by California law. We believe that the law has made a positive difference for consumers while protecting against price increases and addressing a market failure. Again, we applaud your leadership on this critical issue and ensuring that all consumers in our state and nationwide enjoy similar protections.

Please let us know how we can continue to support your efforts.

Sincerely,

Blue Shield of California
Pacific Business Group on Health
SEIU United Healthcare Workers West

Additional Questions for the Record

Additional Questions for the Record

Subcommittee on Health
Hearing on
"No More Surprises: Protecting Patients from Surprise Medical Bills"
June 12, 2019

Sherif Zaafran, MD

The Honorable Michael C. Burgess, M.D.

1. Dr. Zaafran, you mention in your testimony that under a benchmark approach for out-of-network care, "health plans would be greatly incentivized to not renew contracts with practices with existing contracts above the median in-network rate." Have there been any states that have implemented policies that have resulted in declining physician reimbursement?

Thank you, Representative Burgess. Yes, we have seen these concerns realized in California where a benchmark-only approach is being used. The California Medical Association has reported providers are increasingly faced with cancelled contracts and insurance companies are offering dramatically under-market rates for contract renewals, all in an effort to take advantage of a low default one-size-fits-all benchmark approach. Additionally, a recent article in the American Journal of Managed Care provides further evidence the benchmark-only approach in California has shifted negotiating power to insurers, giving them undue leverage during in-network contract discussions. To be certain, dramatic reductions in physician reimbursement imperil our ability to offer economically-viable care, attract and retain high quality physicians to emergency medicine, and ensure we have these physicians available 24/7, every day of the year, including nights, weekends, and holidays.

The Honorable Gus M. Bilirakis

1. How do we reverse perverse incentives to allow more providers to be in-network and care for more patients, which is obviously in their interest to do?

Thank you for this question, Representative Bilirakis. To effectively end surprise billing, we should ensure any solution does not harm the vast portion of the market currently functioning well, one which has brought many providers in-network. As we work to find solutions to encourage even more providers to join networks and insurers to negotiate fairly, we should be sure we are furthering successful market dynamics that result in a level playing field for these negotiations. Ensuring a fair payment standard for unanticipated out-of-network care through an Independent Dispute Resolution process will help establish a basis for providers and payers to work out payment agreements in the future. Ultimately, at some point, most physicians will see out-of-network patients due to Americans traveling for work or vacation, so it is crucial a process exists to resolve impasses over payment in a way that is fair to both physicians and payers, and keeps patients completely out of the middle.

2. One criticism of a benchmark to median rates is that all the contracts above that rate could immediately be brought out-of-network, further lowering the median rate. What long-term effect could this have on access to care, as physicians would be unable to negotiate any rate above the median in their geographic area?

A benchmark-only rate, without the ability to be appealed, could have an incredibly detrimental long-term effect on access to care. A benchmark-only rate could be easily manipulated by insurance companies to drive down in-network reimbursement to unsustainable rates. Physicians at risk of being pushed out-of-network would be forced to accept low default one-size-fits-all rates, regardless of the quality of the care they provide or the complexity of the care. A benchmark rate pays all providers as if they are exactly the same, ignoring the quality initiatives of the physician by underpaying high quality physicians who help reduce avoidable costs such as hospital readmissions, and overpaying those physicians who are not prioritizing quality improvement. Not only would quality suffer, but benchmark rates would make it difficult to provide economically-viable care, leading to staffing shortages, longer wait times, and potentially to facility consolidations and closures. Small, rural, and underserved communities would be hit hardest, as suburban and more populous urban areas could have higher benchmark rates. Furthermore, small and rural hospitals do not have the financial ability to make up for commercial reimbursement cuts from artificial and inadequate benchmark rates given their disproportionately higher rates of uninsured and underfunded Medicaid reimbursement levels compared to other providers.

3. One criticism of the Ruiz-Roe proposal is that it directs the arbiter to look at an independent database of physician charges when deciding which offer is more reasonable. Critics contend that this could allow physicians to raise charges, but a study by Georgetown indicates that physician charges in New York have actually gone down 13% since their law went into effect. Why might that be the case? Could it be because both physicians and insurers are incentivized to be reasonable and come to the table before arbitration?

I believe a key component of the New York model is that it pushes both sides to be reasonable and negotiate a fair reimbursement rate before they even get to arbitration. This is the main reason why other states, including my home state of Texas, are adopting the same model for ending surprise billing. With an Independent Dispute Resolution process, both sides know if they are not reasonable with their offer they will surely lose in this process. As a result, both sides have strong incentives to come to the table with fair offers to have the greatest chance of success. In Texas, for example, our model ensures the stability of the existing market by using previously contracted rates as a key metric in the process. This minimizes disruption in the already contracted market and helps address concerns about increasing costs. Furthermore, as data from New York's experience has shown, once the process has been in place for a few years, it begins to reach a state of equilibrium where neither side is always winning or always losing, a truly optimal outcome.

Additional Questions for the Record

Subcommittee on Health
Hearing on
"No More Surprises: Protecting Patients from Surprise Medical Bills"
June 12, 2019

Rick Sherlock

The Honorable Gus M. Bilirakis

1. Can you share how many air ambulance services operate nationally? Has industry growth grown, flattened, or declined? Of those services operating, what percentage are covered in-network?

   Response: Currently there are ---- emergency air medical bases nationally. Historically, while there was clear industry growth in the 1980s through the turn of the century, that growth rate has slowed since 2005:

   - 1980-1985: 156 %
   - 1985-1990: 193%
   - 1990-1995: 27%
   - 1995-2000: 37%
   - 2000-2005: 88%
   - 2005-2011: 23%
   - 2011-2016: 5%[1]

   Industry growth, over a 30-year period, reflects growth in demand for air medical transport services in response to the continued closures of rural hospitals and trauma centers.

   Following an extended period of slowing growth, 2019 has seen a decline in the number of bases, with 37 having closed since January 1. The substantial gap between Medicare and Medicaid reimbursements and the cost of providing the service has been the main driver of these base closures, which are affecting rural areas and regions that are underserved by hospitals and trauma centers.

   On March 20, 2019, the Government Accountability Office (GAO) published its report, "Air Ambulance: Available Data Show Privately-Insured Patients Are at Financial Risk."[2] GAO reported that "there were 752 bases in the 2012 data and 868 bases in the 2017 data." The report also noted:

   - The added bases "increased the total area served by helicopter bases by 23 percent."
   - "About 60 percent of the new helicopter bases and about half of the new fixed-

[1] Economic & Planning Systems, Inc., "An Economic Analysis of the U.S. Rotary Wing Air Medical Transport Industry", August, 2014, http://medevacfoundation.org/wp-content/uploads/2014/08/Rotary-Wing-AMT-Economic-Benefit-Study-EPS-082114.pdf; and [2016 ADAMS Database].

[2] Government Accountability Office, "Available Data Show Privately-Insured Patients Are at Financial Risk GAO-19-292, Mar 20, 2019, https://www.gao.gov/products/GAO-19-292.

wing bases…were in rural areas."

- "For just under half of the new helicopter bases…the area served overlapped with existing air ambulance coverage by more than 50 percent."
- Emergency air medical service expansion in rural areas helps fill the gap in rural health care created by the closing of rural hospitals.

AAMS' members are actively negotiating with insurance companies to secure in-network contracts where such negotiations are available. Despite that willingness to negotiate in-network rates, some insurers, citing low volumes and infrequent need for transports, have outright refused to even discuss in-network agreements with emergency air medical providers. Even so, our members have managed to increase network participation significantly; one member alone has increased their overall network participation from 2% to almost 30% in the last three years. Overall, AAMS estimates that approximately 40% of commercially insured patients transported by air medical providers are in-network.

2. What are the biggest drivers of lack of network participation?

   Response: AAMS believes the biggest single driver is lack of interest from insurers to enter negotiations. Many of our members have received an outright refusal from some insurers to even discuss going into network; Blue Cross Blue Shield of Illinois, in an email obtained by AAMS, said that "BCBSIL still does not contract with emergency air ambulance providers." We have found this posture in similar communications to members from Arkansas and Texas.

   Our members also report that, when a negotiation is possible, it is often not the rate that is the single biggest issue, but rather the insurers ability to deny payment base on medical necessity. Our members report a 40% medical necessity denial rate, nearly all of which our overturned on appeals- a process that can often take more than 9 months to resolve. We are significantly concerned about these medical necessity denials, as all helicopter air ambulance flights are medical emergencies and all of those flights must be requested by a physician or first-responder. Insurers, by denying those claims based on medical necessity, are questioning decisions made by first responders and doctors in emergency situations. These denials also increase the amount of cost that then must be shifted to the charge of the next patient, thereby increasing costs overall.

3. How do air ambulance companies calculate their rates? Is it based on a reasonable market rate, a government payer rate, or something else?

   Response: While AAMS cannot speak to the business practices of its members, and recognizes that any discussion of how rates are set by its members is strictly prohibited by antitrust laws, AAMS funded an independent cost study of the industry in 2017 that can answer how costs drive charges.[3]

[3] Xcenda, Air Medical Services Cost Study Report, March 24, 2017, https://aams.org/wp-content/uploads/2017/04/Air-Medical-Services-Cost-Study-Report.pdf.

   That study found that the single largest contributor to the cost of providing an air ambulance flight is the unpaid debt from Medicare, Medicaid, and the uninsured. In fact, the mean cost of providing an air ambulance flight when that debt is included was $26,183.00 in 2016. This cost exceeded even the average commercial payment by $2,665.00. This economic model has caused the closure of 37 air medical bases in thus far in 2019, all due to a poor mix of government and commercial payors.

Additional Questions for the Record

Subcommittee on Health
Hearing on
"No More Surprises: Protecting Patients from Surprise Medical Bills"
June 12, 2019

James Gelfand

The Honorable Gus M. Bilirakis

1. The physician community supports a proposal from Rep. Raul Ruiz and Rep. Phil Roe that models a law from New York state. This would create a "baseball-style" arbitration process that incentivizes both parties to come to the table with reasonable offers to bring doctors in network. Georgetown put out a study that says the New York model has reduced out-of-network billing by 34%. As of October 2018, arbitration decisions have been roughly evenly split between providers and payers, with 618 disputes decided in favor of the health plan and 561 decided in favor of the provider. New York has a demonstrably fair process for dispute resolution, can the insurers show how any other solution would result in similar equity between providers and insurers?

ERIC Response: *ERIC does not represent insurance company interests; we represent the large employer plan-sponsors who pay 85% of health insurance costs on behalf of employees, families, and retirees. As you are no doubt aware, over 181 million Americans currently get health insurance through an employer, and this saves the federal government hundreds of billions of dollars per year.*

The Ruiz-Roe proposal, modeled off the New York surprise billing law, would mandate binding arbitration for the entire self-insured market. This would be much more disruptive, in many critical ways, compared to the results of the New York law, which was enacted in the unique legislative environment in the state. New York's health care markets are among the most expensive and highly regulated in the country, with different rules for hospitals, HMOs, and other actors than the rest of the county. As such, attempts to project the results of a New York law on to more than 110 million Americans in self-insured plans across the country, in 50 different states, are an "apples-to-oranges" comparison.

Regardless, the results of the New York law may show a somewhat even split between winners of arbitration. However, in the case of an insurer who loses an arbitration case, the New York law subjects that insurer to potentially unlimited costs. Because the law takes into account provider list prices, which are not market-based (indeed, they are simply invented by providers with no requirement to have any basis on actual costs or economic conditions), any single arbitration

James Gelfand
Page 2

loss could incur extreme costs to the insurer. This directly translates into costs for plan participants, causing premiums, deductibles, copays, and coinsurance to increase.

The Ruiz-Roe legislation would impose a similar system on all 110 million Americans in self-insured plans, as well as on anyone enrolled in a fully-insured plan in a state that does not currently have a comprehensive surprise billing law. It is no surprise that this is an approach favored by providers – it amounts to a government mandate to force insurers and employers to pay potentially unlimited amounts of new money into provider coffers. For this reason, the arbitration approach is highly favored by the private equity hedge funds that own most of the provider firms engaging in egregious surprise billing practices.

For those interested in controlling health care costs and truly protecting patients, a local market-based benchmark is the preferred approach. See ERIC's previously submitted testimony for further details.

2. Under the proposed benchmark, what would prevent insurers from dropping providers out of network and paying everyone that had been in contract above the median the lower benchmark rate? Wouldn't the median rate then drop, so the next year they could pay them even lower?

ERIC Response: *Short answer: market realities. Long answer:*

Employers do not sell health insurance; they provide benefits to meet the needs of beneficiaries – their employees and families. As such, we need robust networks that can handle the volume of care likely to be needed by our beneficiaries in a given plan year. A benefit without sufficient provider networks does not "work." Indeed, if patients cannot obtain care through the benefit, then the costs become incredibly wasteful for an employer.

Employers pay on average more than $15,000 for health care costs per beneficiary, every year. This cost is necessary in order to ensure that the patients receive the care they need, when they need it. If the benefit would not meet the needs of the beneficiaries, a large employer has the option of simply paying the ACA "shared responsibility" penalty, which is $2,000 per employee (and no penalties related to families/dependents or retirees).

Indeed, when an employer chooses an insurance carrier to serve as their self-insured plan's third-party administrator (TPA) and offer a provider network to our beneficiaries, one of the major selling points is the comprehensiveness of the network. Employers compare the networks of various TPAs, and make a selection based on ensuring patients have access to the best providers. An insurance company that emptied out its network in order to lower next year's benchmark would be at a disastrous market disadvantage, likely losing billions of dollars as employers pivot to TPAs that still have comprehensive networks that can handle their volume.

It's no different for fully-insured plans; neither a patient nor a business is likely to choose a plan that cannot meet their needs with a sufficient provider network. The result would be a catastrophic loss of business for the plan attempting to game the system in this manner.

The hyperbolic allegation that employers, TPAs, and insurance companies will cut their own provider networks in half, in order to lower a benchmark rate in future plan years, is a scare tactic. It has been propagated by hedge fund-owned staffing firms, whose current business model is already to stay out of network, and surprise bill unsuspecting patients (who lack provider choice). Congress should not be taken in by these arguments.

the insurer and physician publicly submit unique "final offers" for review by the independent arbiter. The theory behind making the offers public is to encourage the parties to settle outside of the arbitration, as well as to incentivize reasonable bids for review. The ADR/IDR process is particularly important in circumstances where a potential minimum payment standard is insufficient due to factors such as the complexity of the patient's medical condition, the special expertise required, comorbidities, and other extraordinary factors. In addition, the College supports the adoption of the New York statute definition of the usual customary rate:

> "Usual and Customary Cost shall mean the eightieth percentile of all charges for a particular health care service performed by a provider in the same or similar specialty and provided in the same geographical area as reported in a benchmarking database maintained by a nonprofit organization specified by the superintendent. The nonprofit organization shall not be affiliated with any insurer, a corporation, a municipal cooperative health benefit plan, a health maintenance organization, or a student health plan. "

Of note, a May 2019 report from the Georgetown University Health Policy Institute's Center on Health Insurance Reforms concluded that in terms of New York, "...the law has been a success. Consumer complaints have declined dramatically. For the most part, insurers and providers appear to be working out their differences without resorting to arbitration. Further, there is not yet clear evidence that the law's use of UCR as a benchmark price has had broadly inflationary effects." The same report indicated that IDR decisions using the New York model have been relatively even between providers and payers, with 618 disputes decided in favor of the health plan and 561 decided in favor of the provider. Given these compelling results, the College strongly encourages the Committee to include an ADR/IDR process that mirrors the New York model in lieu of establishing an arbitrary payment benchmark.

In fact, the experience of physicians in the state of California reflects the pitfalls of establishing a payment rate tied to Medicare or in-network rates. As was predicted by the California Health Benefits Review Program, "by setting the non-contracted effective rate for potentially surprise professional services, "the new law "put downward pressure on contracted rates among the specialties ...that are most likely to work in non-contracted medical groups within contracted in-network facilities ...". It has also "reduce[d] the negotiated rates for those specialties by setting a ceiling (i.e., based on the Medicare fee schedule) for out-of-network...surprise medical bill payment." According to the California Medical Association, since the passage of the state's surprise medical billing law in late 2016, a substantial number of their member physicians have reported difficulties in renewing contracts with health plans and insurers with which they had longstanding existing contracts for reimbursement greater than 125 percent of the Medicare rate and in obtaining new contracts.

Again, the ACR appreciates the opportunity to provide detailed comments regarding the draft "No Surprises Act," and we look forward collaborating with you to find a federal solution that addresses the issue of surprise medical bills in a comprehensive way that does not compromise access to care through unintended consequences.

If you have any questions and/or would like any additional information regarding the College's comments, please contact Cynthia Moran, ACR's Executive Vice President, Economics, Government Relations and Health Policy, via phone (202-223-1670) or email (cmoran@acr.org).

Sincerely,

William T. Thorwarth, Jr., MD, FACR
Chief Executive Officer

Mr. Thomas Nickels
Page 1

Additional Questions for the Record

Subcommittee on Health
Hearing on
"No More Surprises: Protecting Patients from Surprise Medical Bills"
June 12, 2019

Thomas Nickels

The Honorable Michael C. Burgess, M.D.

1. I think everyone agrees that the patient should be held harmless and that their out-of-pocket costs should be kept to a minimum. Can you explain the existing process that hospitals and insurers go through in balance billing a patient and how you determine how much they must pay?

Answer:

Hospitals and health systems treat all patients who come through their doors, around the clock and regardless of their ability to pay. They work closely with them on their individual bills, including seeking information from their insurer regarding out-of-pocket expenses. Hospitals then share and discuss financial assistance options with the patient. The American Hospital Association provides resources to our members regarding how they can best talk to patients about a hospital's billing process.

For tax-exempt hospitals, Congress has prescribed specific requirements for information that must be included in a Financial Assistance Policy (FAP), and limited the amount an individual eligible for assistance can be expected to pay, typically similar to Medicare pricing. In 2016, tax-exempt hospitals reported that $43.0 billion, 6.4 percent of total hospital expenses, were both devoted to financial assistance for patients and absorbing losses from Medicaid and other means tested government program under payments, on their IRS Form 990 Schedule H. Hospital expenditures include services provided by their employed physicians. Physicians who are not employees typically have no financial assistance obligations.

August 30, 2019

Additional Questions for the Record

Subcommittee on Health
Hearing on
"No More Surprises: Protecting Patients from Surprise Medical Bills"
June 12, 2019

Responses from Jeanette Thornton

The Honorable Michael C. Burgess, M.D.

1. **Ms. Thornton, from the plan perspective, do you anticipate that insurers would behave in a way that would drive down reimbursements?**

The data have been abundantly clear that certain hospital-based provider specialties have increasingly demanded highly inflated reimbursements from patients and payers. Tying out-of-network reimbursements to the locally negotiated rates paid to in-network providers will drive down costs by requiring payments to more closely reflect both the actual cost of providing care and traditional free market forces. Health plans have every incentive to negotiate lower costs that are in the interest of health plan enrollees while ensuring that high quality providers have the necessary incentives to participate in their networks. These market realities will remain should benchmark-based legislation pass.

We do not anticipate any reductions in health plan reimbursement to providers given the larger trends that continue to drive healthcare spending. The Healthcare Cost Institute's (HCCI) 2017 Health Care Cost and Utilization Report provides insightful data on insurer health care spending. HCCI reports that provider price increases drove per-person spending growth among the employer-sponsored health insurance (ESI) population between 2013 and 2017. In fact, while utilization of services declined 0.2% between 2013 and 2017.[1]

a. **Or are there incentives to ensure network adequacy that would prevent this from happening and maintain a physician's ability to negotiate?**

Health plans are required by law to maintain certain network adequacy standards. Beyond the legal requirements, the simple fact is that without ample providers participating in a health plan network, the health plan business is not viable. Health plans need health care providers. They have every incentive to ensure that providers are adequately compensated for their skills and expertise as enrollees value access to high quality providers. The regular course of business for health plans is to routinely negotiate with new and existing providers to develop robust provider networks; physicians will continue to have both the incentive and the ability to negotiate reasonable terms in good faith.

[1] https://www.healthcostinstitute.org/research/annual-reports/entry/2017-health-care-cost-and-utilization-report

Jeanette Thornton Response
Page 2

This is in stark contrast to the status quo and what would remain under an arbitration approach where – particularly for hospital-based providers – there is little, if any, incentive to negotiate. Under both scenarios – the status quo and government-mandated arbitration – hospital-based physicians know they can extract more money by remaining out of network. We firmly believe that when the private market is able to properly function, both sides in a negotiation fare better, as opposed to the market failure that is the status quo. Indeed, we have a clear example from the state of California where – in the nation's largest insurance market – the enactment of a benchmark-based surprise billing law has led to marked increases in provider participation in health plan networks across the board – for all physician groups among all commercial payers in the state. A recent comprehensive study published in AJMC.com, the website of The American Journal of Managed Care, by AHIP, shows that since California passed its legislation to end surprise medical bills in 2016 (AB 72), the number of in-network doctors has increased by 16% and has not threatened provider networks.[2]

2. **I think everyone agrees that the patient should be held harmless and that their out-of-pocket costs should be kept to a minimum. Can you explain the existing process that hospitals and insurers go through in balance billing a patient and how you determine how much they must pay?**

We agree that patients should be held harmless and that their out-of-pocket costs should be limited to what they would have been if they were treated by an in-network provider or hospital. It is critical that policymakers recognize who sends balance bills. Insurers negotiate on behalf of their patient-enrollees and pay on their behalf according to the terms of the contract. Insurers do not bill patients. Health insurance providers are not necessarily aware when a member is balance billed. When a non-participating provider (out-of-network) submits a claim to a health plan, and the health plan adjudicates that claim according to the member's benefits, the interaction between the provider and the payer is complete. Health insurance providers, therefore, do not know if a provider then proceeds to balance bill a patient or for what amount. Health insurance providers are made aware of balance bills when a member contacts the health plan about the receipt of a balance bill through the grievance and appeals process. The way this is cataloged and tracked may vary by insurer and/or market.

Health plans routinely pay in excess of what the contract requires of them in an effort to get the hospital or provider to treat that payment as satisfying the patient's debt. These amounts are often far beyond the actual cost of care and often above in-network rates. For example, Drew Calver's experience receiving a surprise bill has received much public attention. Mr. Calver received a $164,941 bill from the hospital for a four-day hospital stay.[3] The hospital where he was treated was out-of-network with his health plan. Despite being out-of-network, the health plan tried to negotiate with the medical center and ultimately paid more than twice what an independent analysis of the bill determined would have been a reasonable cost. Health plans look to experts and past experience to identify the actual cost of care and what going market rates are

[2] https://www.ajmc.com/contributor/america's-health-insurance-plans/2019/08/can-we-stop-surprise-medical-bills-and-strengthen-provider-networks-california-did
[3] https://www.npr.org/sections/health-shots/2018/08/27/640891882/life-threatening-heart-attack-leaves-teacher-with-108-951-bill

in that region for the services and treatment provided. This process includes comparisons to the in-network rates at those facilities, third-party databases that include other payers, the Medicare rates for the same services, and independent analyses of the cost of care. In Mr. Calver's case, the hospital sent the patient a bill for more than $108,000 despite the health plan paying well above reasonable market rates. A process whereby hospitals or providers may invent charges and stick the patient with an exorbitant bill is not sustainable, nor is a system where good faith negotiations and market-based payments by health plans are not enough to satisfy those inflated bills.

The Honorable Gus M. Bilirakis

1. **Despite the patient no longer receiving a surprise or balance bill, could patients still be harmed by arbitration? If so, how and how could we address?**

Patients would undoubtedly be harmed by an arbitration process. Arbitration is a time consuming, administratively burdensome process that will drive up overall health insurance costs and increase patient premiums and cost sharing. An arbitration process will delay resolution for patients and reduce pricing certainty when setting health insurance rates. Arbitration also places the onus for action on the patient or their health plan, instead of protecting the patient.

We cannot stress enough that independent experts have looked at arbitration proposals and found that not only will this fail to rein in health spending, it will likely increase the cost of health care in the United States. This is a time when every effort by every stakeholder in health care must be focused on reducing the unsustainable cost of care. Arbitration proposals that would increase health costs by even a single dollar take us in the wrong direction.

Instead of arbitration, legislation that addresses surprise medical bills should focus on applying free market principles that avoid government-rate setting and look to negotiations between doctors and health insurance providers. This benchmark approach is known to reduce health costs and increase network participation by providers. A fair and reasonable benchmark based on existing market rates will result in transparency for patients, health plans, and providers.

2. **Have there been any observable trends in surprise or balance billing? Are some places or patients more likely to see surprise or balance billing than others – if so, why?**

Certain physician specialties such as anesthesiologists, radiologists, pathologists, and emergency physicians are more likely to balance bill than their peers. For these specialties there is little need to participate in health plan networks as these physicians will always see a steady flow of patients. In terms of the magnitude of these balance bills relative to Medicare anesthesiologists charge an average of 5.8 times that of Medicare rates, radiologists charge 4.5 times, and pathologists and emergency physicians at least 4 times. In many places these rates are even higher.

Surprise billing is also more common at hospitals that use outside staffing firms to staff their emergency departments. For example, in a National Bureau of Economic Research paper published in 2017, researchers found that once EmCare, a large physician staffing firm, took over the management of emergency department services at a hospital, out-of-network billing rates increased over 80 percent. This increased insurer payments by 122 percent and patient cost sharing by 83 percent.[4] There is a direct link between the influx of private-equity owned physician staffing firms buying emergency departments and other hospital practices and them taking providers out-of-network and electing to code services at a higher reimbursement rate. There is a reason surprise billing is not a widespread problem at every hospital; it is a significant problem where these physician staffing firms have identified surprise billing as a profit-earning strategy.

Another trend important to highlight is that the prevalence of out of network billing has been increasing; among emergency room visits for example, surprise medical bills increased from 32.3% in 2010 to 42.8% in 2016, and the financial responsibility associated with these bills increased from a mean of $220 in 2010 to a mean of $628 in 2016.[5] This trend is not by accident and eliminating the financial incentive to remain out of network – accomplishable by requiring payments to be based on negotiated network rates – would help halt this trend and rein in health costs for patients nationwide.

3. **Patients in the same location can have a different risk for receiving a surprise bill depending on which insurance plan they have: What differentiates these plans? Does federal law ensure that networks provide adequate and transparent choices for patients?**

Patients who are in plans governed by the Employee Retirement Income Security Act (ERISA) are preempt from state laws regulating insurance. For example, if a patient resides in a state that has enacted surprise medical legislation yet is covered by an ERISA-governed plan the state's legislation on surprise medical billing will not apply to this individual. As such, patients in the same location may experience varying levels of risk of receiving a surprise medical bill depending on whether their plan is provided through a self-funded plan covered by ERISA versus a plan that is fully-insured and covered under state insurance law and regulation. These plans could be offered through the individual health insurance market (on or off Exchange), the small group health insurance market, or be plans sold strictly to large employers.

Health plans are subject to strict licensure requirements in order to sell health plans in the various states, and a key requirement is having an adequate provider network. Health plans use provider networks as a tool to improve quality and control costs. Through selectively contracting with credentialed providers, health plans can create networks that provide consumers with lower cost, high-quality care. When contracting with providers health plans must negotiate rates and set up contracts with each provider separately.

---

[4] Cooper, Z.; Morton, F.; Shekita, N. January 2018. Surprise! Out-of-Network Billing for Emergency Care in the United States. *National Bureau of Economic Research*. Retrieved from: https://www.nber.org/papers/w23623.pdf
[5] Sun, E.; Mello, M.; Moshfegh, J.; & Baker, L. August 2019. Assessment of Out-of-Network Billing for Privately Insured Patients Receiving Care in In-Network Hospitals. *JAMA Internal Medicine*.

Jeanette Thornton Response
Page 5

Different types of plans allow consumers to decide what type of network flexibility best fit their needs; Preferred Provider Organizations (PPOs) and Health Maintenance Organizations (HMOs) are two examples of plans that give consumers different network flexibility options. It's important to highlight that we see similar rates of surprise billing in both broad PPO networks and narrow HMO networks.

Finally, it is worth noting that the state of Texas has some of the strongest network adequacy laws in the country and yet its residents are more likely to receive a surprise medical bill than residents of any other state.

4. Can you discuss some perverse incentives that could lead to the creation of narrow, inadequate networks?

When it comes to health plan networks, narrow does not mean inadequate. Consumers have a number of choices when deciding which plan works best for them whether that be a PPO with a broader network or an HMO with a more limited network. Individual consumers and employers often elect a more limited network as a means of restraining costs and our members offer options for large provider networks or less expensive options depending on the needs and choice of the consumer. The problem we see with surprise billing is not one of network adequacy, and academic experts have reached that very conclusion.[6] We do, however, see a real problem in terms of provider participation. Hospital-based providers have recognized and exploited a market failure wherein they need not participate in networks to see patients and by not participating they can charge more money. Regardless of the network flexibility choices, all plans are subject to strict licensure requirements based on the state they are operating in--one of those requirements being adequate provider networks.

Under a benchmark approach to surprise billing, networks will continue to be adequate and held to the same standards they are now. We also know from experience in California – the nation's largest insurance market – that a benchmark approach results in increased provider participation in health plan networks, including marked increases among hospital-based physicians. A recent comprehensive study published in AJMC.com, the website of The American Journal of Managed Care, by AHIP, shows that since California passed its legislation to end surprise medical bills in 2016 (AB 72), the number of in-network doctors has increased by 16% and has not threatened provider networks.[7] A benchmark reimbursement approach works for consumers and physicians alike.

---

[6] https://www.brookings.edu/blog/usc-brookings-schaeffer-on-health-policy/2019/05/10/the-relationship-between-network-adequacy-and-surprise-billing/
[7] https://www.ajmc.com/contributor/america's-health-insurance-plans/2019/08/can-we-stop-surprise-medical-bills-and-strengthen-provider-networks-california-did

Chapter 2

Ban Surprise Billing Act*

House of Representatives

Mr. SCOTT of Virginia, from the Committee on Education and Labor, submitted the following report

[To accompany H.R. 5800]

[Including cost estimate of the Congressional Budget Office]

The Committee on Education and Labor, to whom was referred the bill (H.R. 5800) to end surprise medical billing and increase transparency in health coverage, having considered the same, reports favorably thereon with an amendment and recommends that the bill as amended do pass.

The amendment is as follows:

Strike all after the enacting clause and insert the following:

SECTION 1. SHORT TITLE.

This Act may be cited as the "Ban Surprise Billing Act."

SECTION 2. PREVENTING SURPRISE MEDICAL BILLS.

(a) PUBLIC HEALTH SERVICE ACT AMENDMENTS.—Section 2719A of the Public Health Service Act (42 U.S.C. 300gg–19a) is amended—

(1) by amending subsection (b) to read as follows:

"(b) COVERAGE OF EMERGENCY SERVICES.—

"(1) IN GENERAL.—If a group health plan, or a health insurance issuer offering group or individual health insurance coverage, provides or covers any benefits with respect to services in an emergency department of a hospital or with respect to emergency services in an independent freestanding emergency department (as defined in paragraph (3)(D)), the plan or issuer shall cover emergency services (as defined in paragraph (3)(C))—

"(A) without the need for any prior authorization determination;

* This is an edited, reformatted and augmented version of House of Representatives; 116th Congress, 2d Session, Publication No. Rept. 116–615, Part 1, dated December 2, 2020.

In: Putting an End to Surprise Medical Billing
Editor: Danial E. Tackett
ISBN: 979-8-88697-296-2

"(B) whether the health care provider furnishing such services is a participating provider or a participating emergency facility, as applicable, with respect to such services;

"(C) in a manner so that, if such services are provided to a participant, beneficiary, or enrollee by a nonparticipating provider or a nonparticipating emergency facility—

"(i) such services will be provided without imposing any requirement under the plan or coverage for prior authorization of services or any limitation on coverage that is more restrictive than the requirements or limitations that apply to emergency services received from participating providers and participating emergency facilities with respect to such plan or coverage, respectively;

"(ii)the cost-sharing requirement (expressed as a copayment amount or coinsurance rate) is not greater than the requirement that would apply if such services were provided by a participating provider or a participating emergency facility;

"(iii) such cost-sharing requirement is calculated as if the total amount that would have been charged for such services by such participating provider or participating emergency facility were equal to the recognized amount (as defined in paragraph (3)(H)) for such services, plan or coverage, and year;

"(iv) the group health plan or health insurance issuer, respectively, pays to such provider or facility, respectively the amount by which the recognized amount for such services and year involved exceeds the cost-sharing amount for such services (as determined in accordance with clauses (ii) and (iii)) and year; and

"(v) any cost-sharing payments made by the participant, beneficiary, or enrollee with respect to such emergency services so furnished shall be counted toward any in-network deductible or out-of-pocket maximums applied under the plan or coverage, respectively (and such in-network deductible and out-of-pocket maximums shall be applied) in the same manner as if such cost-sharing payments were made with respect to emergency services furnished by a participating provider or a participating emergency facility; and

"(D) without regard to any other term or condition of such coverage (other than exclusion or coordination of benefits, or an affiliation or waiting period, permitted under section 2704 of this Act, including as incorporated pursuant to section 715 of the Employee Retirement Income Security Act of 1974 and section 9815 of the Internal Revenue Code of 1986, and other than applicable cost-sharing).

"(2) AUDIT PROCESS AND REGULATIONS FOR MEDIAN CONTRACTED RATES.— "

"(A) AUDIT PROCESS.—

"(i) IN GENERAL.—Not later than July 1, 2021, the Secretary, in consultation with appropriate State agencies and the Secretary of Labor and the Secretary of the Treasury, shall establish through rulemaking a process, in accordance with clause (ii), under which group health plans and health insurance issuers offering health insurance coverage in the group or individual market are audited by the Secretary or applicable State authority to ensure that—

"(I) such plans and coverage are in compliance with the requirement of applying a median contracted rate under this section; and "(II) such median contracted rate so applied satisfies the definition under paragraph (3)(E) with respect to the year involved, including with respect to a group health plan or health insurance issuer described in clause (ii) of such paragraph (3)(E).

"(ii) AUDIT SAMPLES.—Under the process established pursuant to clause (i), the Secretary—

"(I) shall conduct audits described in such clause, with respect to a year (beginning with 2022), of a sample with respect to such year of claims data from not more than 25 group health plans and health insurance issuers offering health insurance coverage in the group or individual market; and

"(II) may audit any group health plan or health insurance issuer offering health insurance coverage in the group or individual market if the Secretary has received any complaint about such plan or coverage, respectively, that involves the compliance of the plan or coverage, respectively, with either of the requirements described in subclauses (I) and (II) of such clause.

"(iii) REPORTS.—Beginning for 2022, the Secretary shall annually submit to Congress a report on the number of plans and issuers with respect to which audits were conducted during such year pursuant to this subparagraph.

"(B) RULEMAKING.—Not later than July 1, 2021, the Secretary, in consultation with the Secretary of Labor and the Secretary of the Treasury, shall establish through rulemaking—

"(i) the methodology the group health plan or health insurance issuer offering health insurance coverage in the group or individual market shall use to determine the median contracted rate, differentiating by line of business;

"(ii) the information such plan or issuer, respectively, shall share with the nonparticipating provider or nonparticipating facility, as applicable, when making such a determination;

"(iii) the geographic regions applied for purposes of this subparagraph, taking into account access to items and services in rural and underserved areas, including health professional shortage areas, as defined in section 332; and "(iv) a process to receive complaints of violations of the requirements described in subclauses (I) and (II) of subparagraph (A)(i) by group health plans and health insurance issuers offering health insurance coverage in the group or individual market.

Such rulemaking shall take into account payments that are made by such plan or issuer, respectively, that are not on a fee-for-service basis. Such methodology may account for relevant payment adjustments that take into account quality or facility type (including higher acuity settings and the case-mix of various facility types) that are otherwise taken into account for purposes of determining payment amounts with respect to participating facilities. In carrying out clause (iii), the Secretary shall consult with the National Association of Insurance Commissioners to establish the geographic regions under such clause and shall periodically update such regions, as appropriate.

"(3) DEFINITIONS.—In this part:

"(A) EMERGENCY DEPARTMENT OF A HOSPITAL.—The term 'emergency department of a hospital' includes a hospital outpatient department that provides emergency services.

"(B) EMERGENCY MEDICAL CONDITION.—The term 'emergency medical condition' means a medical condition manifesting itself by acute symptoms of sufficient severity (including severe pain) such that a prudent layperson, who possesses an average knowledge of health and medicine, could reasonably expect the absence of immediate medical attention to result in a condition described in clause (i), (ii), or (iii) of section 1867(e)(1)(A) of the Social Security Act.

"(C) EMERGENCY SERVICES.—

"(i) IN GENERAL.—The term 'emergency services', with respect to an emergency medical condition, means—

"(I) a medical screening examination (as required under section 1867 of the Social Security Act, or as would be required under such section if such section applied to an independent freestanding emergency department) that is within the capability of the emergency department of a hospital or of an independent freestanding emergency department, as applicable, including ancillary services routinely available to the emergency department to evaluate such emergency medical condition; and

"(II) within the capabilities of the staff and facilities available at the hospital or the independent freestanding emergency department, as applicable, such further medical examination and treatment as are required under section 1867 of such Act, or as would be required under such section if such section applied to an independent freestanding emergency department, to stabilize the patient.

"(ii) INCLUSION OF CERTAIN SERVICES OUTSIDE OF EMERGENCY DEPARTMENT.—

"(I) IN GENERAL.—For purposes of this subsection and section 2799A–1, in the case of an individual enrolled in a group health plan or health insurance coverage offered by a health insurance issuer in the group or individual market who is furnished services described in clause (i) by a participating or nonparticipating provider or a participating or nonparticipating emergency facility to stabilize such individual with respect to an emergency medical condition, the term 'emergency services' shall include, unless each of the conditions described in subclause (II) are met, in addition to the items and services described in clause (i), items and services for which benefits are provided or covered under the plan or coverage, respectively, furnished by a nonparticipating provider or nonparticipating facility, regardless of the department of the hospital in which such individual is furnished such items or services, if, after such stabilization but during such visit in which such individual is so stabilized, the provider or facility determines that such items or services are needed.

"(II) CONDITIONS.—For purposes of subclause (I), the conditions described in this subclause, with respect to an individual who is stabilized and furnished additional items and services described in subclause (I) after such stabilization by a provider or facility described in subclause (I), are the following:

"(aa) Such a provider or facility determines such individual is able to travel using nonmedical transportation or non-emergency medical transportation.

"(bb) Such provider furnishing such additional items and services satisfies the notice and consent criteria of section 2799A–2(d) with respect to such items and services.

"(cc) Such an individual is in a condition to receive (as determined in accordance with guidance issued by the Secretary) the information described in section 2799A–2 and to provide informed consent under such section, in accordance with applicable State law.

"(D) INDEPENDENT FREESTANDING EMERGENCY DEPARTMENT.—The term 'independent freestanding emergency department' means a facility that—

"(i) is geographically separate and distinct and licensed separately from a hospital under applicable State law; and

"(ii) provides any emergency services (as defined in subparagraph (C)).

"(E) MEDIAN CONTRACTED RATE.—

"(i) IN GENERAL.—The term 'median contracted rate' means, subject to clauses (ii) and (iii), with respect to a sponsor of a group health plan and health insurance issuer offering health insurance coverage in the group or individual market—

"(I) for an item or service furnished during 2022, the median of the contracted rates recognized by the plan or issuer, respectively (determined with respect to all such plans of such sponsor or all such coverage offered by such issuer that are offered within the same line of business as the plan or coverage) as the total maximum payment (including the cost-sharing amount imposed for such item or service and the amount to be paid by the plan or issuer, respectively) under such plans or coverage, respectively, on January 31, 2019, for the same or a similar item or service that is provided by a provider in the same or similar specialty and provided in the geographic region in which the item or service is furnished, consistent with the methodology established by the Secretary under paragraph (2)(B), increased by the percentage increase in the consumer price index for all urban consumers (United States city average) over 2019, such percentage increase over 2020, and such percentage increase over 2021; and

"(II) for an item or service furnished during 2023 or a subsequent year, the median contracted rate determined under this clause for such an item or service furnished in the previous year, increased by the percentage increase in the consumer price index for all urban consumers (United States city average) over such previous year.

"(ii) NEW PLANS AND COVERAGE.—The term 'median contracted rate' means, with respect to a sponsor of a group health plan or health insurance issuer offering health insurance coverage in the group or individual market in a geographic region in which such sponsor or issuer, respectively, did not offer any group health plan or health insurance coverage during 2019—

"(I) for the first year in which such group health plan or health insurance coverage, respectively, is offered in such region, a rate (determined in accordance with a methodology established by the Secretary) for items and services that are covered by such plan and furnished during such first year; and

"(II) for each subsequent year such group health plan or health insurance coverage, respectively, is offered in such region, the median contracted rate determined under this clause for such items and services furnished in the previous year, increased by the percentage increase in the consumer price index for all urban consumers (United States city average) over such previous year.

"(iii) INSUFFICIENT INFORMATION; NEWLY COVERED ITEMS AND SERVICES.—In the case of a sponsor of a group health plan or health insurance issuer offering health insurance coverage in the group or individual market that does not have sufficient information to calculate the median of the contracted rates described in clause (i)(I) in 2019 (or, in the case of a newly covered item or service (as defined in clause (iv)(III)), in the first coverage year (as defined in clause (iv)(I)) for such item or service with respect to such plan or coverage) for an item or service (including with respect to provider type, or amount, of claims for items or services (as determined by the Secretary) provided in a particular geographic region (other than in a case with respect to which clause (ii) applies)) the term 'median contracted rate'—

"(I) for an item or service furnished during 2022 (or, in the case of a newly covered item or service, during the first coverage year for such item or service with respect to such plan or coverage), means such rate for such item or service determined by the sponsor or issuer, respectively, through use of any database that is determined, in accordance with rulemaking described in paragraph (2)(B), to not have any conflicts of interest and to have sufficient information reflecting allowed amounts paid to a health care provider or facility for relevant services furnished in the applicable geographic region (such as a State all-payer claims database);

"(II) for an item or service furnished in a subsequent year (before the first sufficient information year (as defined in clause (iv)(II)) for such item or service with respect to such plan or coverage), means the rate determined under subclause (I) or this subclause, as applicable, for such item or service for the year previous to such subsequent year, increased by the percentage increase in the consumer price index for all urban consumers (United States city average) over such previous year;

"(III) for an item or service furnished in the first sufficient information year for such item or service with respect to such plan or coverage, has the meaning given the term median contracted rate in clause (i)(I), except that in applying such clause to such item or service, the reference to 'furnished during 2022' shall be treated as a reference to furnished during such first sufficient information year, the reference to 'in 2019' shall be treated as a reference to such sufficient information year, and the increase described in such clause shall not be applied; and

"(IV) for an item or service furnished in any year subsequent to the first sufficient information year for such item or service with respect to such plan or coverage, has the meaning given such term in clause (i)(II), except that in applying such clause to such item or service, the reference to 'furnished during 2023 or a subsequent year' shall be treated as a reference to furnished during the year after such first sufficient information year or a subsequent year.

"(iv) DEFINITIONS.—For purposes of this subparagraph:

"(I) FIRST COVERAGE YEAR.—The term 'first coverage year' means, with respect to a group health plan or health insurance coverage offered by a health insurance issuer in the group or individual market and an item or service for which coverage is not offered in 2019 under such plan or coverage, the first year after 2019 for which coverage for such item or service is offered under such plan or health insurance coverage.

"(II) FIRST SUFFICIENT INFORMATION YEAR.—The term 'first sufficient information year' means, with respect to a group health plan or health insurance coverage offered by a health insurance issuer in the group or individual market—

"(aa) in the case of an item or service for which the plan or coverage does not have sufficient information to calculate the median of the contracted rates described in clause (i)(I) in 2019, the first year subsequent to 2022 for which the sponsor or issuer has such sufficient information to calculate the median of such contracted rates in the year previous to such first subsequent year; and

"(bb) in the case of a newly covered item or service, the first year subsequent to the first coverage year for such item or service with respect to such plan or coverage for which the sponsor or issuer has sufficient information to calculate the median of the contracted rates described in clause (i)(I) in the year previous to such first subsequent year.

"(III) NEWLY COVERED ITEM OR SERVICE.—The term 'newly covered item or service' means, with respect to a group health plan or health insurance issuer offering health insurance coverage in the group or individual market, an item or service for which coverage was not offered in 2019 under such plan or coverage, but is offered under such plan or coverage in a year after 2019.

"(F) NONPARTICIPATING EMERGENCY FACILITY; PARTICIPATING EMERGENCY FACILITY.—

"(i) NONPARTICIPATING EMERGENCY FACILITY.—The term 'nonparticipating emergency facility' means, with respect to an item or service and a group health plan or health insurance coverage offered by a health insurance issuer in the group or individual market, an emergency department of a hospital, or an independent freestanding emergency department, that does not have a contractual relationship directly or indirectly with the plan or issuer, respectively, for furnishing such item or service under the plan or coverage, respectively.

"(ii) PARTICIPATING EMERGENCY FACILITY.—The term 'participating emergency facility' means, with respect to an item or service and a group health plan or health insurance coverage offered by a health insurance issuer in the group or individual market, an emergency department of a hospital, or an independent freestanding emergency department, that has a contractual relationship directly or indirectly with the plan or issuer, respectively, with respect to the furnishing of such an item or service at such facility.

"(G) NONPARTICIPATING PROVIDERS; PARTICIPATING PROVIDERS.—

"(i) NONPARTICIPATING PROVIDER.—The term 'nonparticipating provider' means, with respect to an item or service and a group health plan or health insurance coverage offered by a health insurance issuer in the group or individual market, a physician or other health care provider who is acting within the scope of practice of that provider's license or certification under applicable State law and who does not have a contractual relationship with the plan or issuer, respectively, for furnishing such item or service under the plan or coverage, respectively.

"(ii) PARTICIPATING PROVIDER.—The term 'participating provider' means, with respect to an item or service and a group health plan or health insurance coverage offered by a health insurance issuer in the group or individual market, a physician or other health care provider who is acting within the scope of practice of that provider's license or certification under applicable State law and who has a contractual relationship with the plan or issuer, respectively, for furnishing such item or service under the plan or coverage, respectively.

"(H) RECOGNIZED AMOUNT.—The term 'recognized amount' means, with respect to an item or service furnished by a nonparticipating provider or emergency facility during a year and a group health plan or health insurance coverage offered by a health insurance issuer in the group or individual market—

"(i) subject to clause (iii), in the case of such item or service furnished in a State that has in effect a specified State law with respect to such plan, coverage, or issuer, respectively, such a nonparticipating provider or emergency facility, and such an item or service, the amount determined in accordance with such law;

"(ii) subject to clause (iii), in the case of such item or service furnished in a State that does not have in effect a specified State law, with respect to such plan, coverage, or issuer, respectively, such a nonparticipating provider or emergency facility, and such an item or service, an amount that is the median contracted rate (as defined in subparagraph (E)) for such year and determined in accordance with rulemaking described in paragraph (2)(B)) for such item or service; or

"(iii) in the case of such item or service furnished in a State with an All-Payer Model Agreement under section 1115A of the Social Security Act, the amount that the State approves under such system for such item or service so furnished.

"(I) SPECIFIED STATE LAW.—The term 'specified State law' means, with respect to a State, an item or service furnished by a nonparticipating provider or emergency facility during a year and a group health plan or health insurance coverage offered by a health insurance issuer in the group or individual market, a State law that provides for a method for determining the amount of payment that is required to be covered by such a plan, coverage, or issuer, respectively (to the extent such State law applies to such plan, coverage, or issuer, subject to section 514 of the Employee Retirement Income Security Act of 1974) in the case of a participant, beneficiary, or enrollee covered under such plan or coverage and receiving such item or service from such a nonparticipating provider or emergency facility.

"(J) STABILIZE.—The term 'to stabilize', with respect to an emergency medical condition (as defined in subparagraph (B)), has the meaning give in section 1867(e)(3) of the Social Security Act (42 U.S.C. 1395dd(e)(3))."; and

(2) by adding at the end the following new subsections:

"(e) COVERAGE OF NON-EMERGENCY SERVICES PERFORMED BY NON-PARTICIPATING PROVIDERS AT CERTAIN PARTICIPATING FACILITIES.—

"(1) IN GENERAL.—In the case of items or services (other than emergency services to which subsection (b) applies) for which any benefits are provided or covered by a group health plan or health insurance issuer offering health insurance coverage in the group or individual market furnished to a participant, beneficiary, or enrollee of such plan or coverage by a nonparticipating provider (as defined in subsection (b)(3)(G)(i)) (and who, with respect to such items and services, has not satisfied the notice and consent criteria of section 2799A–2(d)) with respect to a visit (as defined by the Secretary in accordance with paragraph (2)(B)) at a participating health care facility (as defined in paragraph (2)(A)), with respect to such plan or coverage, respectively, the plan or coverage, respectively—

"(A) shall not impose on such participant, beneficiary, or enrollee a cost-sharing amount (expressed as a copayment amount or coinsurance rate) for such items and services so furnished that is greater than the cost-sharing amount that would apply under such plan or coverage, respectively, had such items or services been furnished by a participating provider (as defined in subsection (b)(3)(G)(ii));

"(B) shall calculate such cost-sharing amount as if the total amount that would have been charged for such items and services by such participating provider were equal to the recognized amount (as defined in subsection (b)(3)(H)) for such items and services, plan or coverage, and year;

"(C) shall pay to such provider furnishing such items and services to such participant, beneficiary, or enrollee the amount by which the recognized amount (as defined in subsection (b)(3)(H)) for such items and services and year involved exceeds the cost-sharing amount imposed under the plan or coverage, respectively, for such items and services (as determined in accordance with subparagraphs (A) and (B)); and

"(D) shall count toward any in-network deductible and in-network out-of-pocket maximums (as applicable) applied under the plan or coverage, respectively, any cost-sharing payments made by the participant, beneficiary, or enrollee (and such in-network deductible and out-of-pocket maximums shall be applied) with respect to such items and services so furnished in the same manner as if such cost-sharing payments were with respect to items and services furnished by a participating provider.

"(2) DEFINITIONS.—In this section:

"(A) PARTICIPATING HEALTH CARE FACILITY.—

"(i) IN GENERAL.—The term 'participating health care facility' means, with respect to an item or service and a group health plan or health insurance issuer offering health insurance coverage in the group or individual market, a health care facility described in clause (ii) that has a contractual relationship with the plan or issuer, respectively, with respect to the furnishing of such an item or service at the facility.

"(ii) HEALTH CARE FACILITY DESCRIBED.—A health care facility described in this clause, with respect to a group health plan or health insurance coverage offered in the group or individual market, is each of the following:

"(I) A hospital (as defined in 1861(e) of the Social Security Act).

"(II) A hospital outpatient department.

"(III) A critical access hospital (as defined in section 1861(mm) of such Act).

"(IV) An ambulatory surgical center (as defined in section 1833(i)(1)(A) of such Act).

"(V) Any other facility that provides items or services for which coverage is provided under the plan or coverage, respectively.

"(B) VISIT.—The term 'visit' shall, with respect to items and services furnished to an individual at a participating health care facility, include equipment and devices, telemedicine services, imaging services, laboratory services, and such other items and services as the Secretary may specify, regardless of whether or not the provider furnishing such items or services is at the facility.

"(f) AIR AMBULANCE SERVICES.—

"(1) IN GENERAL.—In the case of a participant, beneficiary, or enrollee in a group health plan or health insurance coverage offered in the group or individual market who receives air ambulance services from a nonparticipating provider (as defined in subsection (b)(3)(G)) with respect to such plan or coverage, if such services would be covered if provided by a participating provider (as defined in such section) with respect to such plan or coverage—

"(A) the cost-sharing requirement (expressed as a copayment amount, coinsurance rate, or deductible) with respect to such services shall be the same requirement that would apply if such services were provided by such a participating provider, and any coinsurance or deductible shall be based on rates that would apply for such services if they were furnished by such a participating provider;

"(B) such cost-sharing amounts shall be counted toward the in-network deductible and in-network out-of-pocket maximum amount under the plan or coverage for the plan year (and such in-network deductible shall be applied) with respect to such items and services so furnished in the same manner as if such cost-sharing payments were with respect to items and services furnished by a participating provider; and

"(C) the plan or coverage shall pay to such provider furnishing such services to such participant, beneficiary, or enrollee the amount by which the recognized amount (as defined in and determined pursuant to subsection (b)(3)(H)(ii)) for such services and year involved exceeds the cost-sharing amount imposed under the plan or coverage, respectively, for such services (as determined in accordance with subparagraphs (A) and (B)).

"(2) AIR AMBULANCE SERVICE DEFINED.—For purposes of this section, the term 'air ambulance service' means medical transport by helicopter or airplane for patients.

"(g) CERTAIN ACCESS FEES TO CERTAIN DATABASES.—In the case of a sponsor of a group health plan or health insurance issuer offering health insurance coverage in the group or individual market that, pursuant to subsection (b)(3)(E)(iii), uses a database described in such subsection to determine a rate to apply under such subsection for an item or service by reason of having insufficient information described in such subsection with respect to such item or service, such sponsor or issuer shall cover the cost for access to such database."

(b) ERISA AMENDMENTS.—

(1) IN GENERAL.—Subpart B of part 7 of subtitle B of title I of the Employee Retirement Income Security Act of 1974 (29 U.S.C. 1185 et seq.) is amended by adding at the end the following:

"SEC. 716. CONSUMER PROTECTIONS.

"(a) CHOICE OF HEALTH CARE PROFESSIONAL.—If a group health plan or health insurance issuer offering group health insurance coverage requires or provides for designation by a participant or beneficiary of a participating primary care provider, then the plan or issuer shall permit each participant or beneficiary to designate any participating primary care provider who is available to accept such individual.

"(b) COVERAGE OF EMERGENCY SERVICES.—

"(1) IN GENERAL.—If a group health plan, or a health insurance issuer offering group health insurance coverage, provides or covers any benefits with respect to services in an emergency department of a hospital or with respect to emergency services in an independent freestanding emergency department (as defined in paragraph (3)(D)), the plan or issuer shall cover emergency services (as defined in paragraph (3)(C))—

"(A) without the need for any prior authorization determination;

"(B) whether the health care provider furnishing such services is a participating provider or a participating emergency facility, as applicable, with respect to such services;

"(C) in a manner so that, if such services are provided to a participant or beneficiary by a nonparticipating provider or a nonparticipating emergency facility—

"(i) such services will be provided without imposing any requirement under the plan for prior authorization of services or any limitation on coverage that is more restrictive than the requirements or limitations that apply to emergency services received from participating providers and participating emergency facilities with respect to such plan or coverage, respectively;

"(ii) the cost-sharing requirement (expressed as a copayment amount or coinsurance rate) is not greater than the requirement that would apply if such services were provided by a participating provider or a participating emergency facility;

"(iii) such cost-sharing requirement is calculated as if the total amount that would have been charged for such services by such participating provider or participating emergency facility were equal to the recognized amount (as defined in paragraph (3)(H)) for such services, plan or coverage, and year;

"(iv) the group health plan or health insurance issuer, respectively, pays to such provider or facility, respectively, the amount by which the recognized amount for such services and year involved exceeds the cost-sharing amount for such services (as determined in accordance with clauses (ii) and (iii)) and year; and

"(v) any cost-sharing payments made by the participant or beneficiary with respect to such emergency services so furnished shall be counted toward any in-network deductible or out-of-pocket maximums applied under the plan or coverage, respectively (and such in-network deductible and out-of-pocket maximums shall be applied) in the same manner as if such cost-sharing payments were made with respect to emergency services furnished by a participating provider or a participating emergency facility; and

"(D) without regard to any other term or condition of such coverage (other than exclusion or coordination of benefits, or an affiliation or waiting period, permitted under section 2704 of the Public Health Service Act, including as incorporated pursuant to section 715 of this Act and section 9815 of the Internal Revenue Code of 1986, and other than applicable cost-sharing).

"(2) AUDIT PROCESS AND REGULATIONS FOR MEDIAN CONTRACTED RATES.— "

"(A) AUDIT PROCESS.—

"(i) IN GENERAL.—Not later than July 1, 2021, the Secretary, in consultation with appropriate State agencies and the Secretary of Health and Human Services and the Secretary of the Treasury, shall establish through rulemaking a process, in accordance with clause (ii), under which group health plans and health insurance issuers offering health insurance coverage in the group market are audited by the Secretary or applicable State authority to ensure that—

"(I) such plans and coverage are in compliance with the requirement of applying a median contracted rate under this section; and "(II) such median contracted rate so applied satisfies the definition under paragraph (3)(E) with respect to the year involved, including with respect to a group health plan or health insurance issuer described in clause (ii) of such paragraph (3)(E).

"(ii) AUDIT SAMPLES.—Under the process established pursuant to clause (i), the Secretary—

"(I) shall conduct audits described in such clause, with respect to a year (beginning with 2022), of a sample with respect to such year of claims data from not more than 25 group health plans and health insurance issuers offering health insurance coverage in the group market; and

"(II) may audit any group health plan or health insurance issuer offering health insurance coverage in the group market if the Secretary has received any complaint about such plan or coverage, respectively, that involves the compliance of the plan or coverage, respectively, with either of the requirements described in subclauses and (II) of such clause.

"(iii) REPORTS.—Beginning for 2022, the Secretary shall annually submit to Congress information on the number of plans and issuers with respect to which audits were conducted during such year pursuant to this subparagraph.

"(B) RULEMAKING.—Not later than July 1, 2021, the Secretary, in consultation with the Secretary of the Treasury and the Secretary of Health and Human Services, shall establish through rulemaking—

"(i) the methodology the group health plan or health insurance issuer offering health insurance coverage in the group market shall use to determine the median contracted rate, differentiating by line of business;

"(ii) the information such plan or issuer, respectively, shall share with the nonparticipating provider or nonparticipating facility, as applicable, when making such a determination;

"(iii) the geographic regions applied for purposes of this subparagraph, taking into account access to items and services in rural and underserved areas, including health professional shortage areas, as defined in section 332 of the Public Health Service Act; and

"(iv) a process to receive complaints of violations of the requirements described in subclauses (I) and (II) of paragraph (2)(A)(i) by group health plans and health insurance issuers offering health insurance coverage in the group market.

Such rulemaking shall take into account payments that are made by such plan or issuer, respectively, that are not on a fee-for-service basis. Such methodology may account for relevant payment adjustments that take into account quality or facility type (including higher acuity settings and the case-mix of various facility types) that are otherwise taken into account for purposes of determining payment amounts with respect to participating facilities. In carrying out clause (iii), the Secretary shall consult with the National Association of Insurance Commissioners to establish the geographic regions under such clause and shall periodically update such regions, as appropriate.

"(3) DEFINITIONS.—In this section:

"(A) EMERGENCY DEPARTMENT OF A HOSPITAL.—The term 'emergency department of a hospital' includes a hospital outpatient department that provides emergency services.

"(B) EMERGENCY MEDICAL CONDITION.—The term 'emergency medical condition' means a medical condition manifesting itself by acute symptoms of sufficient severity (including severe pain) such that a prudent layperson, who possesses an average knowledge of health and medicine, could reasonably expect the absence of immediate medical attention to result in a condition described in clause (i), (ii), or (iii) of section 1867(e)(1)(A) of the Social Security Act.

"(C) EMERGENCY SERVICES.—

"(i) IN GENERAL.—The term 'emergency services', with respect to an emergency medical condition, means—

"(I) a medical screening examination (as required under section 1867 of the Social Security Act, or as would be required under such section if such section applied to an independent freestanding emergency department) that is within the capability of the emergency department of a hospital or of an independent freestanding emergency department, as applicable, including ancillary services routinely available to the emergency department to evaluate such emergency medical condition; and

"(II) within the capabilities of the staff and facilities available at the hospital or the independent freestanding emergency department, as applicable, such further medical examination and treatment as are required under section 1867 of such Act, or as would be required under such section if such section applied to an independent freestanding emergency department, to stabilize the patient.

"(ii) INCLUSION OF CERTAIN SERVICES OUTSIDE OF EMERGENCY DEPARTMENT.—

"(I) IN GENERAL.—For purposes of this subsection and section 2799A–1, in the case of an individual enrolled in a group health plan or health insurance coverage offered by a health insurance issuer in the group or individual market who is furnished services described in clause (i) by a participating or nonparticipating provider or a participating or nonparticipating emergency facility to stabilize such individual with respect to an emergency medical condition, the term 'emergency services' shall include, unless each of the conditions described in subclause (II) are met, in addition to the items and services described in clause (i), items and services for which benefits are provided or covered under the plan or coverage, respectively, furnished by a nonparticipating provider or nonparticipating facility, regardless of the department of the hospital in which such individual is furnished such items or services, if, after such stabilization but during such visit in which such individual is so stabilized, the provider or facility determines that such items or services are needed.

"(II) CONDITIONS.—For purposes of subclause (I), the conditions described in this subclause, with respect to an individual who is stabilized and furnished additional items and services described in subclause (I) after such stabilization by a provider or facility described in subclause (I), are the following:

"(aa) Such a provider or facility determines such individual is able to travel using nonmedical transportation or non-emergency medical transportation.

"(bb) Such provider furnishing such additional items and services satisfies the notice and consent criteria of section 2799A–2(d) of the Public Health Service Act with respect to such items and services.

"(cc) Such an individual is in a condition to receive (as determined in accordance with guidance issued by the Secretary) the information described in section 2799A–2 of the Public Health Service Act and to provide informed consent under such section, in accordance with applicable State law.

"(D) INDEPENDENT FREESTANDING EMERGENCY DEPARTMENT.—The term 'independent freestanding emergency department' means a facility that—

"(i) is geographically separate and distinct and licensed separately from a hospital under applicable State law; and

"(ii)provides any emergency services (as defined in subparagraph (C)).

"(E) MEDIAN CONTRACTED RATE.—

"(i) IN GENERAL.—The term 'median contracted rate' means, subject to clauses (ii) and (iii), with respect to a sponsor of a group health plan and health insurance issuer offering health insurance coverage in the group market—

"(I) for an item or service furnished during 2022, the median of the contracted rates recognized by the plan or issuer, respectively (determined with respect to all such plans of such sponsor or all such coverage offered by such issuer that are offered within the same line of business as the plan or coverage) as the total maximum payment (including the cost-sharing amount imposed for such item or service and the amount to be paid by such plan or such issuer, respectively) under such plans or coverage, respectively, on January 31, 2019, for the same or a similar item or service that is provided by a provider in the same or similar specialty and provided in the geographic region in which the item or service is furnished, consistent with the methodology established by the Secretary under paragraph (2)(B), increased by the percentage increase in the consumer price index for all urban consumers (United States city average) over 2019, such percentage increase over 2020, and such percentage increase over 2021; and

"(II) for an item or service furnished during 2023 or a subsequent year, the median contracted rate determined under this clause for such an item or service furnished in the previous year, increased by the percentage increase in the consumer price index for all urban consumers (United States city average) over such previous year.

"(ii) NEW PLANS AND COVERAGE.—The term 'median contracted rate' means, with respect to a sponsor of a group health plan or health insurance issuer offering health insurance coverage in the group market in a geographic region in which such sponsor or issuer, respectively, did not offer any group health plan or health insurance coverage during 2019—

"(I) for the first year in which such group health plan or health insurance coverage, respectively, is offered in such region, a rate (determined in accordance with a methodology established by the Secretary) for items and services that are covered by such plan and furnished during such first year; and

"(II) for each subsequent year such group health plan or health insurance coverage, respectively, is offered in such region, the median contracted rate determined under this clause for such items and services furnished in the previous year, increased by the percentage increase in the consumer price index for all urban consumers (United States city average) over such previous year.

"(iii) INSUFFICIENT INFORMATION; NEWLY COVERED ITEMS AND SERVICES.—In the case of a sponsor of a group health plan or health insurance issuer offering health insurance coverage in the group market that does not have sufficient information to calculate the median of the contracted rates described in clause (i)(I) in 2019 (or, in the case of a newly covered item or service (as defined in clause (iv)(III)), in the first coverage year (as defined in clause (iv)(I)) for such item or service with respect to such plan or coverage) for an item or service (including with respect to provider type, or amount, of claims for items or services (as determined by the Secretary) provided in a particular geographic region (other than in a case with respect to which clause (ii) applies)) the term 'median contracted rate'—

"(I) for an item or service furnished during 2022 (or, in the case of a newly covered item or service, during the first coverage year for such item or service with respect to such plan or coverage), means such rate for such item or service determined by the sponsor or issuer, respectively, through use of any database that is determined, in accordance with rulemaking described in paragraph (2)(B), to not have any conflicts of interest and to have sufficient information reflecting allowed amounts paid to a health care provider or facility for relevant services furnished in the applicable geographic region (such as a State all-payer claims database);

"(II) for an item or service furnished in a subsequent year (before the first sufficient information year (as defined in clause (iv)(II)) for such item or service with respect to such plan or coverage), means the rate determined under subclause (I) or this subclause, as applicable, for such item or service for the year previous to such subsequent year, increased by the percentage increase in the consumer price index for all urban consumers (United States city average) over such previous year;

"(III) for an item or service furnished in the first sufficient information year for such item or service with respect to such plan or coverage, has the meaning given the term median contracted rate in clause (i)(I), except that in applying such clause to such item or service, the reference to 'furnished during 2022' shall be treated as a reference to furnished during such first sufficient information year, the reference to 'in 2019' shall be treated as a reference to such sufficient information year, and the increase described in such clause shall not be applied; and

"(IV) for an item or service furnished in any year subsequent to the first sufficient information year for such item or service with respect to such plan or coverage, has the meaning given such term in clause (i)(II), except that in applying such clause to such item or service, the reference to 'furnished during 2023 or a subsequent year' shall be treated as a reference to furnished during the year after such first sufficient information year or a subsequent year.

"(iv) DEFINITIONS.—For purposes of this subparagraph:

"(I) FIRST COVERAGE YEAR.—The term 'first coverage year' means, with respect to a group health plan or health insurance coverage offered by a health insurance issuer in the group market and an item or service for which coverage is not offered in 2019 under such plan or coverage, the first year after 2019 for which coverage for such item or service is offered under such plan or health insurance coverage.

"(II) FIRST SUFFICIENT INFORMATION YEAR.—The term 'first sufficient information year' means, with respect to a group health plan or health insurance coverage offered by a health insurance issuer in the group market—

"(aa) in the case of an item or service for which the plan or coverage does not have sufficient information to calculate the median of the contracted rates described in clause (i)(I) in 2019, the first year subsequent to 2022 for which such sponsor or issuer has such sufficient information to calculate the median of such contracted rates in the year previous to such first subsequent year; and

"(bb) in the case of a newly covered item or service, the first year subsequent to the first coverage year for such item or service with respect to such plan or coverage for which the sponsor or issuer has sufficient information to calculate the median of the contracted rates described in clause (i)(I) in the year previous to such first subsequent year.

"(III) NEWLY COVERED ITEM OR SERVICE.—The term 'newly covered item or service' means, with respect to a group health plan or health insurance issuer offering health insurance coverage in the group market, an item or service for which coverage was not offered in 2019 under such plan or coverage, but is offered under such plan or coverage in a year after 2019.

"(F) NONPARTICIPATING EMERGENCY FACILITY; PARTICIPATING EMERGENCY FACILITY.—

"(i) NONPARTICIPATING EMERGENCY FACILITY.—The term 'nonparticipating emergency facility' means, with respect to an item or service and a group health plan or health insurance coverage offered by a health insurance issuer in the group market, an emergency department of a hospital, or an independent freestanding emergency department, that does not have a contractual relationship directly or indirectly with the plan or issuer, respectively, for furnishing such item or service under the plan or coverage, respectively.

"(ii) PARTICIPATING EMERGENCY FACILITY.—The term 'participating emergency facility' means, with respect to an item or service and a group health plan or health insurance coverage offered by a health insurance issuer in the group market, an emergency department of a hospital, or an independent freestanding emergency department, that has a contractual relationship directly or indirectly with the plan or issuer, respectively, with respect to the furnishing of such an item or service at such facility.

"(G) NONPARTICIPATING PROVIDERS; PARTICIPATING PROVIDERS.—

"(i) NONPARTICIPATING PROVIDER.—The term 'nonparticipating provider' means, with respect to an item or service and a group health plan or health insurance coverage offered by a health insurance issuer in the group market, a physician or other health care provider who is acting within the scope of practice of that provider's license or certification under applicable State law and who does not have a contractual relationship with the plan or issuer, respectively, for furnishing such item or service under the plan or coverage, respectively.

"(ii) PARTICIPATING PROVIDER.—The term 'participating provider' means, with respect to an item or service and a group health plan or health insurance coverage offered by a health insurance issuer in the group market, a physician or other health care provider who is acting within the scope of practice of that provider's license or certification under applicable State law and who has a contractual relationship with the plan or issuer, respectively, for furnishing such item or service under the plan or coverage, respectively.

"(H) RECOGNIZED AMOUNT.—The term 'recognized amount' means, with respect to an item or service furnished by a nonparticipating provider or emergency facility during a year and a group health plan or health insurance coverage offered by a health insurance issuer in the group market—

"(i) subject to clause (iii), in the case of such item or service furnished in a State that has in effect a specified State law with respect to such plan, coverage, or issuer, respectively, such a nonparticipating provider or emergency facility, and such an item or service, the amount determined in accordance with such law;

"(ii) subject to clause (iii), in the case of such item or service furnished in a State that does not have in effect a specified State law, with respect to such plan, coverage, or issuer, respectively, such a nonparticipating provider or emergency facility, and such an item or service, an amount that is the median contracted rate (as defined in subparagraph (E)) for such year and determined in accordance with rulemaking described in paragraph (2)(B)) for such item or service; or

"(iii) in the case of such item or service furnished in a State with an All-Payer Model Agreement under section 1115A of the Social Security Act, the amount that the State approves under such system for such item or service so furnished.

"(I) SPECIFIED STATE LAW.—The term 'specified State law' means, with respect to a State, an item or service furnished by a nonparticipating provider or emergency facility during a year and a group health plan or health insurance coverage offered by a health insurance issuer in the group market, a State law that provides for a method for determining the amount of payment that is required to be covered by such a plan, coverage, or issuer, respectively (to the extent such State law applies to such plan, coverage, or issuer, subject to section 514) in the case of a participant or beneficiary covered under such plan or coverage and receiving such item or service from such a nonparticipating provider or emergency facility.

"(J) STABILIZE.—The term 'to stabilize', with respect to an emergency medical condition (as defined in subparagraph (B)), has the meaning give in section 1867(e)(3) of the Social Security Act (42 U.S.C. 1395dd(e)(3)).

"(c) ACCESS TO PEDIATRIC CARE.—

"(1) PEDIATRIC CARE.—In the case of a person who has a child who is a participant or beneficiary under a group health plan, or health insurance coverage offered by a health insurance issuer in the group market, if the plan or issuer requires or provides for the designation of a participating primary care provider for the child, the plan or issuer shall permit such person to designate a physician (allopathic or osteopathic) who specializes in pediatrics as the child's primary care provider if such provider participates in the network of the plan or issuer.

"(2) CONSTRUCTION.—Nothing in paragraph (1) shall be construed to waive any exclusions of coverage under the terms and conditions of the plan or health insurance coverage with respect to coverage of pediatric care.

"(d) PATIENT ACCESS TO OBSTETRICAL AND GYNECOLOGICAL CARE.—

"(1) GENERAL RIGHTS.—

"(A) DIRECT ACCESS.—A group health plan, or health insurance issuer offering group health insurance coverage, described in paragraph (2) may not require authorization or referral by the plan, issuer, or any person (including a primary care provider described in paragraph (2)(B)) in the case of a female participant or beneficiary who seeks coverage for obstetrical or gynecological care provided by a participating health care professional who specializes in obstetrics or gynecology. Such professional shall agree to otherwise adhere to such plan's or issuer's policies and procedures, including procedures regarding referrals and obtaining prior authorization and providing services pursuant to a treatment plan (if any) approved by the plan or issuer.

"(B) OBSTETRICAL AND GYNECOLOGICAL CARE.—A group health plan or health insurance issuer described in paragraph (2) shall treat the provision of obstetrical and gynecological care, and the ordering of related obstetrical and gynecological items and services, pursuant to the direct access described under subparagraph (A), by a participating health care professional who specializes in obstetrics or gynecology as the authorization of the primary care provider.

"(2) APPLICATION OF PARAGRAPH.—A group health plan, or health insurance issuer offering group health insurance coverage, described in this paragraph is a group health plan or coverage that—

"(A) provides coverage for obstetric or gynecologic care; and

"(B) requires the designation by a participant or beneficiary of a participating primary care provider.

"(3) CONSTRUCTION.—Nothing in paragraph (1) shall be construed to—

"(A) waive any exclusions of coverage under the terms and conditions of the plan or health insurance coverage with respect to coverage of obstetrical or gynecological care; or

"(B) preclude the group health plan or health insurance issuer involved from requiring that the obstetrical or gynecological provider notify the primary care health care professional or the plan or issuer of treatment decisions.

"(e) COVERAGE OF NON-EMERGENCY SERVICES PERFORMED BY NONPARTICIPATING PROVIDERS AT CERTAIN PARTICIPATING FACILITIES.—

"(1) IN GENERAL.—In the case of items or services (other than emergency services to which subsection (b) applies) for which any benefits are provided or covered by a group health plan or health insurance issuer offering health insurance coverage in the group market furnished to a participant or beneficiary of such plan or coverage by a nonparticipating provider (as defined in subsection (b)(3)(G)(i)) (and who, with respect to such items and services, has not satisfied the notice and consent criteria of section 2799A–2(d) of the Public Health Service Act) with respect to a visit (as defined by the Secretary in accordance with paragraph (2)(B)) at a participating health care facility (as defined in paragraph (2)(A)), with respect to such plan or coverage, respectively, the plan or coverage, respectively—

"(A) shall not impose on such participant or beneficiary a cost-sharing amount (expressed as a copayment amount or coinsurance rate) for such items and services so furnished that is greater than the cost-sharing amount that would apply under such plan or coverage, respectively, had such items or services been furnished by a participating provider (as defined in subsection (b)(3)(G)(ii));

"(B) shall calculate such cost-sharing amount as if the total amount that would have been charged for such items and services by such participating provider were equal to the recognized amount (as defined in subsection (b)(3)(H)) for such items and services, plan or coverage, and year;

"(C) shall pay to such provider furnishing such items and services to such participant or beneficiary the amount by which the recognized amount (as defined in subsection (b)(3)(H)) for such items and services and year involved exceeds the cost-sharing amount imposed under the plan or coverage, respectively, for such items and services (as determined in accordance with subparagraphs (A) and (B)); and

"(D) shall count toward any in-network deductible and in-network out-of-pocket maximums (as applicable) applied under the plan or coverage, respectively, any cost-sharing payments made by the participant or beneficiary (and such in-network deductible and out-of-pocket maximums shall be applied) with respect to such items and services so furnished in the same manner as if such cost-sharing payments were with respect to items and services furnished by a participating provider.

"(2) DEFINITIONS.—In this section:

"(A) PARTICIPATING HEALTH CARE FACILITY.—

"(i) IN GENERAL.—The term 'participating health care facility' means, with respect to an item or service and a group health plan or health insurance issuer offering health insurance coverage in the group market, a health care facility described in clause (ii) that has a contractual relationship with the plan or issuer, respectively, with respect to the furnishing of such an item or service at the facility.

"(ii) HEALTH CARE FACILITY DESCRIBED.—A health care facility described in this clause, with respect to a group health plan or health insurance coverage offered in the group market, is each of the following:

"(I) A hospital (as defined in 1861(e) of the Social Security Act).

"(II) A hospital outpatient department.

"(III) A critical access hospital (as defined in section 1861(mm) of such Act).

"(IV) An ambulatory surgical center (as defined in section 1833(i)(1)(A) of such Act).

"(V) Any other facility that provides items or services for which coverage is provided under the plan or coverage, respectively.

"(B) VISIT.—The term 'visit' shall, with respect to items and services furnished to an individual at a participating health care facility, include equipment and devices, telemedicine services, imaging services, laboratory services, and such other items and services as the Secretary may specify, regardless of whether or not the provider furnishing such items or services is at the facility.

"(f) AIR AMBULANCE SERVICES.—

"(1) IN GENERAL.—In the case of a participant or beneficiary in a group health plan or health insurance coverage offered in the group market who receives air ambulance services from a nonparticipating provider (as defined in subsection (b)(3)(G)) with respect to such plan or coverage, if such services would be covered if provided by a participating provider (as defined in such subsection) with respect to such plan or coverage—

"(A) the cost-sharing requirement (expressed as a copayment amount, coinsurance rate, or deductible) with respect to such services shall be the same requirement that would apply if such services were provided by such a participating provider, and any coinsurance or deductible shall be based on rates that would apply for such services if they were furnished by such a participating provider;

"(B) such cost-sharing amounts shall be counted toward the in-network deductible and in-network out-of-pocket maximum amount under the plan or coverage for the plan year (and such in-network deductible shall be applied) with respect to such items and services so furnished in the same manner as if such cost-sharing payments were with respect to items and services furnished by a participating provider; and

"(C) the plan or coverage shall pay to such provider furnishing such services to such participant or beneficiary the amount by which the recognized amount (as defined in and determined pursuant to subsection (b)(3)(H)(ii)) for such services and year involved exceeds the cost-sharing amount imposed under the plan or coverage, respectively, for such services (as determined in accordance with subparagraphs (A) and (B)).

"(2) AIR AMBULANCE SERVICE DEFINED.—For purposes of this section, the term 'air ambulance service' means medical transport by helicopter or airplane for patients.

"(g) CERTAIN ACCESS FEES TO CERTAIN DATABASES.—In the case of a sponsor of a group health plan or health insurance issuer offering health insurance coverage in the group market that, pursuant to subsection (b)(3)(E)(iii), uses a database described in such subsection to determine a rate to apply under such subsection for an item or service by reason of having insufficient information described in such subsection with respect to such item or service, such sponsor or issuer shall cover the cost for access to such database."

(2) CLERICAL AMENDMENT.—The table of contents of the Employee Retirement Income Security Act of 1974 is amended by inserting after the item relating to section 714 the following:

"Sec. 715. Additional market reforms.
"Sec. 716. Consumer protections."

(c) IRC AMENDMENTS.—

(1) IN GENERAL.—Subchapter B of chapter 100 of the Internal Revenue Code of 1986 is amended by adding at the end the following:

"SEC. 9816. CONSUMER PROTECTIONS.

"(a) CHOICE OF HEALTH CARE PROFESSIONAL.—If a group health plan requires or provides for designation by a participant or beneficiary of a participating primary care provider, then the plan shall permit each participant or beneficiary to designate any participating primary care provider who is available to accept such individual.

"(b) COVERAGE OF EMERGENCY SERVICES.—

"(1) IN GENERAL.—If a group health plan provides or covers any benefits with respect to services in an emergency department of a hospital or with respect to emergency services in an independent freestanding emergency department (as defined in paragraph (3)(D)), the plan shall cover emergency services (as defined in paragraph (3)(C))—

"(A) without the need for any prior authorization determination;

"(B) whether the health care provider furnishing such services is a participating provider or a participating emergency facility, as applicable, with respect to such services;

"(C) in a manner so that, if such services are provided to a participant or beneficiary by a nonparticipating provider or a nonparticipating emergency facility—

"(i) such services will be provided without imposing any requirement under the plan for prior authorization of services or any limitation on coverage that is more restrictive than the requirements or limitations that apply to emergency services received from participating providers and participating emergency facilities with respect to such plan;

"(ii) the cost-sharing requirement (expressed as a copayment amount or coinsurance rate) is not greater than the requirement that would apply if such services were provided by a participating provider or a participating emergency facility;

"(iii) such cost-sharing requirement is calculated as if the total amount that would have been charged for such services by such participating provider or participating emergency facility were equal to the recognized amount (as defined in paragraph (3)(H)) for such services, plan, and year;

"(iv) the group health plan pays to such provider or facility, respectively, the amount by which the recognized amount for such services and year involved exceeds the cost-sharing amount for such services (as determined in accordance with clauses (ii) and (iii)) and year; and

"(v) any cost-sharing payments made by the participant or beneficiary with respect to such emergency services so furnished shall be counted toward any in-network deductible or out-of-pocket maximums applied under the plan (and such in-network deductible and out-of-pocket maximums shall be applied) in the same manner as if such cost-sharing payments were made with respect to emergency services furnished by a participating provider or a participating emergency facility; and

"(D) without regard to any other term or condition of such coverage (other than exclusion or coordination of benefits, or an affiliation or waiting period, permitted under section 2704 of this Act, including as incorporated pursuant to section 715 of the Employee Retirement Income Security Act of 1974 and section 9815 of this Act, and other than applicable cost-sharing).

"(2) AUDIT PROCESS AND REGULATIONS FOR MEDIAN CONTRACTED RATES.—

"(A) AUDIT PROCESS.—

"(i) IN GENERAL.—Not later than July 1, 2021, the Secretary, in consultation with appropriate State agencies and the Secretary of Health and Human Services and the Secretary of Labor, shall establish through rulemaking a process, in accordance with clause (ii), under which group health plans are audited by the Secretary or applicable State authority to ensure that—

"(I) such plans are in compliance with the requirement of applying a median contracted rate under this section; and

"(II) such median contracted rate so applied satisfies the definition under paragraph (3)(E) with respect to the year involved, including with respect to a group health plan described in clause (ii) of such paragraph (3)(E).

"(ii) AUDIT SAMPLES.—Under the process established pursuant to clause (i), the Secretary—

"(I) shall conduct audits described in such clause, with respect to a year (beginning with 2022), of a sample with respect to such year of claims data from not more than 25 group health plans; and

"(II) may audit any group health plan if the Secretary has received any complaint about such plan or coverage, respectively, that involves the compliance of the plan with either of the requirements described in subclauses (I) and (II) of such clause.

"(iii) REPORTS.—Beginning for 2022, the Secretary shall annually submit to Congress a report on the number of plans and issuers with respect to which audits were conducted during such year pursuant to this subparagraph.

"(B) RULEMAKING.—Not later than July 1, 2021, the Secretary, in consultation with the Secretary of Labor and the Secretary of Health and Human Services, shall establish through rulemaking—

"(i) the methodology the group health plan shall use to determine the median contracted rate, differentiating by line of business;

"(ii) the information such plan or issuer, respectively, shall share with the nonparticipating provider or nonparticipating facility, as applicable, when making such a determination;

"(iii) the geographic regions applied for purposes of this subparagraph, taking into account access to items and services in rural and underserved areas, including health professional shortage areas, as defined in section 332 of the Public Health Service Act; and

"(iv) a process to receive complaints of violations of the requirements described in subclauses (I) and (II) of paragraph (2)(A)(i) by group health plans.

Such rulemaking shall take into account payments that are made by such plan that are not on a fee-for-service basis. Such methodology may account for relevant payment adjustments that take into account quality or facility type (including higher acuity settings and the case-mix of various facility types) that are otherwise taken into account for purposes of determining payment amounts with respect to participating facilities. In carrying out clause (iii), the Secretary shall consult with the National Association of Insurance Commissioners to establish the geographic regions under such clause and shall periodically update such regions, as appropriate.

"(3) DEFINITIONS.—In this section:

"(A) EMERGENCY DEPARTMENT OF A HOSPITAL.—The term 'emergency department of a hospital' includes a hospital outpatient department that provides emergency services.

"(B) EMERGENCY MEDICAL CONDITION.—The term 'emergency medical condition' means a medical condition manifesting itself by acute symptoms of sufficient severity (including severe pain) such that a prudent layperson, who possesses an average knowledge of health and medicine, could reasonably expect the absence of immediate medical attention to result in a condition described in clause (i), (ii), or (iii) of section 1867(e)(1)(A) of the Social Security Act.

"(C) EMERGENCY SERVICES.—

"(i) IN GENERAL.—The term 'emergency services', with respect to an emergency medical condition, means—

"(I) a medical screening examination (as required under section 1867 of the Social Security Act, or as would be required under such section if such section applied to an independent freestanding emergency department) that is within the capability of the emergency department of a hospital or of an independent freestanding emergency department, as applicable, including ancillary services routinely available to the emergency department to evaluate such emergency medical condition; and

"(II) within the capabilities of the staff and facilities available at the hospital or the independent freestanding emergency department, as applicable, such further medical examination and treatment as are required under section 1867 of such Act, or as would be required under such section if such section applied to an independent freestanding emergency department, to stabilize the patient.

"(ii) INCLUSION OF CERTAIN SERVICES OUTSIDE OF EMERGENCY DEPARTMENT.—

"(I) IN GENERAL.—For purposes of this subsection and section 2799A–1, in the case of an individual enrolled in a group health plan or health insurance coverage offered by a health insurance issuer in the group or individual market who is furnished services described in clause (i) by a participating or nonparticipating provider or a participating or nonparticipating emergency facility to stabilize such individual with respect to an emergency medical condition, the term 'emergency services' shall include, unless each of the conditions described in subclause (II) are met, in addition to the items and services described in clause (i), items and services for which benefits are provided or covered under the plan or coverage, respectively, furnished by a nonparticipating provider or nonparticipating facility, regardless of the department of the hospital in which such individual is furnished such items or services, if, after such stabilization but during such visit in which such individual is so stabilized, the provider or facility determines that such items or services are needed.

"(II) CONDITIONS.—For purposes of subclause (I), the conditions described in this subclause, with respect to an individual who is stabilized and furnished additional items and services described in subclause (I) after such stabilization by a provider or facility described in subclause (I), are the following:

"(aa) Such a provider or facility determines such individual is able to travel using nonmedical transportation or non-emergency medical transportation.

"(bb) Such provider furnishing such additional items and services satisfies the notice and consent criteria of section 2799A–2(d) of the Public Health Service Act with respect to such items and services.

"(cc) Such an individual is in a condition to receive (as determined in accordance with guidance issued by the Secretary) the information described in section 2799A–2 of the Public Health Service Act and to provide informed consent under such section, in accordance with applicable State law.

"(D) INDEPENDENT FREESTANDING EMERGENCY DEPARTMENT.—The term 'independent freestanding emergency department' means a facility that—

"(i) is geographically separate and distinct and licensed separately from a hospital under applicable State law; and

"(ii) provides any emergency services (as defined in subparagraph (C)).

"(E) MEDIAN CONTRACTED RATE.—

"(i) IN GENERAL.—The term 'median contracted rate' means, subject to clauses (ii) and (iii), with respect to a sponsor of a group health plan—

"(I) for an item or service furnished during 2022, the median of the contracted rates recognized by the plan (determined with respect to all such plans of such sponsor that are offered within the same line of business as the total maximum payment (including the cost-sharing amount imposed for such item or service and the amount to be paid by the plan) under such plans on January 31, 2019 for the same or a similar item or service that is provided by a provider in the same or similar specialty and provided in the geographic region in which the item or service is furnished, consistent with the methodology established by the Secretary under paragraph (2)(B), increased by the percentage increase in the consumer price index for all urban consumers (United States city average) over 2019, such percentage increase over 2020, and such percentage increase over 2021; and

"(II) for an item or service furnished during 2023 or a subsequent year, the median contracted rate determined under this clause for such an item or service furnished in the previous year, increased by the percentage increase in the consumer price index for all urban consumers (United States city average) over such previous year.

"(ii) NEW PLANS AND COVERAGE.—The term 'median contracted rate' means, with respect to a sponsor of a group health plan in a geographic region in which such sponsor, respectively, did not offer any group health plan or health insurance coverage during 2019—

"(I) for the first year in which such group health plan is offered in such region, a rate (determined in accordance with a methodology established by the Secretary) for items and services that are covered by such plan and furnished during such first year; and

"(II) for each subsequent year such group health plan is offered in such region, the median contracted rate determined under this clause for such items and services furnished in the previous year, increased by the percentage increase in the consumer price index for all urban consumers (United States city average) over such previous year.

"(iii) INSUFFICIENT INFORMATION; NEWLY COVERED ITEMS AND SERVICES.—In the case of a sponsor of a group health plan that does not have sufficient information to calculate the median of the contracted rates described in clause (i)(I) in 2019 (or, in the case of a newly covered item or service (as defined in clause (iv)(III)), in the first coverage year (as defined in clause (iv)(I)) for such item or service with respect to such plan) for an item or service (including with respect to provider type, or amount, of claims for items or services (as determined by the Secretary) provided in a particular geographic region (other than in a case with respect to which clause (ii) applies)) the term 'median contracted rate'—

"(I) for an item or service furnished during 2022 (or, in the case of a newly covered item or service, during the first coverage year for such item or service with respect to such plan), means such rate for such item or service determined by the sponsor through use of any database that is determined, in accordance with rulemaking described in paragraph (2)(B), to not have any conflicts of interest and to have sufficient information reflecting allowed amounts paid to a health care provider or facility for relevant services furnished in the applicable geographic region (such as a State all-payer claims database);

"(II) for an item or service furnished in a subsequent year (before the first sufficient information year (as defined in clause (iv)(II)) for such item or service with respect to such plan), means the rate determined under subclause (I) or this subclause, as applicable, for such item or service for the year previous to such subsequent year, increased by the percentage increase in the consumer price index for all urban consumers (United States city average) over such previous year;

"(III) for an item or service furnished in the first sufficient information year for such item or service with respect to such plan, has the meaning given the term median contracted rate in clause (i)(I), except that in applying such clause to such item or service, the reference to 'furnished during 2022' shall be treated as a reference to furnished during such first sufficient information year, the reference to 'on January 31, 2019' shall be treated as a reference to in such sufficient information year, and the increase described in such clause shall not be applied; and

"(IV) for an item or service furnished in any year subsequent to the first sufficient information year for such item or service with respect to such plan, has the meaning given such term in clause (i)(II), except that in applying such clause to such item or service, the reference to 'furnished during 2023 or a subsequent year' shall be treated as a reference to furnished during the year after such first sufficient information year or a subsequent year.

"(iv) DEFINITIONS.—For purposes of this subparagraph:

"(I) FIRST COVERAGE YEAR.—The term 'first coverage year' means, with respect to a group health plan and an item or service for which coverage is not offered in 2019 under such plan or coverage, the first year after 2019 for which coverage for such item or service is offered under such plan.

"(II) FIRST SUFFICIENT INFORMATION YEAR.—The term 'first sufficient information year' means, with respect to a group health plan—

"(aa) in the case of an item or service for which the plan does not have sufficient information to calculate the median of the contracted rates described in clause (i)(I) in 2019, the first year subsequent to 2022 for which such sponsor has such sufficient information to calculate the median of such contracted rates in the year previous to such first subsequent year; and

"(bb) in the case of a newly covered item or service, the first year subsequent to the first coverage year for such item or service with respect to such plan for which the sponsor has sufficient information to calculate the median of the contracted rates described in clause (i)(I) in the year previous to such first subsequent year.

"(III) NEWLY COVERED ITEM OR SERVICE.—The term 'newly covered item or service' means, with respect to a group health plan, an item or service for which coverage was not offered in 2019 under such plan or coverage, but is offered under such plan or coverage in a year after 2019.

"(F) NONPARTICIPATING EMERGENCY FACILITY; PARTICIPATING EMERGENCY FACILITY.—

"(i) NONPARTICIPATING EMERGENCY FACILITY.—The term 'nonparticipating emergency facility' means, with respect to an item or service and a group health plan, an emergency department of a hospital, or an independent freestanding emergency department, that does not have a contractual relationship directly or indirectly with the plan for furnishing such item or service under the plan.

"(ii) PARTICIPATING EMERGENCY FACILITY.—The term 'participating emergency facility' means, with respect to an item or service and a group health plan, an emergency department of a hospital, or an independent freestanding emergency department, that has a contractual relationship directly or indirectly with the plan, with respect to the furnishing of such an item or service at such facility.

"(G) NONPARTICIPATING PROVIDERS; PARTICIPATING PROVIDERS.—

"(i) NONPARTICIPATING PROVIDER.—The term 'nonparticipating provider' means, with respect to an item or service and a group health plan, a physician or other health care provider who is acting within the scope of practice of that provider's license or certification under applicable State law and who does not have a contractual relationship with the plan or issuer, respectively, for furnishing such item or service under the plan.

"(ii) PARTICIPATING PROVIDER.—The term 'participating provider' means, with respect to an item or service and a group health plan, a physician or other health care provider who is acting within the scope of practice of that provider's license or certification under applicable State law and who has a contractual relationship with the plan for furnishing such item or service under the plan.

"(H) RECOGNIZED AMOUNT.—The term 'recognized amount' means, with respect to an item or service furnished by a nonparticipating provider or emergency facility during a year and a group health plan—

"(i) subject to clause (iii), in the case of such item or service furnished in a State that has in effect a specified State law with respect to such plan; such a nonparticipating provider or emergency facility; and such an item or service, the amount determined in accordance with such law;

"(ii) subject to clause (iii), in the case of such item or service furnished in a State that does not have in effect a specified State law, with respect to such plan; such a nonparticipating provider or emergency facility; and such an item or service, an amount that is the median contracted rate (as defined in subparagraph (E)) for such year and determined in accordance with rulemaking described in paragraph (2)(B)) for such item or service; or

"(iii) in the case of such item or service furnished in a State with an All-Payer Model Agreement under section 1115A of the Social Security Act, the amount that the State approves under such system for such item or service so furnished.

"(I) SPECIFIED STATE LAW.—The term 'specified State law' means, with respect to a State, an item or service furnished by a nonparticipating provider or emergency facility during a year and a group health plan, a State law that provides for a method for determining the amount of payment that is required to be covered by such a plan (to the extent such State law applies to such plan, subject to section 514 of the Employee Retirement Income Security Act of

1974) in the case of a participant or beneficiary covered under such plan and receiving such item or service from such a nonparticipating provider or emergency facility.

"(J) STABILIZE.—The term 'to stabilize', with respect to an emergency medical condition (as defined in subparagraph (B)), has the meaning give in section 1867(e)(3) of the Social Security Act (42 U.S.C. 1395dd(e)(3)).

"(c) ACCESS TO PEDIATRIC CARE.—

"(1) PEDIATRIC CARE.—In the case of a person who has a child who is a participant or beneficiary under a group health plan, if the plan requires or provides for the designation of a participating primary care provider for the child, the plan shall permit such person to designate a physician (allopathic or osteopathic) who specializes in pediatrics as the child's primary care provider if such provider participates in the network of the plan or issuer.

"(2) CONSTRUCTION.—Nothing in paragraph (1) shall be construed to waive any exclusions of coverage under the terms and conditions of the plan with respect to coverage of pediatric care.

"(d) PATIENT ACCESS TO OBSTETRICAL AND GYNECOLOGICAL CARE.— "

(1) GENERAL RIGHTS.—

"(A) DIRECT ACCESS.—A group health plan described in paragraph (2) may not require authorization or referral by the plan or any person (including a primary care provider described in paragraph (2)(B)) in the case of a female participant or beneficiary who seeks coverage for obstetrical or gynecological care provided by a participating health care professional who specializes in obstetrics or gynecology. Such professional shall agree to otherwise adhere to such plan's policies and procedures, including procedures regarding referrals and obtaining prior authorization and providing services pursuant to a treatment plan (if any) approved by the plan.

"(B) OBSTETRICAL AND GYNECOLOGICAL CARE.—A group health plan described in paragraph (2) shall treat the provision of obstetrical and gynecological care, and the ordering of related obstetrical and gynecological items and services, pursuant to the direct access described under subparagraph (A), by a participating health care professional who specializes in obstetrics or gynecology as the authorization of the primary care provider.

"(2) APPLICATION OF PARAGRAPH.—A group health plan described in this paragraph is a group health plan that—

"(A) provides coverage for obstetric or gynecologic care; and

"(B) requires the designation by a participant or beneficiary of a participating primary care provider.

"(3) CONSTRUCTION.—Nothing in paragraph (1) shall be construed to—

"(A) waive any exclusions of coverage under the terms and conditions of the plan with respect to coverage of obstetrical or gynecological care; or

"(B) preclude the group health plan involved from requiring that the obstetrical or gynecological provider notify the primary care health care professional or the plan of treatment decisions.

"(e) COVERAGE OF NON-EMERGENCY SERVICES PERFORMED BY NONPARTICIPATING PROVIDERS AT CERTAIN PARTICIPATING FACILITIES.—

"(1) IN GENERAL.—In the case of items or services (other than emergency services to which subsection (b) applies) for which any benefits are provided or covered by a group health plan furnished to a participant or beneficiary of such plan by a nonparticipating provider (as defined in subsection (b)(3)(G)(i)) (and who, with respect to such items and services, has not satisfied the notice and consent criteria of section 2799A–2(d) of the Public Health Service Act) with respect to a visit (as defined by the Secretary in accordance with paragraph (2)(B)) at a participating health care facility (as defined in paragraph (2)(A)), with respect to such plan, the plan—

"(A) shall not impose on such participant or beneficiary a cost-sharing amount (expressed as a copayment amount or coinsurance rate) for such items and services so furnished that is greater than the cost-sharing amount that would apply under such plan had such items or services been furnished by a participating provider (as defined in subsection (b)(3)(G)(ii));

"(B) shall calculate such cost-sharing amount as if the total amount that would have been charged for such items and services by such participating provider were equal to the recognized amount (as defined in subsection (b)(3)(H)) for such items and services, plan, and year;

"(C) shall pay to such provider furnishing such items and services to such participant or beneficiary the amount by which the recognized amount (as defined in subsection (b)(3)(H)) for such items and services and year involved exceeds the cost-sharing amount imposed under the plan for such items and services (as determined in accordance with subparagraphs (A) and (B)); and

"(D) shall count toward any in-network deductible and in-network out-of-pocket maximums (as applicable) applied under the plan, any cost-sharing payments made by the participant or beneficiary (and such in-network deductible shall be applied) with respect to such items and services so furnished in the same manner as if such cost-sharing payments were with respect to items and services furnished by a participating provider.

"(2) DEFINITIONS.—In this section:

"(A) PARTICIPATING HEALTH CARE FACILITY.—

"(i) IN GENERAL.—The term 'participating health care facility' means, with respect to an item or service and a group health plan, a health care facility described in clause (ii) that has a contractual relationship with the plan, with respect to the furnishing of such an item or service at the facility.

"(ii) HEALTH CARE FACILITY DESCRIBED.—A health care facility described in this clause, with respect to a group health plan, is each of the following:

"(I) A hospital (as defined in 1861(e) of the Social Security Act).

"(II) A hospital outpatient department.

"(III) A critical access hospital (as defined in section 1861(mm) of such Act).

"(IV) An ambulatory surgical center (as defined in section 1833(i)(1)(A) of such Act).

"(V) Any other facility that provides items or services for which coverage is provided under the plan or coverage, respectively.

"(B) VISIT.—The term 'visit' shall, with respect to items and services furnished to an individual at a participating health care facility, include equipment and devices, telemedicine services, imaging services, laboratory services, and such other items and services as the Secretary may specify, regardless of whether or not the provider furnishing such items or services is at the facility.

"(f) AIR AMBULANCE SERVICES.—

"(1) IN GENERAL.—In the case of a participant or beneficiary in a group health plan who receives air ambulance services from a nonparticipating provider (as defined in subsection (b)(3)(G)) with respect to such plan or coverage, if such services would be covered if provided by a participating provider (as defined in such subsection) with respect to such plan—

"(A) the cost-sharing requirement (expressed as a copayment amount, coinsurance rate, or deductible) with respect to such services shall be the same requirement that would apply if such services were provided by such a participating provider, and any coinsurance or deductible shall be based on rates that would apply for such services if they were furnished by such a participating provider;

"(B) such cost-sharing amounts shall be counted toward the in-network deductible and in-network out-of-pocket maximum amount under the plan for the plan year (and such in-network deductible shall be applied) with respect to such items and services so furnished in the same manner as if such cost-sharing payments were with respect to items and services furnished by a participating provider; and

"(C) the plan or coverage shall pay to such provider furnishing such services to such participant or beneficiary the amount by which the recognized amount (as defined in and determined pursuant to subsection (b)(3)(H)(ii)) for such services and year involved exceeds the cost-sharing amount imposed under the plan for such services (as determined in accordance with subparagraphs (A) and (B)).

"(2) AIR AMBULANCE SERVICE DEFINED.—For purposes of this section, the term 'air ambulance service' means medical transport by helicopter or airplane for patients.

"(g) CERTAIN ACCESS FEES TO CERTAIN DATABASES.—In the case of a sponsor of a group health plan that, pursuant to subsection (b)(3)(E)(iii), uses a database described in such subsection to determine a rate to apply under such subsection for an item or service by reason of having insufficient information described in such subsection with respect to such item or service, such sponsor shall cover the cost for access to such database."

(2) CLERICAL AMENDMENT.—The table of sections for subchapter B of chapter 100 of the Internal Revenue Code of 1986 is amended by adding at the end the following new item:

"Sec. 9815. Additional market reforms.
"Sec. 9816. Consumer protections."

(d) ADDITIONAL APPLICATION PROVISIONS.—

(1) APPLICATION TO FEHB.—

(A) IN GENERAL.—Section 8902 of title 5, United States Code, is amended by adding at the end the following new subsection:

"(p) Each contract under this chapter shall require the carrier to comply with requirements described in the provisions of section 2719A of the Public Health Service Act and sections 2730 and 2731 of such Act, sections 716, 717, and 718 of the Employee Retirement Income Security Act of 1974, sections 9816, 9817, and 9818 of the Internal Revenue Code of 1986 (as applicable), and section 2(d) of the Ban Surprise Billing Act in the same manner as such provisions apply to a group health plan or health insurance issuer offering health insurance coverage, as described in such sections. The provisions of sections 2799A–1, 2799A–2, 2799A–3, and 2799A–4 of the Public Health Service Act shall apply to a health care provider and facility and an air ambulance provider described in such respective sections with respect to a participant, beneficiary, or enrollee in a health benefits plan under this chapter in the same manner as such provisions apply to such a provider and facility with respect to an enrollee in a group health plan or health insurance coverage offered by a health insurance issuer in the group or individual market, as described in such sections."

(B) EFFECTIVE DATE.—The amendment made by this paragraph shall apply with respect to contracts entered into or renewed for contract years beginning on or after January 1, 2022.

(2) APPLICATION TO GRANDFATHERED PLANS.—Section 1251(a) of the Patient Protection and Affordable Care Act (42 U.S.C. 18011(a)) is amended by adding at the end the following:

"(5) APPLICATION OF ADDITIONAL PROVISIONS.—Subsections (b), (e), (f), (g), and (h) of section 2719A of the Public Health Service Act shall apply to grandfathered health plans for plan years beginning on or after January 1, 2022."

(3) COORDINATION.—The Secretary of the Treasury, the Secretary of Health and Human Services, and the Secretary of Labor shall ensure, through the execution of an interagency memorandum of understanding among such Secretaries, that—

(A) regulations, rulings, and interpretations issued by such Secretaries relating to the same matter over which 2 or more such Secretaries have responsibility under this title (and the amendments made by this title) are administered so as to have the same effect at all times; and

(B) coordination of policies relating to enforcing the same requirements through such Secretaries in order to have a coordinated enforcement strategy that avoids duplication of enforcement efforts and assigns priorities in enforcement.

(4) RULE OF CONSTRUCTION.—Nothing in this title, including the amendments made by this title may be construed as modifying, reducing, or eliminating—

(A) the protections under section 222 of the Indian Health Care Improvement Act (25 U.S.C. 1621u) and under subpart I of part 136 of title 42, Code of Federal Regulations (or any successor regulation), against payment liability for a patient who receives contract health services that are authorized by the Indian Health Service; or

(B) the requirements under section 1866(a)(1)(U) of the Social Security Act (42 U.S.C. 1395cc(a)(1)(U)).

(e) EFFECTIVE DATE.—The amendments made by this section shall apply with respect to plan years beginning on or after January 1, 2022.

SECTION 3. PREVENTING CERTAIN CASES OF BALANCE BILLING.

(a) IN GENERAL.—Title XXVII of the Public Health Service Act (42 U.S.C. 300gg et seq.) is amended by adding at the end the following new part:

"PART D—HEALTH CARE PROVIDER REQUIREMENTS

"SEC. 2799A–1. BALANCE BILLING IN CASES OF EMERGENCY SERVICES.

"(a) IN GENERAL.—In the case of a participant, beneficiary, or enrollee with benefits under a group health plan or health insurance coverage offered by a health insurance issuer in the group or individual market who is furnished during a plan year beginning on or after January 1, 2022, emergency services for which any benefit is provided under such plan or coverage with respect to an emergency medical condition with respect to a visit at an emergency department of a hospital or an independent freestanding emergency department—

"(1) in the case that the hospital or independent freestanding emergency department is a nonparticipating emergency facility, the emergency department of a hospital or independent freestanding emergency department shall not hold the participant, beneficiary, or enrollee liable for a payment amount for such emergency services so furnished that is more than the cost-sharing amount for such services (as determined in accordance with clauses (ii) and (iii) of section 2719A(b)(1)(C), section 716(b)(1)(C) of the Employee Retirement Income Security Act of 1974, and section 9816(b)(1)(C) of the Internal Revenue Code of 1986, as applicable); and

"(2) in the case that such services are furnished by a nonparticipating provider, the health care provider shall not hold such participant, beneficiary, or enrollee liable for a payment amount for an emergency service furnished to such individual by such provider with respect to such emergency medical condition and visit for which the individual receives emergency services at the hospital or emergency department that is more than the cost-sharing amount for such services furnished by the provider (as determined in accordance with clauses (ii) and (iii) of section 2719A(b)(1)(C), section 716(b)(1)(C) of the Employee Retirement Income Security Act of 1974, and section 9816(b)(1)(C) of the Internal Revenue Code of 1986, as applicable).

"(b) DEFINITION.—In this section, the term 'visit' shall have such meaning as applied to such term for purposes of section 2719A(e).

"SEC. 2799A–2. BALANCE BILLING IN CASES OF NON-EMERGENCY SERVICES PERFORMED BY NONPARTICIPATING PROVIDERS AT CERTAIN PARTICIPATING FACILITIES.

"(a) IN GENERAL.—Subject to subsection (b), in the case of a participant, beneficiary, or enrollee with benefits under a group health plan or health insurance coverage offered by a health insurance issuer in the group or individual market who is furnished during a plan year beginning on or after January 1, 2022, items or services (other than emergency services to which section 2799A–1 applies) for which any benefit is provided under such plan or coverage at a participating health care facility by a nonparticipating provider, such provider shall not bill, and shall not hold liable, such participant, beneficiary, or enrollee for a payment amount for such an item or service furnished by such provider with respect to a visit at such facility that is more than the cost-sharing amount for such item or service (as determined in accordance with subparagraphs (A) and (B) of section 2719A(e)(1), section 716(e)(1) of the Employee Retirement Income Security Act of 1974, and section 9816(e)(1) of the Internal Revenue Code of 1986, as applicable).

"(b) EXCEPTION.—

"(1) IN GENERAL.—Subsection (a) shall not apply with respect to items or services (other than ancillary services described in paragraph (2)) furnished by a nonparticipating provider to a participant, beneficiary, or enrollee of a group health plan or health insurance coverage offered by a health insurance issuer in the group or individual market, if the provider satisfies the notice and consent criteria of subsection (d).

"(2) ANCILLARY SERVICES DESCRIBED.—For purposes of paragraph (1), ancillary services described in this paragraph are, with respect to a participating health care facility—

"(A) subject to paragraph (3), items and services related to emergency medicine, anesthesiology, pathology, radiology, and neonatology, whether or not provided by a physician or non-physician practitioner, and items and services provided by assistant surgeons, hospitalists, and intensivists;

"(B) subject to paragraph (3), diagnostic services (including radiology and laboratory services);

"(C) items and services provided by such other specialty practitioners, as the Secretary specifies through rulemaking; and

"(D) items and services provided by a nonparticipating provider if there is no participating provider who can furnish such item or service at such facility.

"(3) EXCEPTION.—The Secretary may, through rulemaking, establish a list (and update such list) of advanced diagnostic laboratory tests, which shall not be included as an ancillary service described in paragraph (2) and with respect to which subsection (a) would apply.

"(c) CLARIFICATION.—In the case of a nonparticipating provider that satisfies the notice and consent criteria of subsection (d) with respect to an item or service (referred to in this subsection as a 'covered item or service'), such notice and consent criteria may not be construed as applying with respect to any item or service that is furnished as a result of unforeseen, urgent medical needs that arise at the time such covered item or service is furnished. For purposes of the previous sentence, a covered item or service shall not include an ancillary service described in subsection (b)(2).

"(d) NOTICE AND CONSENT TO BE TREATED BY A NONPARTICIPATING PROVIDER OR NONPARTICIPATING FACILITY.—

"(1) IN GENERAL.—A nonparticipating provider or nonparticipating facility satisfies the notice and consent criteria of this subsection, with respect to items or services furnished by the provider or facility to a participant, beneficiary, or enrollee of a group health plan or health insurance coverage offered by a health insurance issuer in the group or individual market, if the provider (or, if applicable, the participating health care facility on behalf of such provider) or nonparticipating facility—

"(A) provides to the participant, beneficiary, or enrollee (or to an authorized representative of the participant, beneficiary, or enrollee) on the date on which the individual is furnished such items or services and, in the case that the participant, beneficiary, or enrollee makes an appointment to be furnished such items or services, on such date the appointment is made—

"(i) an oral explanation of the written notice described in clause (ii); and

"(ii) a written notice in paper or electronic form (and including electronic notification, as practicable) specified by the Secretary, not later than July 1, 2021, through guidance (which shall be updated as determined necessary by the Secretary) that—

"(I) contains the information required under paragraph (2);

"(II) clearly states that consent to receive such items and services from such nonparticipating provider or nonparticipating facility is optional and that the participant, beneficiary, or enrollee may instead seek care from a participating provider or at a participating facility, with respect to such plan or coverage, as applicable, in which case the cost-sharing responsibility of the participant, beneficiary, or enrollee would not exceed such responsibility that would apply with respect to such an item or service that is furnished by a participating provider or participating facility, as applicable with respect to such plan;

"(III) is available in the 15 most common languages in the geographic region of the applicable facility and, in the case the primary language of the beneficiary, participant, or enrollee, respectively, is not one of such 15 language, makes a good faith effort to also provide such notice orally in such primary language of the beneficiary, participant, or enrollee; and

"(IV) is signed and dated by the participant, beneficiary, or enrollee (or by an authorized representative of the participant, beneficiary, or enrollee) and, with respect to items or services to be furnished by such a provider that are not poststabilization services described in section 2719A(b)(3)(C)(ii), is so signed and dated not less than 72 hours prior to the participant, beneficiary, or enrollee being furnished such items or services by such provider; and

"(B) obtains from the participant, beneficiary, or enrollee (or from such an authorized representative) the consent described in paragraph (3) to be treated by a nonparticipating provider or nonparticipating facility.

"(2) INFORMATION REQUIRED UNDER WRITTEN NOTICE.—For purposes of paragraph (1)(A)(ii)(I), the information described in this paragraph, with respect to a nonparticipating provider or nonparticipating facility and a participant, beneficiary, or enrollee of a group health plan or health insurance coverage offered by a health insurance issuer in the group or individual market, is each of the following:

"(A) Notification, as applicable, that the health care provider is a nonparticipating provider with respect to the health plan or the health care facility is a nonparticipating facility with respect to the health plan.

"(B) Notification of the good faith estimated amount that such provider or facility may charge the participant, beneficiary, or enrollee for such items and services involved, including a notification that the provision of such estimate or consent to be treated under paragraph (3) does not constitute a contract with respect to the charges estimated for such items and services.

"(C) In the case of a participating facility and a nonparticipating provider, a list of any participating providers at the facility who are able to furnish such items and services involved and notification that the participant, beneficiary, or enrollee may be referred, at their option, to such a participating provider.

"(D) Information about whether prior authorization or other care management limitations may be required in advance of receiving such items or services at the facility.

"(3) CONSENT DESCRIBED TO BE TREATED BY A NONPARTICIPATING PROVIDER OR NONPARTICIPATING FACILITY.—For purposes of paragraph (1)(B), the consent described in this paragraph, with respect to a participant, beneficiary, or enrollee of a group health plan or health insurance coverage offered by a health insurance issuer in the group or individual market who is to be furnished items or services by a nonparticipating provider or nonparticipating facility, is a document specified by the Secretary through rulemaking, in consultation with the Secretary of Labor, that—

"(A) acknowledges that the participant, beneficiary, or enrollee has been—

"(i) provided with a written good faith estimate and an oral explanation of the charge that may be applied for the items or services anticipated to be furnished by such provider or facility; and

"(ii) informed that the payment of such charge by the participant, beneficiary, or enrollee may not accrue toward meeting any limitation that the plan or coverage places on cost-sharing, including an explanation that such payment may not apply to an in-network deductible applied under the plan or coverage; and

"(B) documents the consent of the participant, beneficiary, or enrollee to be furnished such item or services by such provider or facility.

"(4) RULE OF CONSTRUCTION.—The consent described in paragraph (3), with respect to a participant, beneficiary, or enrollee of a group health plan or health insurance coverage offered by a health insurance issuer in the group or individual market, shall constitute only consent to the receipt of the information provided pursuant to this subsection and shall not constitute a contractual agreement of the participant, beneficiary, or enrollee to any estimated charge or amount included in such information.

"(e) RETENTION OF CERTAIN DOCUMENTS.—A nonparticipating facility (with respect to such facility or any nonparticipating provider at such facility) or a participating facility (with respect to nonparticipating providers at such facility) that obtains from a participant, beneficiary, or enrollee of a group health plan or health insurance coverage offered by a health insurance issuer in the group or individual market (or an authorized representative of such participant, beneficiary, or enrollee) a written notice in accordance with subsection (d)(1)(A)(ii), with respect to furnishing an item or service to such participant, beneficiary, or enrollee, shall retain such notice for at least a 2-year period after the date on which such item or service is so furnished.

"(f) DEFINITIONS.—In this section:

"(1) The terms 'nonparticipating provider' and 'participating provider' have the meanings given such terms, respectively, in subsection (b)(3) of section 2719A.

"(2) The term 'participating health care facility' has the meaning given such term in subsection (e)(2) of section 2719A.

"(3) The term 'nonparticipating facility' means—

"(A) with respect to emergency services (as defined in section 2719A(b)(3)(C)(i)) and a group health plan or health insurance coverage offered by a health insurance issuer in the group or individual market, an emergency department of a hospital, or an independent freestanding emergency department, that does not have a contractual relationship with the plan or issuer, respectively, with respect to the furnishing of such services under the plan or coverage, respectively; and

"(B) with respect to services described in section 2719A(b)(3)(C)(ii) and a group health plan or health insurance coverage offered by a health insurance issuer in the group or individual market, a hospital or an independent freestanding emergency department, that does not have a contractual relationship with the plan or issuer, respectively, with respect to the furnishing of such services under the plan or coverage, respectively.

"(4) The term 'participating facility' means—

"(A) with respect to emergency services (as defined in clause (i) of section 2719A(b)(3)(C)) that are not described in clause (ii) of such section and a group health plan or health insurance coverage offered by a health insurance issuer in the group or individual market, an emergency department of a hospital, or an independent freestanding emergency department, that has a contractual relationship with the plan or issuer, respectively, with respect to the furnishing of such services under the plan or coverage, respectively; and

"(B) with respect to services that pursuant to clause (ii) of section 2719A(b)(3)(C) are included as emergency services (as defined in clause (i) of such section) and a group health plan or health insurance coverage offered by a health insurance issuer in the group or individual market, a hospital or an independent freestanding emergency department, that has a contractual relationship with the plan or coverage, respectively, with respect to the furnishing of such services under the plan or coverage, respectively.

"SEC. 2799A–3. PROVIDER REQUIREMENT WITH RESPECT TO PUBLIC PROVISION OF INFORMATION.

"(a) IN GENERAL.—Each health care provider and health care facility shall make publicly available, and (if applicable) post on a public website of such provider or facility and provide to individuals who are participants, beneficiaries, or enrollees of a group health plan or health insurance coverage offered by a health insurance issuer in the group or individual market a one-page notice in plain language containing information on—

"(1) the requirements and prohibitions of such provider or facility under sections 2799A–1, 2799A–2, and 2799A–4 (relating to prohibitions on balance billing in certain circumstances);

"(2) if provided for under applicable State law, any other requirements on such provider or facility regarding the amounts such provider or facility may, with respect to an item or service, charge a participant, beneficiary, or enrollee of a group health plan or health insurance coverage offered by a health insurance issuer in the group or individual market with respect to which such provider or facility does not have a contractual relationship for furnishing such item or service under the plan or coverage, respectively, after receiving payment from the plan or coverage, respectively, for such item or service and any applicable cost-sharing payment from such participant, beneficiary, or enrollee; and "(3) information on contacting appropriate State and Federal agencies in the case that an individual believes that such provider or facility has violated any requirement described in paragraph (1) or (2) with respect to such individual.

"(b) GUIDANCE.—Not later than 6 months after the date of the enactment of this section, the Secretary, in consultation with the Secretary of Labor, shall issue guidance on the requirements for the notice under this section.

"SEC. 2799A–4. AIR AMBULANCE SERVICES.

"In the case of a participant, beneficiary, or enrollee with benefits under a group health plan or health insurance coverage offered by a health insurance issuer in the group or individual market who is furnished on or after January 1, 2022, air ambulance services from a nonparticipating provider (as defined in section 2719A(b)(3)(G)) with respect to such plan or coverage, such provider shall not bill, and shall not hold liable, such participant, beneficiary, or enrollee for a payment amount for such service furnished by such provider that is more than the cost-sharing amount for such service (as determined in accordance with paragraphs (1) and (2) of section 2719A(f), section 716(f) of the Employee Retirement Income Security Act of 1974, or section 9816(f) of the Internal Revenue Code of 1986, as applicable).

"SEC. 2799A–5. ENFORCEMENT.

"(a) STATE ENFORCEMENT.—

"(1) STATE AUTHORITY.—Each State may require a provider or health care facility (including a provider of air ambulance services) subject to the requirements of this part (except section 2799A–5) to satisfy such requirements applicable to the provider or facility.

"(2) FAILURE TO IMPLEMENT REQUIREMENTS.—In the case of a determination by the Secretary that a State has failed to substantially enforce the requirements specified in paragraph (1) with respect to applicable providers and facilities in the State, the Secretary shall enforce such requirements under subsection (b) insofar as they relate to violations of such requirements occurring in such State.

"(3) NOTIFICATION OF SECRETARY OF LABOR.—A State may notify the Secretary of Labor of instances of violations of sections 2799A–1, 2799A–2, or 2799A–4 with respect to participants or beneficiaries under a group health plan or health insurance coverage offered by a health insurance issuer in the group market and any enforcement actions taken against providers or facilities as a result of such violations, including the disposition of any such enforcement actions.

"(b) SECRETARIAL ENFORCEMENT AUTHORITY.—

"(1) IN GENERAL.—If a provider or facility is found to be in violation of a requirement specified in subsection (a)(1) by the Secretary, the Secretary may apply a civil monetary penalty with respect to such provider or facility (including, as applicable, a provider of air ambulance services) in an amount not to exceed $10,000 per violation. The provisions of subsections (c) (with the exception of the first sentence of paragraph (1) of such subsection), (d), (e), (g), (h), (k), and (l) of section 1128A of the Social Security Act shall apply to a civil monetary penalty or assessment under this subsection in the same manner as such provisions apply to a penalty, assessment, or proceeding under subsection (a) of such section.

"(2) LIMITATION.—The provisions of paragraph (1) shall apply to enforcement of a provision (or provisions) specified in subsection (a)(1) only as provided under subsection (a)(2).

"(3) COMPLAINT PROCESS.—The Secretary shall, through rulemaking conducted in consultation with the Secretary of Labor, establish a process to re ceive consumer complaints of violations of such provisions and resolve such complaints within 60 days of receipt of such complaints. Such process shall provide that the Secretary of Labor be informed of complaints by participants or beneficiaries under a group health plan or health insurance coverage offered by a health insurance issuer in the group market and any enforcement actions against providers resulting from such complaints, including the disposition of any such enforcement actions.

"(4) EXCEPTION.—The Secretary may waive the penalties described under paragraph (1) with respect to a facility or provider (including a provider of air ambulance services) who does not knowingly violate, and should not have reasonably known it violated, sections 2799A–1, 2799A–2, or 2799A–4 with respect to a participant, beneficiary, or enrollee, if such facility or provider, within 30 days of the violation, withdraws the bill that was in violation of such provision and reimburses the health plan or participant, beneficiary, or enrollee, as applicable, in an amount equal to the difference between the amount billed and the amount allowed to be billed under the provision, plus interest, at an interest rate determined by the Secretary.

"(5) HARDSHIP EXEMPTION.—The Secretary may establish a hardship exemption to the penalties under this subsection.

"(c) CONTINUED APPLICABILITY OF STATE LAW.—The sections specified in subsection (a)(1) shall not be construed to supersede any provision of State law which establishes, implements, or continues in effect any requirement or prohibition except to the extent that such requirement or prohibition prevents the application of a requirement or prohibition of such a section."

(b) SECRETARY OF LABOR INVESTIGATIVE AUTHORITY.—

(1) IN GENERAL.—Part 5 of subtitle B of title I of the Employee Retirement Income Security Act of 1974 (29 U.S.C. 1131 et seq.) is amended by adding at the end the following new section:

"SEC. 522. INVESTIGATIVE AUTHORITY REGARDING VIOLATIONS OF CERTAIN HEALTH CARE PROVIDER REQUIREMENTS; COMPLAINT PROCESS.

"(a) INVESTIGATIVE AUTHORITY.—Upon receiving a notice from a State or the Secretary of Health and Human Services of violations of sections 2799A–1, 2799A–2, or 2799A–4 of the Public Health Service Act, the Secretary of Labor shall have the power to conduct an investigation to identify patterns of such violations with respect to participants or beneficiaries under a group health plan or health insurance coverage offered in connection with a group health plan by a health insurance issuer in the group market. The Secretary may assist States, the Secretary of Health and Human Services, plans, or issuers to ensure that appropriate measures have been taken to correct such violations retrospectively and prospectively with respect to participants or beneficiaries under a group health plan or health insurance coverage offered in connection with a group health plan by a health insurance issuer in the group market.

"(b) COMPLAINT PROCESS.—Not later than January 1, 2022, the Secretary shall establish a process under which the Secretary—

"(1) may receive complaints from participants and beneficiaries of group health plans or health insurance coverage offered in connection with such plans relating to alleged violations of the sections specified in subsection (a); and

"(2) transmits such complaints to States or the Secretary of Health and Human Services (as determined appropriate by the Secretary) for potential enforcement actions."

(2) TECHNICAL AMENDMENT.—The table of contents in section 1 of the Employee Retirement Income Security Act of 1974 (29 U.S.C. 1001 et seq.) is amended by inserting after the item relating to section 521 the following new item:

"Sec. 522. Investigative authority regarding violations of certain health care provider requirements; complaint process."

(c) DISCLOSURE OF CERTAIN PROTECTIONS AGAINST BALANCE BILLING.—Section 716 of the Employee Retirement Income Security Act of 1974, as added by section 2, is further amended by adding at the end the following new subsection:

"(h) DISCLOSURE OF CERTAIN PROTECTIONS AGAINST BALANCE BILLING.—Each group health plan and health insurance issuer offering group health insurance coverage shall make publicly available, and (if applicable) post on a public website of such plan or issuer—

"(1) information in plain language on—

"(A) the requirements and prohibitions applied under sections 2799A–1, 2799A–2 and 2799A–4 of the Public Health Service Act (relating to prohibitions on balance billing in certain circumstances);

"(B) if provided for under applicable State law, any other requirements on providers and facilities regarding the amounts such providers and facilities may, with respect to an item or service, charge a participant, beneficiary, or enrollee of such plan or coverage with respect to which such a provider or facility does not have a contractual relationship for furnishing such item or service under the plan or coverage after receiving payment from the plan or coverage for such item or service and any applicable cost-sharing payment from such participant, beneficiary, or enrollee; and

"(C) the requirements applied under subsections (b), (e), and (f); and

"(2) information on contacting appropriate State and Federal agencies in the case that an individual believes that such a provider or facility has violated any requirement described in paragraph (1) with respect to such individual."

SECTION 4. INDEPENDENT DISPUTE RESOLUTION PROCESS.

(a) ESTABLISHMENT.—

(1) IN GENERAL.—Not later than 1 year after the date of the enactment of this section, the Secretary of Health and Human Services, the Secretary of Labor, and the Secretary of the Treasury (in this section referred to as the "Secretaries") shall jointly establish by regulation an independent dispute resolution process (in this section referred to as the "IDR process") under which, with respect to a payment made by a group health plan or health insurance issuer offering health insurance coverage in the group or individual market pursuant to subsection (b)(1), (e)(1), or (f)(1) of section 2719A of the Public Health Service Act, section 716 of the Employee Retirement Income Security Act of 1974, or section 9816 of the Internal Revenue Code of 1986 (as applicable) using the recognized amount (as defined in and determined pursuant to section 2719A(b)(3)(H)(ii) of the Public Health Service Act or subsection (b)(3)(H)(ii) of section 716 of the Employee Retirement Income Security Act of 1974 or section 9816 of the Internal Revenue Code of 1986, as applicable) to a nonparticipating provider (as defined in subparagraph (G) of section 2719A(b)(3) of the Public Health Service Act or subparagraph (G) of subsection (b)(3) of section 716 of the Employee Retirement Income Security Act of 1974 or section 9816 of the Internal Revenue Code of 1986, as applicable) or a nonparticipating emergency facility (as defined in subparagraph (F) of such section 2719A(b)(3) or such subsection (b)(3) of such section 716 or such section 9816, as applicable) with respect to an item or service (or, in the case of payment made under section 2719A(f)(1) of the Public Health Service Act or subsection (f)(1) of section 716 of the Employee Retirement Income Security Act of 1974 or section 9816 of the Internal Revenue Code of 1986, as applicable, with respect to air ambulance services) furnished by such provider or facility—

(A) subject to subparagraph (B), the nonparticipating provider, nonparticipating emergency facility, or group health plan or health insurance issuer, respectively, may, not later than the date specified in paragraph (2), submit a request that such payment should be increased or decreased; and

(B) in the case a settlement described in subsection (d)(2) is not reached with respect to such request, an entity certified and selected under subsection (c) shall determine in accordance with such paragraph an alternative payment to be applied, with respect to such request.

(2) DATE SPECIFIED.—For purposes of paragraph (1)(A), the date specified in this paragraph is—

(A) in the case of a request described in such paragraph (1)(A) being submitted by a nonparticipating provider or nonparticipating emergency facility, with respect to items and services (or air ambulance services) described in paragraph (1), the date that is 30 days after the applicable date described in subsection (b)(2)(A)(ii); or

(B) in the case of such a request filed by a group health plan or health insurance issuer, the date that is 30 days after the date of the submission of the notice described in subsection (b)(1)(B)(ii).

(3) CLARIFICATION.—A nonparticipating provider may not, with respect to an item or service (or air ambulance service) furnished by such provider, submit a request under the IDR process if such provider is exempt from the requirement under subsection (a) of section 2799A–2 of the Public Health Service Act with respect to such item or service pursuant to subsection (e) of such section.

(b) REQUIREMENTS FOR REQUESTS TO BE ELIGIBLE FOR SUBMISSION UNDER IDR PROCESS.—

(1) TIMING REQUIREMENTS.—A request may not be submitted under the IDR process, with respect to items and services (or air ambulance services) furnished by a nonparticipating provider or nonparticipating emergency facility for which a group health plan or health insurance issuer offering health insurance coverage in the group or individual market made a payment pursuant to subsection (b)(1), (e)(1), or (f)(1) of section 2719A of the Public Health Service Act or subsection (b)(1), (e)(1), or (f)(1) of section 716 of the Employee Retirement Income Security Act of 1974 or section 9816 of the Internal Revenue Code of 1986 (as applicable) unless—

(A) in the case such request is being submitted by the nonparticipating provider or nonparticipating emergency facility—

(i) the provider or facility, respectively, filed, not later than 30 days after the date such payment is received by the provider or facility, respectively, an appeal under the appeals process of the group health plan or health insurance issuer, the subject of which includes the payment for such items and services (or air ambulance services); and

(ii) such request is not submitted before the sooner of the date on which such appeal has been resolved or the date that is 30 days after the date on which such appeal is so filed; or

(B) in the case such request is being submitted by the group health plan or health insurance issuer—

(i) the group health plan or health insurance issuer, respectively, not later than 30 days after such provider or facility, respectively, receives such payment, submits to such provider or facility, respectively, a notice that such plan or issuer, respectively, disputes the amount of such payment with respect to such items and services (or air ambulance services); and

(ii) such request is not submitted before the date that is 30 days after the date of the submission of such notice.

(2) MINIMUM MEDIAN CONTRACTED RATE.—A request may not be submitted under the IDR process, with respect to items and services (or air ambulance services) furnished in a geographic area by a nonparticipating provider or nonparticipating emergency facility for which a group health plan or health insurance issuer offering health insurance coverage in the group or individual market made a payment pursuant to subsection (b)(1), (e)(1), or (f)(1) of section 2719A of the Public Health Service Act or subsection (b)(1), (e)(1), or (f)(1) of section 716 of the Employee Retirement Income Security Act of 1974 or section 9816 of the Internal Revenue Code of 1986 (as applicable) unless—

(A) in the case such item or service is furnished during 2022, the median contracted rate (as defined in subsection (b)(3)(E) of section 2719A of the Public Health Service Act or subsection (b)(3)(E) of section 716 of the Employee Retirement Income Security Act of 1974 or section 9816 of the Internal Revenue Code of 1986 (as applicable)) for such year under such plan or such coverage with respect to each such item or service furnished by such a provider or such a facility in such area is at least $750 (or, in the case of air ambulance services, is at least $25,000); or

(B) in the case such item or service (or air ambulance services) is furnished during a subsequent year, the median contracted rate (as so defined) for such year under such plan or such coverage with respect to each such item or service furnished by such a provider or such a facility in such area is at least the amount applied under this paragraph for the previous year, increased by the percentage increase in the consumer price index for all urban consumers (United States city average) over such previous year.

(3) LIMITATION ON BATCHING OF ITEMS AND SERVICES IN A REQUEST.—A request may not be submitted under the IDR process by a nonparticipating provider, nonparticipating emergency facility, or a group health plan or health insurance issuer offering health insurance coverage in the group or individual market, with respect to multiple items and services (or multiple air ambulance services), unless—

(A) all such items and services (or air ambulance services) included in such request are furnished by the same provider or facility;

(B) payment for all such items and services (or air ambulance services) made pursuant to subsection (b)(1), (e)(1), or (f)(1) of section 2719A of the Public Health Service Act or subsection (b)(1), (e)(1), or (f)(1) of section 716 of the Employee Retirement Income Security Act of 1974 or section 9816 of the Internal Revenue Code of 1986 (as applicable) was made by a single group health plan or health insurance coverage;

(C) all such items and services (or air ambulance services) are related to the treatment of the same condition; and

(D) all such items and services were furnished during the 30-day period following the date on which the first item or service (or air ambulance service) included in such request was furnished.

(c) IDR ENTITIES.—

(1) PROCESS OF CERTIFICATION.—The process described in subsection (a) shall include a certification process under which eligible entities may be certified to carry out the IDR process.

(2) CERTIFICATION.—

(A) IN GENERAL.—An entity wishing to participate in the IDR process under this section shall request certification from the Secretaries. The Secretaries shall determine whether or not to certify applicant entities, taking into consideration whether the entity is unbiased and unaffiliated with health insurance issuers, group health plans, health care facilities, and health care providers and free of conflicts of interest, in accordance with the Secretaries' rulemaking on determining criteria for conflicts of interest.

(B) ELIGIBLE ENTITIES.—For purposes of this section, an eligible entity is an entity that is a nongovernmental entity and that agrees to comply with the fee limitations described in subparagraph (C).

(C) FEE LIMITATIONS.—For purposes of subparagraph (B), the fee limitations described in this subparagraph are limitations established by the Secretaries for the amount a certified IDR entity may charge a nonparticipating provider, nonparticipating emergency facility, group health plan, or health insurance issuer offering heath insurance coverage in the group or individual market for services furnished by such entity with respect to the resolution of a specified request of such provider, facility, plan, or issuer under the process described in subsection (a).

(3) SELECTION OF CERTIFIED IDR ENTITY.—The group health plan or health insurance issuer offering health insurance coverage in the group or individual market and the nonparticipating provider or the nonparticipating emergency facility (as applicable) involved in a request submitted under the IDR process shall agree on a certified IDR entity to resolve such request. In the case that such plan or issuer (as applicable) and such provider or facility (as applicable) cannot so agree, such an entity shall be selected by the Secretaries at random, in accordance with a manner and timeline specified by the Secretaries.

(d) PAYMENT DETERMINATION.—

(1) TIMING.—A certified IDR entity selected under subsection (c)(3) with respect to a request under the IDR process shall, subject to paragraph (2), not later than 30 days after being so selected, determine the alternative payment that should be made for items and services (or air ambulance services) included in such request in accordance with paragraph (3).

(2) SETTLEMENT.—

(A) IN GENERAL.—If such entity determines that a settlement between the group health plan or issuer, as applicable, and the provider or facility, as applicable, is likely with respect to a request under the IDR process, the entity may direct the parties to attempt, for a period not to exceed 10 days, a good faith negotiation for a settlement of such request.

(B) TIMING.—The period for a settlement described in subparagraph (A) shall accrue toward the 30-day period described in paragraph (1).

(3) DETERMINATION OF ALTERNATIVE PAYMENT.—

(A) IN GENERAL.—The group health plan or health insurance issuer offering health insurance coverage in the group or individual market (as applicable) and the nonparticipating provider or nonparticipating emergency facility (as applicable) involved shall, with respect to a request under the IDR process, each submit to the certified IDR entity selected under subsection (c)(3) for such request a final offer to be considered for the alternative payment to be applied with respect to items and services (or air ambulance services) which are the subject of the request. Such entity shall determine, in accordance with subparagraph (B), which such offer is the most reasonable and will be applied as the alternative payment.

(B) CONSIDERATIONS IN DETERMINATION.—

(i) IN GENERAL.—In determining which final offer is the alternative payment to be applied, the certified IDR entity selected under subsection (c)(3) for such request shall consider—

(I) the median contracted rates (as defined in subsection (b)(3)(E) of section 2719A of the Public Health Service Act or subsection (b)(3)(E) of section 716 of the Employee Retirement Income Security Act of 1974 or section 9816 of the Internal Revenue Code of 1986 (as applicable)) for the applicable year for items or services (or air ambulance services) that are comparable to the items and services (or air ambulance services) included in the request and that are furnished in the same geographic area (as defined by the Secretaries for purposes of such subsection) as such items and services (or air ambulance services) (not including any facility fees with respect to such rates); and

(II) in the case of items and services (other than air ambulances services), each circumstance described in clause (ii) with respect to which information is submitted by either party or, in the case of air ambulance services, each circumstance described in clause (iii) with respect to which information is submitted by either party.

(ii) ADDITIONAL CIRCUMSTANCES FOR CERTAIN ITEMS AND SERVICES.— For purposes of clause (i)(II), the circumstances described in this clause are, with respect to items and services (other than air ambulance services) included in the request under the IDR process of a nonparticipating provider, nonparticipating emergency facility, group health plan, or health insurance issuer the following:

(I) The level of training, education, experience, and quality and outcomes measurements of the provider or facility that furnished such items and services (such as those endorsed by the consensusbased entity authorized under section 1890 of the Social Security Act).

(II) The market share held by the provider or facility, or the plan or issuer, in the geographic area in which the item or service was provided.

(III) Any other extenuating circumstances with respect to the furnishing of such items and services that relate to the acuity of the individual receiving such items and services or the complexity of furnishing such items and services to such individual.

(IV) A demonstration of good faith efforts (or lack of good faith efforts) made by the provider or facility (as applicable) or the plan or issuer (as applicable).

(iii) ADDITIONAL CIRCUMSTANCES FOR AIR AMBULANCE SERVICES.—For purposes of clause (i)(II), the circumstances described in this clause are, with respect to air ambulance services included in the request under the IDR process of a nonparticipating provider, group health plan, or health insurance issuer the following:

(I) The quality and outcomes measurements of the provider that furnished such services.

(II) Any other extenuating circumstances with respect to the furnishing of such services that relate to the acuity of the individual receiving such services or the complexity of furnishing such services to such individual.

(III) The training, education, experience, and quality of the medical personnel that furnished such services.

(IV) Ambulance vehicle type, including the clinical capability level of such vehicle.

(V) Population density of the pick up location (such as urban, suburban, rural, or frontier).

(iv) PROHIBITION ON CONSIDERATION OF BILLED CHARGES.—In determining which final offer is the alternative payment amount to be applied with respect to items and services (or air ambulance services) furnished by a provider or facility and included in the request under the IDR process, the certified IDR entity selected under subsection (c)(3) with respect to such request shall not consider the amount that would have been billed by such provider or facility with respect to such items and services had the provisions of section 2799A–1, 2799A–2, or 2799A–4 of the Public Health Service Act (as applicable) not applied.

(C) EFFECTS OF DETERMINATION.—

(i) IN GENERAL.—A determination of a certified IDR entity under subparagraph (A) shall be binding.

(ii) LIMITATION ON CERTAIN SUBSEQUENT IDR CLAIMS.—In the case of a determination of a certified IDR entity under subparagraph (A), with respect to a request submitted under subsection (a)(1)(A) and the two parties involved with such request, the party that submitted such initial request may not submit during the 90-day period following such determination a subsequent request under such subsection involving the same other party to such request with respect to such an item or service (or air ambulance service) that was the subject of such initial request.

(D) COSTS OF INDEPENDENT DISPUTE RESOLUTION PROCESS.—In the case of a request made by a nonparticipating provider, nonparticipating emergency facility, group health plan, or health insurance issuer offering health insurance coverage in the group or individual market and submitted to a certified IDR entity—

(i) if such entity makes a determination with respect to such request under subparagraph (A), the party whose offer is not chosen under such clause shall be responsible for paying all fees charged by such entity; and

(ii) if the parties reach a settlement with respect to such request prior to such a determination, each party shall pay half of all fees charged by such entity, unless the parties otherwise agree.

(E) PAYMENT.—Not later than 30 days after the date on which a determination described in subparagraph (B) is made with respect to a request under the IDR process of a nonparticipating provider, nonparticipating emergency facility, group health plan, or health insurance issuer offering health insurance coverage in the group or individual market—

(i) in the case that the alternative payment determined to be applied is greater than the amount paid with respect to such request, such plan or issuer (as applicable) shall pay directly to the provider or facility (as applicable) the difference between such alternative payment and the amount so paid; and

(ii) in the case that the alternative payment determined to be applied is less than the amount paid with respect to such request, such provider or facility (as applicable) shall pay directly to the plan or issuer (as applicable) the difference between the amount so paid and such alternative payment.

(e) PUBLICATION OF INFORMATION RELATING TO DISPUTES.—

(1) PUBLICATION OF INFORMATION.—For 2022 and each subsequent year, the Secretaries shall make available on the public website of the Department of Health and Human Services, the Department of Labor, and the Department of the Treasury—

(A) the number of requests submitted under the IDR process during such year;

(B) the practice size of the providers and facilities submitting requests under the IDR process during such year;

(C) the number of such requests with respect to which a final determination was made under subsection (d)(3)(A);

(D) the average response time under the process, after the first sign of billing discrepancies between the providers, facilities, group health plans, and health insurance issuers involved in the process during such year; information comparing the average period for resolving such a billing discrepancy between such a provider, facility, plan, or issuer during such year and the average period for resolving such a discrepancy between such parties during the most recent year before the date of the enactment of this Act; and

(F) the information described in paragraph (2) for each request with respect to which such a determination was so made.

(2) INFORMATION WITH RESPECT TO REQUESTS.—For purposes of paragraph (1), the information described in this paragraph is, with respect to a request under the IDR process of a nonparticipating provider, nonparticipating

emergency facility, group health plan, or health insurance issuer offering health insurance coverage in the group or individual market—

(A) a description of each item and service (or air ambulance service) included in such request;

(B) the geography in which the items and services (or air ambulance services) included in such request were provided;

(C) the amount of the offer submitted under subsection (d)(3)(A) by the group health plan or health insurance issuer (as applicable) and by the nonparticipating provider or nonparticipating emergency facility (as applicable) expressed as a percentage of the median contracted rate;

(D) whether the offer selected by the certified IDR entity under such subsection to be the alternative payment applied was the offer submitted by such plan or issuer (as applicable) or by such provider or facility (as applicable) and the amount of such offer so selected expressed as a percentage of the median contracted rate;

(E) the category and practice specialty of each such provider or facility involved in furnishing such items and services (or, in the case of air ambulance services, the ambulance vehicle type, including the clinical capability level of such vehicle); and the identity of the group health plan or health insurance issuer, provider, or facility, with respect to the request.

(3) IDR ENTITY REQUIREMENTS.—For 2022 and each subsequent year, an IDR entity, as a condition of certification as an IDR entity, shall submit to the Secretaries such information as the Secretaries determine necessary for the Secretaries to carry out the provisions of this subsection.

(f) ENFORCEMENT.—

(1) IN GENERAL.—Any health care provider, health care facility, group health plan, or health insurance issuer offering group or individual health insurance coverage that violates a provision of this section shall be subject to a civil monetary penalty in an amount not to exceed $10,000 for each such violation.

(2) APPLICATION.—The provisions of section 1128A of the Social Security Act (other than subsections (a) and (b) and the first sentence of subsection (c)(1)) shall apply with respect to a civil monetary penalty imposed under this subsection in the same manner as such provisions apply with respect to a penalty or proceeding under subsection (a) of such section, except that any reference to "the Secretary" in such provisions shall be treated as a reference to "the Secretaries."

(g) DEFINITIONS.—In this subsection, the terms "group health plan," "group market," "health insurance issuer," "health insurance coverage," "individual health insurance coverage," "group health insurance coverage," and "individual market" have the meanings given such terms, respectively, in section 2791 of the Public Health Service Act.

(h) REPORT.—Not later than December 31, 2023, the Comptroller General of the United States shall conduct a study and submit to Congress a report on the IDR process established under this section. Such study and report shall include an analysis of potential financial relationships between providers and facilities that utilize the IDR process and private equity investment firms.

SECTION 5. ADVISORY COMMITTEE ON GROUND AMBULANCE AND PATIENT BILLING.

(a) IN GENERAL.—Not later than 60 days after the date of enactment of this Act, the Secretary of Labor, Secretary of Health and Human Services, and the Secretary of the Treasury (the Secretaries) shall jointly establish an advisory committee for the purpose of reviewing options to improve the disclosure of charges and fees for ground ambulance services, better inform consumers of insurance options for such services, and protect consumers from balance billing.

(b) COMPOSITION OF THE ADVISORY COMMITTEE.—The advisory committee shall be composed of the following members:

(1) The Secretary of Labor, or the Secretary's designee.

(2) The Secretary of Health and Human Services, or the Secretary's designee.

(3) The Secretary of the Treasury, or the Secretary's designee.

(4) One representative, to be appointed jointly by the Secretaries, for each of the following:

(A) Each relevant Federal agency, as determined by the Secretaries.

(B) State insurance regulators.

(C) Health insurance providers.

(D) Patient advocacy groups.

(E) Consumer advocacy groups.

(F) State and local governments.

(G) Physician specializing in emergency, trauma, cardiac, or stroke.

(5) Three representatives, to be appointed jointly by the Secretaries, to represent the various segments of the ground ambulance industry.

(6) Up to an additional 2 representatives otherwise not described in paragraphs (1) through (5), as determined necessary and appropriate by the Secretaries.

(c) CONSULTATION.—The advisory committee shall, as appropriate, consult with relevant experts and stakeholders, including those not otherwise included under subsection (b), while conducting the review described in subsection (a).

(d) RECOMMENDATIONS.—The advisory committee shall make recommendations with respect to disclosure of charges and fees for ground ambulance services and insurance coverage, consumer protection and enforcement authorities of the Departments of Labor, Health and Human Services, and the Treasury and State authorities, and the prevention of balance billing to consumers. The recommendations shall address, at a minimum—

(1) options, best practices, and identified standards to prevent instances of balance billing;

(2) steps that can be taken by State legislatures, State insurance regulators, State attorneys general, and other State officials as appropriate, consistent with current legal authorities regarding consumer protection; and

(3) legislative options for Congress to prevent balance billing.

(e) REPORT.—Not later than 180 days after the date of the first meeting of the advisory committee, the advisory committee shall submit to the Secretaries, and the Committees on Education and Labor, Energy and Commerce, and Ways and Means of the House of Representatives and the Committees on Finance and Health, Education, Labor, and Pensions a report containing the recommendations made under subsection (d).

SECTION 6. IMPROVING PROVIDER DIRECTORIES.

(a) PHSA.—Part A of title XXVII of the Public Health Service Act (42 U.S.C. 300gg et seq.) is amended by adding at the end the following new section:

"SEC. 2730. PROTECTING PATIENTS AND IMPROVING THE ACCURACY OF PROVIDER DIRECTORY INFORMATION.

"(a) NETWORK STATUS OF PROVIDERS.—

"(1) IN GENERAL.—Beginning on the date that is one year after the date of enactment of this section, a group health plan or a health insurance issuer offering group or individual health insurance coverage shall—

"(A) establish business processes to ensure that all enrollees in such plan or coverage receive proof of a health care provider's network status, based on what a plan or issuer knows or should know—

"(i) upon a telephone inquiry by an enrollee—

"(I) through a written electronic communication from the plan or issuer to the enrollee, as soon as practicable and not later than 1 business day after such inquiry is made by such participant, beneficiary, or enrollee for such information;

"(II) through an oral communication from the plan or issuer to the enrollee, as soon as practicable and not later than 1 business day after such inquiry is made by such enrollee for such information, which communication shall be documented by such plan or issuer, and such documentation shall be kept in the enrollee's file for a minimum of 2 years; and

"(ii) in real-time through an online health care provider directory search tool maintained by the plan or issuer; and

"(B) include in any print directory—

"(i) a disclosure that the information included in the directory is accurate as of the date of the last data update and that enrollees or prospective enrollees should consult the group health plan's or issuer's electronic provider directory on its website or call a specified customer service telephone number to obtain the most current provider directory information; and

"(ii) a list of the categories of providers of ancillary services for which the plan or coverage has no in-network providers.

"(2) GROUP HEALTH PLAN AND HEALTH INSURANCE ISSUER BUSINESS PROCESSES.—Beginning on the date that is one year after the date of the enactment of this section, a group health plan or a health insurance issuer offering group or individual health insurance coverage shall establish business processes to—

"(A) verify and update, at least once every 90 days, the provider directory information for all providers included in the online health care provider directory search tool described in paragraph (1)(A)(ii); and

"(B) remove any provider from such online directory search tool if such provider has not verified the directory information within the previous 6 months or the plan or issuer has been unable to verify the provider's network participation.

"(b) COST-SHARING LIMITATIONS.—A group health plan or a health insurance issuer offering group or individual health insurance coverage shall not apply, and shall ensure that no provider applies, cost-sharing to an enrollee for treatment or services provided by a health care provider in excess of the normal cost-sharing applied for such treatment or services provided in-network (including any balance bill issued by the health care provider involved), if such enrollee, or health care provider referring such enrollee, demonstrates (based on the electronic, written information described in subsection (a)(1)(A)(i)(I), the oral confirmation described in subsection (a)(1)(A)(i)(II) received by the enrollee not more than 30 days before the date the treatment or services were received, or a copy of the online provider directory described in subsection (a)(1)(A)(ii) on a date not more than 30 days before the date the treatment or services were received), that the enrollee relied on the information described in subsection (a)(1) for which such enrollee provides such documentation, that indicated that the provider is an in-network provider, if the provider was out-of-network at the time the treatment or service involved was received.

"(c) DEFINITION.—For purposes of this section, the term 'provider directory information' includes the names, addresses, specialty, and telephone numbers of individual health care providers, and the names, addresses, and telephone numbers of each medical group, clinic, or facility contracted to participate in any of the networks of the group health plan or health insurance coverage involved.

"(d) RULE OF CONSTRUCTION.—Nothing in this section shall be construed to preempt any provision of State law relating to health care provider directories."

(b) ERISA.—Subpart B of part 7 of subtitle B of title I of the Employee Retirement Income Security Act of 1974 (29 U.S.C. 1185 et seq.), as amended by section 2, is further amended by adding at the end the following:

"SEC. 717. PROTECTING PATIENTS AND IMPROVING THE ACCURACY OF PROVIDER DIRECTORY INFORMATION.

"(a) NETWORK STATUS OF PROVIDERS.—

"(1) IN GENERAL.—Beginning on the date that is one year after the date of enactment of this section, a group health plan (or health insurance coverage offered in connection with such a plan) shall—

"(A) establish business processes to ensure that all participants and beneficiaries in such plan or coverage receive proof of a health care provider's network status, based on what a plan or issuer of such coverage knows or should know—

"(i) upon a telephone inquiry by a participant or beneficiary—

"(I) through a written electronic communication from the plan or issuer to the participant or beneficiary, as soon as practicable and not later than 1 business day after such inquiry is made by such participant or beneficiary for such information;

"(II) through an oral communication from the plan or issuer to the participant or beneficiary, as soon as practicable and not later than 1 business day after such inquiry is made by such participant or beneficiary for such information, which communication shall be documented by such plan or issuer, and such documentation shall be kept in the participant's or beneficiary's file for a minimum of 5 years; and

"(ii) in real-time through an online health care provider directory search tool maintained by the plan or issuer; and

"(B) include in any print directory—

"(i) a disclosure that the information included in the directory is accurate as of the date of the last data update and that participants or beneficiaries or prospective participants or beneficiaries should consult the group health plan's or issuer's electronic provider directory on its website or call a specified customer service telephone number to obtain the most current provider directory information; and

"(ii) a list of the categories of providers of ancillary services for which the plan or coverage has no in-network providers.

"(2) GROUP HEALTH PLAN AND HEALTH INSURANCE ISSUER BUSINESS PROCESSES.—Beginning on the date that is one year after the date of enactment of this section, a group health plan (or health insurance coverage offered in connection with such a plan) shall establish business processes to—

"(A) verify and update, at least once every 90 days, the provider directory information for all providers included in the online health care provider directory search tool described in paragraph (1)(A)(ii); and

"(B) remove any provider from such online directory search tool if such provider has not verified the directory information within the previous 6 months or the plan or issuer has been unable to verify the provider's network participation.

"(b) COST-SHARING LIMITATIONS.—A group health plan (or health insurance coverage offered in connection with such a plan) shall not apply, and shall ensure that no provider applies, cost-sharing to a participant or beneficiary for treatment or services provided by a health care provider in excess of the normal cost-sharing applied for such treatment or services provided in-network (including any balance bill issued by the health care provider involved), if such participant or beneficiary, or health care provider referring such participant or beneficiary, demonstrates (based on the electronic, written information described in subsection (a)(1)(A)(i)(I), the oral confirmation described in subsection (a)(1)(A)(i)(II) received by the participant or beneficiary not more than 30 days before the date the treatment or services were received, or a copy of the online provider directory described in subsection (a)(1)(A)(ii) on a date not more than 30 days before the date the treatment or services were received), that the participant or beneficiary relied on the information described in subsection (a)(1) for which such participant or beneficiary provides such documentation, that indicated that the provider is an in-network provider, if the provider was out-of-network at the time the treatment or service involved was received.

"(c) DEFINITION.—For purposes of this section, the term 'provider directory information' includes the names, addresses, specialty, and telephone numbers of individual health care providers, and the names, addresses, and telephone numbers of each medical group, clinic, or facility contracted to participate in any of the networks of the group health plan or health insurance coverage involved."

(c) IRC.—Subchapter B of chapter 100 of the Internal Revenue Code of 1986, as amended by section 2, is further amended by adding at the end the following:

"SEC. 9817. PROTECTING PATIENTS AND IMPROVING THE ACCURACY OF PROVIDER DIRECTORY INFORMATION.

"(a) NETWORK STATUS OF PROVIDERS.—

"(1) IN GENERAL.—Beginning on the date that is one year after the date of enactment of this section, a group health plan shall—

"(A) establish business processes to ensure that all participants or beneficiaries in such plan receive proof of a health care provider's network status, based on what a plan or issuer knows or should know—

"(i) upon a telephone inquiry by a participant or beneficiary—

"(I) through a written electronic communication from the plan to the participant or beneficiary, as soon as practicable and not later than 1 business day after such inquiry is made by such participant or beneficiary for such information;

"(II) through an oral communication from the plan to the participant or beneficiary, as soon as practicable and not later than 1 business day after such inquiry is made by such participant or beneficiary for such information, which communication shall be documented by such plan, and such documentation shall be kept in the participant's or beneficiary's file for a minimum of 2 years; and

"(ii) in real-time through an online health care provider directory search tool maintained by the plan; and

"(B) include in any print directory—

"(i) a disclosure that the information included in the directory is accurate as of the date of the last data update and that participants or beneficiaries or prospective participants or beneficiaries should consult the group health plan's electronic provider directory on its website or call a specified customer service telephone number to obtain the most current provider directory information; and

"(ii) a list of the categories of providers of ancillary services for which the plan or coverage has no in-network providers.

"(2) GROUP HEALTH PLAN BUSINESS PROCESSES.—Beginning on the date that is one year after the date of enactment of this section, a group health plan shall establish business processes to—

"(A) verify and update, at least once every 90 days, the provider directory information for all providers included in the online health care provider directory search tool described in paragraph (1)(A)(ii); and

"(B) remove any provider from such online directory search tool if such provider has not verified the directory information within the previous 6 months or the plan or issuer has been unable to verify the provider's network participation.

"(b) COST-SHARING LIMITATIONS.—A group health plan shall not apply, and shall ensure that no provider applies, cost-sharing to a participant or beneficiary for treatment or services provided by a health care provider in excess of the normal cost-sharing applied for such treatment or services provided in-network (including any balance bill issued by the health care provider involved), if such participant or beneficiary, or health care provider referring such participant or beneficiary, demonstrates (based on the electronic, written information described in subsection (a)(1)(A)(i)(I), the oral confirmation described in subsection (a)(1)(A)(i)(II) received by the participant or beneficiary not more than 30 days before the date the treatment or services were received, or a copy of the online provider directory described in subsection (a)(1)(A)(ii) on a date not more than 30 days before the date the treatment or services were received), that the participant or beneficiary relied on the information described in subsection (a)(1) for which such participant or beneficiary provides such documentation, that indicated that the provider is an in-network provider, if the provider was out-of-network at the time the treatment or service involved was received.

"(c) DEFINITION.—For purposes of this section, the term 'provider directory information' includes the names, addresses, specialty, and telephone numbers of individual health care providers, and the names, addresses, and telephone numbers of each medical group, clinic, or facility contracted to participate in any of the networks of the group health plan involved.

"(d) RULE OF CONSTRUCTION.—Nothing in this section shall be construed to preempt any provision of State law relating to health care provider directories."

(d) CLERICAL AMENDMENTS.—

(1) ERISA.—The table of contents in section 1 of the Employee Retirement Income Security Act of 1974 (29 U.S.C. 1001 et seq.), as amended by section 2, is further amended by inserting after the item relating to section 716 the following new item:

"Sec. 717. Protecting patients and improving the accuracy of provider directory information."

(2) IRC.—The table of sections for subchapter B of chapter 100 of the Internal Revenue Code of 1986, as amended by section 2, is further amended by adding at the end the following new item:

"Sec. 9817. Protecting patients and improving the accuracy of provider directory information."

(e) PROVIDER REQUIREMENTS.—Part D of title XXVII of the Public Health Service Act (42 U.S.C. 300gg et seq.), as added by section 3, is amended—
(1) by redesignating section 2799A–5 as section 2799A–7; and
(2) by inserting after section 2799A–4 the following new section:

"SEC. 2799A–5. PROVIDER REQUIREMENTS TO PROTECT PATIENTS AND IMPROVE THE ACCURACY OF PROVIDER DIRECTORY INFORMATION.

"(a) PROVIDER BUSINESS PROCESSES.—A health care provider shall have in place business processes to ensure the timely provision of provider directory information to a group health plan or a health insurance issuer offering group or individual health insurance coverage to support compliance by such plans or issuers with section 2730(a)(1), section 717(a)(1) of the Employee Retirement Income Security Act of 1974, or section 9817(a)(1) of the Internal Revenue Code of 1986 (as applicable). Such providers shall submit provider directory information to a plan or issuers, at a minimum—
"(1) when the provider begins a network agreement with a plan or with an issuer with respect to certain coverage;
"(2) when the provider terminates a network agreement with a plan or with an issuer with respect to certain coverage;
"(3) when there are material changes to the content of provider directory information described in section 2730(a)(1), section 717(a)(1) of the Employee Retirement Income Security Act of 1974, or section 9817(a)(1) of the Internal Revenue Code of 1986 (as applicable); and
"(4) every 90 days throughout the duration of the network agreement with a plan or issuer.
"(b) ENFORCEMENT.—
"(1) CIVIL PENALTIES.—
"(A) IN GENERAL.—Subject to paragraph (2), a health care provider that violates a requirement under subsection (a) or takes actions that prevent a group health plan or health insurance issuer from complying with subsection (a)(1) or (b) of sections 2730, 717 of the Employee Retirement Income Security Act of 1974, or 9817 of the Internal Revenue Code of 1986 (as applicable) shall be subject to a civil monetary penalty of not more than $10,000 for each act constituting such violation.

"(B) SAFE HARBOR.—The Secretary may waive the penalty described under paragraph (1) with respect to a health care provider that unknowingly violates section 2730(b)(1), section 717(b)(1) of the Employee Retirement Income Security Act of 1974, or section 9817(b)(1) of the Internal Revenue Code of 1986 (as applicable) with respect to an enrollee if such provider rescinds the bill involved and, if applicable, reimburses the enrollee within 30 days of the date on which the provider billed the enrollee in violation of such subsection.

"(C) PROCEDURE.—The provisions of section 1128A of the Social Security Act, other than subsections (a) and (b) and the first sentence of subsection (c)(1) of such section, shall apply to civil money penalties under this subsection in the same manner as such provisions apply to a penalty or proceeding under section 1128A of the Social Security Act.

"(2) REFUNDS TO ENROLLEES.—If a health care provider submits a bill to an enrollee based on cost-sharing for treatment or services provided by the health care provider that is in excess of the normal cost-sharing applied for such treatment or services provided in-network, as prohibited under section 2730(b), section 717(b) of the Employee Retirement Income Security Act of 1974, or section 9817(b) of the Internal Revenue Code of 1986 (as applicable) and the enrollee pays such bill, the provider shall reimburse the enrollee for the full amount paid by the enrollee in excess of the in-network cost-sharing amount for the treatment or services involved, plus interest, at an interest rate determined by the Secretary.

"(c) LIMITATION.—Nothing in this section shall prohibit a provider from requiring in the terms of a contract, or contract termination, with a group health plan or health insurance issuer—

"(1) that the plan or issuer remove, at the time of termination of such contract, the provider from a directory of the plan or issuer described in section 2730(a)(1), section 717(a)(1) of the Employee Retirement Income Security Act of 1974, or section 9817(a)(1) of the Internal Revenue Code of 1986 (as applicable); or

"(2) that the plan or issuer bear financial responsibility, including under section 2730(b), section 717(b) of the Employee Retirement Income Security Act of 1974, or section 9817(b) of the Internal Revenue Code of 1986 (as applicable) for providing inaccurate network status information to an enrollee.

"(d) DEFINITION.—For purposes of this section, the term 'provider directory information' includes the names, addresses, specialty, and telephone numbers of individual health care providers, and the names, addresses, and telephone numbers of each medical group, clinic, or facility contracted to participate in any of the networks of the group health plan or health insurance coverage involved.

"(e) RULE OF CONSTRUCTION.—Nothing in this section shall be construed to preempt any provision of State law relating to health care provider directories."

SECTION 7. INCREASING TRANSPARENCY IN HEALTH COVERAGE.

(a) DISCLOSURE OF DIRECT AND INDIRECT COMPENSATION FOR BROKERS AND CONSULTANTS TO EMPLOYER-SPONSORED HEALTH PLANS AND ENROLLEES IN PLANS ON THE INDIVIDUAL MARKET.—

(1) GROUP HEALTH PLANS.—Section 408(b)(2) of the Employee Retirement Income Security Act of 1974 (29 U.S.C. 1108(b)(2)) is amended—

(A) by striking "(2) Contracting or making" and inserting "(2)(A) Contracting or making"; and

(B) by adding at the end the following:

"(B)(i) No contract or arrangement for services between a covered plan and a covered service provider, and no extension or renewal of such a contract or arrangement, is reasonable within the meaning of this paragraph unless the requirements of this subparagraph are met.

"(ii)(I) For purposes of this subparagraph:

"(aa) The term 'covered plan' means a group health plan as defined section 733(a).

"(bb) The term 'covered service provider' means a service provider that enters into a contract or arrangement with the covered plan and reasonably expects $1,000 (or such amount as the Secretary may establish in regulations to account for inflation since the date of the enactment of the Ban Surprise Billing Act, as appropriate) or more in compensation, direct or indirect, to be received in connection with providing one or more of the following services, pursuant to the contract or arrangement, regardless of whether such services will be performed, or such compensation received, by the covered service provider, an affiliate, or a subcontractor:

"(AA) Brokerage services, for which the covered service provider, an affiliate, or a subcontractor reasonably expects to receive indirect compensation or direct compensation described in item (dd), provided to a covered plan with respect to selection of insurance products (including vision and dental), recordkeeping services, medical management vendor, benefits administration (including vision and dental), stop-loss insurance, pharmacy benefit management services, wellness services, transparency tools and vendors, group purchasing organization preferred vendor panels, disease management vendors and products, compliance services, employee assistance programs, or third party administration services.

"(BB) Consulting, for which the covered service provider, an affiliate, or a subcontractor reasonably expects to receive indirect compensation or direct compensation described in item (dd), related to the development or implementation of plan design, insurance or insurance product selection (including vision and dental), recordkeeping, medical management, benefits administration selection (including vision and dental), stop-loss insurance, pharmacy benefit management services, wellness design and management services, transparency tools, group purchasing organization agreements and services, participation in and services from preferred vendor panels, disease management, compliance services, employee assistance programs, or third party administration services.

"(cc) The term 'affiliate', with respect to a covered service provider, means an entity that directly or indirectly (through one or more intermediaries) controls, is controlled by, or is under common control with, such provider, or is an officer, director, or employee of, or partner in, such provider.

"(dd)(AA) The term 'compensation' means anything of monetary value, but does not include non-monetary compensation valued at $250 (or such amount as the Secretary may establish in regulations to account for inflation since the date of enactment of the Ban Surprise Billing Act, as appropriate) or less, in the aggregate, during the term of the contract or arrangement.

"(BB) The term 'direct compensation' means compensation received directly from a covered plan.

"(CC) The term 'indirect compensation' means compensation received from any source other than the covered plan, the plan sponsor, the covered service provider, or an affiliate. Compensation received from a subcontractor is indirect compensation, unless it is received in connection with services performed under a contract or arrangement with a subcontractor.

"(ee) The term 'responsible plan fiduciary' means a fiduciary with authority to cause the covered plan to enter into, or extend or renew, the contract or arrangement.

"(ff) The term 'subcontractor' means any person or entity (or an affiliate of such person or entity) that is not an affiliate of the covered service provider and that, pursuant to a contract or arrangement with the covered service provider or an affiliate, reasonably expects to receive $1,000 (or such amount as the Secretary may establish in regulations to account for inflation since the date of enactment of the Ban Surprise Billing Act, as appropriate) or more in compensation for performing one or more services described in item (bb) under a contract or arrangement with the covered plan.

"(II) For purposes of this subparagraph, a description of compensation or cost may be expressed as a monetary amount, formula, or a per capita charge for each enrollee or, if the compensation or cost cannot reasonably be expressed in such terms, by any other reasonable method, including a disclosure that additional compensation may be earned but may not be calculated at the time of contract if such a disclosure includes a description of the circumstances under which the additional compensation may be earned and a reasonable and good faith estimate if the covered service provider cannot otherwise readily describe compensation or cost and explains the methodology and assumptions used to prepare such estimate. Any such description shall contain sufficient information to permit evaluation of the reasonableness of the compensation or cost.

"(III) No person or entity is a 'covered service provider' within the meaning of subclause (I)(bb) solely on the basis of providing services as an affiliate or a subcontractor that is performing one or more of the services described in subitem (AA) or (BB) of such subclause under the contract or arrangement with the covered plan.

"(iii) A covered service provider shall disclose to a responsible plan fiduciary, in writing, the following:

"(I) A description of the services to be provided to the covered plan pursuant to the contract or arrangement.

"(II) If applicable, a statement that the covered service provider, an affiliate, or a subcontractor will provide, or reasonably expects to provide, services pursuant to the contract or arrangement directly to the covered plan as a fiduciary (within the meaning of section 3(21)).

"(III) A description of all direct compensation, either in the aggregate or by service, that the covered service provider, an affiliate, or a subcontractor reasonably expects to receive in connection with the services described in subclause (I).

"(IV)(aa) A description of all indirect compensation that the covered service provider, an affiliate, or a subcontractor reasonably expects to receive in connection with the services described in subclause (I)—

"(AA) including compensation from a vendor to a brokerage firm based on a structure of incentives not solely related to the contract with the covered plan; and

"(BB) not including compensation received by an employee from an employer on account of work performed by the employee.

"(bb) A description of the arrangement between the payer and the covered service provider, an affiliate, or a subcontractor, as applicable, pursuant to which such indirect compensation is paid.

"(cc) Identification of the services for which the indirect compensation will be received, if applicable.

"(dd) Identification of the payer of the indirect compensation.

"(V) A description of any compensation that will be paid among the covered service provider, an affiliate, or a subcontractor, in connection with the services described in subclause (I) if such compensation is set on a transaction basis (such as commissions, finder's fees, or other similar incentive compensation based on business placed or retained), including identification of the services for which such compensation will be paid and identification of the payers and recipients of such compensation (including the status of a payer or recipient as an affiliate or a subcontractor), regardless of whether such compensation also is disclosed pursuant to subclause (III) or (IV).

"(VI) A description of any compensation that the covered service provider, an affiliate, or a subcontractor reasonably expects to receive in connection with termination of the contract or arrangement, and how any prepaid amounts will be calculated and refunded upon such termination.

"(iv) A covered service provider shall disclose to a responsible plan fiduciary, in writing a description of the manner in which the compensation described in clause (iii), as applicable, will be received.

"(v)(I) A covered service provider shall disclose the information required under clauses (iii) and (iv) to the responsible plan fiduciary not later than the date that is reasonably in advance of the date on which the contract or arrangement is entered into, and extended or renewed.

"(II) A covered service provider shall disclose any change to the information required under clause (iii) and (iv) as soon as practicable, but not later than 60 days from the date on which the covered service provider is informed of such change, unless such disclosure is precluded due to extraordinary circumstances beyond the covered service provider's control, in which case the information shall be disclosed as soon as practicable.

"(vi)(I) Upon the written request of the responsible plan fiduciary or covered plan administrator, a covered service provider shall furnish any other information relating to the compensation received in connection with the contract or arrangement that is required for the covered plan to comply with the reporting and disclosure requirements under this Act.

"(II) The covered service provider shall disclose the information required under clause (iii)(I) reasonably in advance of the date upon which such responsible plan fiduciary or covered plan administrator states that it is required to comply with the applicable reporting or disclosure requirement, unless such disclosure is precluded due to extraordinary circumstances beyond the covered service provider's control, in which case the information shall be disclosed as soon as practicable.

"(vii) No contract or arrangement will fail to be reasonable under this subparagraph solely because the covered service provider, acting in good faith and with reasonable diligence, makes an error or omission in disclosing the information required pursuant to clause (iii) (or a change to such information disclosed pursuant to clause (v)(II)) or clause (vi), provided that the covered service provider discloses the correct information to the responsible plan fiduciary as soon as practicable, but not later than 30 days from the date on which the covered service provider knows of such error or omission.

"(viii)(I) Pursuant to subsection (a), subparagraphs (C) and (D) of section 406(a)(1) shall not apply to a responsible plan fiduciary, notwithstanding any failure by a covered service provider to disclose information required under clause (iii), if the following conditions are met:

"(aa) The responsible plan fiduciary did not know that the covered service provider failed or would fail to make required disclosures and reasonably believed that the covered service provider disclosed the information required to be disclosed.

"(bb) The responsible plan fiduciary, upon discovering that the covered service provider failed to disclose the required information, requests in writing that the covered service provider furnish such information.

"(cc) If the covered service provider fails to comply with a written request described in subclause (II) within 90 days of the request, the responsible plan fiduciary notifies the Secretary of the covered service provider's failure, in accordance with subclauses (II) and (III).

"(II) A notice described in subclause (I)(cc) shall contain—

"(aa) the name of the covered plan;

"(bb) the plan number used for the annual report on the covered plan;

"(cc) the plan sponsor's name, address, and employer identification number;

"(dd) the name, address, and telephone number of the responsible plan fiduciary;

"(ee) the name, address, phone number, and, if known, employer identification number of the covered service provider;

"(ff) a description of the services provided to the covered plan;

"(gg) a description of the information that the covered service provider failed to disclose;

"(hh) the date on which such information was requested in writing from the covered service provider; and

"(ii)a statement as to whether the covered service provider continues to provide services to the plan.

"(III) A notice described in subclause (I)(cc) shall be filed with the Department not later than 30 days following the earlier of—

"(aa) The covered service provider's refusal to furnish the information requested by the written request described in subclause (I)(bb); or

"(bb) 90 days after the written request referred to in subclause (I)(cc) is made.

"(IV) If the covered service provider fails to comply with the written request under subclause (I)(bb) within 90 days of such request, the responsible plan fiduciary shall determine whether to terminate or continue the contract or arrangement under section 404. If the requested information relates to future services and is not disclosed promptly after the end of the 90-day period, the responsible plan fiduciary shall terminate the contract or arrangement as expeditiously as possible, consistent with such duty of prudence.

"(ix) Nothing in this subparagraph shall be construed to supersede any provision of State law that governs disclosures by parties that provide the services described in this section, except to the extent that such law prevents the application of a requirement of this section."

(2) APPLICABILITY OF EXISTING REGULATIONS.—Nothing in the amendments made by paragraph (1) shall be construed to affect the applicability of section 2550.408b–2 of title 29, Code of Federal Regulations (or any successor regulations), with respect to any applicable entity other than a covered plan or a covered service provider (as defined in section 408(b)(2)(B)(ii) of the Employee Retirement Income Security Act of 1974, as amended by paragraph (1)).

(3) INDIVIDUAL MARKET COVERAGE.—Subpart 1 of part B of title XXVII of the Public Health Service Act (42 U.S.C. 300gg–41 et seq.) is amended by adding at the end the following:

"SEC. 2746. DISCLOSURE TO ENROLLEES OF INDIVIDUAL MARKET COVERAGE.

"(a) IN GENERAL.—A health insurance issuer offering individual health insurance coverage shall make disclosures to enrollees in such coverage, as described in subsection (b), and reports to the Secretary, as described in subsection (c), regarding direct or indirect compensation provided to an agent or broker associated with enrolling individuals in such coverage.

"(b) DISCLOSURE.—A health insurance issuer described in subsection (a) shall disclose to an enrollee the amount of direct or indirect compensation provided to an agent or broker for services provided by such agent or broker associated with plan selection and enrollment. Such disclosure shall be—

"(1) made prior to the individual finalizing plan selection; and

"(2) included on any documentation confirming the individual's enrollment.

"(c) REPORTING.—A health insurance issuer described in subsection (a) shall annually report to the Secretary, prior to the beginning of open enrollment, any direct or indirect compensation provided to an agent or broker associated with enrolling individuals in such coverage.

"(d) RULEMAKING.—Not later than 1 year after the date of enactment of the Ban Surprise Billing Act, the Secretary shall finalize, through notice-and-comment rulemaking, the form and manner in which issuers described in subsection (a) are required to make the disclosures described in subsection (b) and the reports described in subsection (c). Such rulemaking may also include adjustments to notice requirements to reflect the different processes for plan renewals, in order to provide enrollees with full, timely information."

(4) TRANSITION RULE.—No contract executed prior to the effective date described in paragraph (5) by a group health plan subject to the requirements of section 408(b)(2)(B) of the Employee Retirement Income Security Act of 1974 (as amended by paragraph (1)) or by a health insurance issuer subject to the requirements of section 2746 of the Public Health Service Act (as added by paragraph (3)) shall be subject to the requirements of such section 408(b)(2)(B) or such section 2746, as applicable.

(5) EFFECTIVE DATE.—The amendments made by paragraphs (1) and (3) shall apply beginning one year after the date of enactment of this Act.

(b) STANDARDIZED REPORTING FORMAT.—Section 716 of the Employee Retirement Income Security Act of 1974, as added by section 2 and amended by section 3(c), is further amended by adding at the end the following new subsection:

"(i) STANDARDIZED REPORTING FORMAT.—

"(1) IN GENERAL.—Not later than 1 year after the date of enactment of this subsection, the Secretary shall establish a standardized reporting format for the reporting, by group health plans (or health insurance coverage offered in connection with such a plan) to State All Payer Claims Databases, of medical claims, pharmacy claims, dental claims, and eligibility and provider files that are collected from private and public payers, and shall provide guidance to States on the process by which States may collect such data from such plans or coverage in the standardized reporting format.

"(2) DEFINITION.—In this subsection, the term 'State All Payer Claims Database' means, with respect to a State, a database that may include medical claims, pharmacy claims, dental claims, and eligibility and provider files, which are collected from private and public payers."

SECTION 8. ACCESS TO COST-SHARING INFORMATION.

(a) INSURER AND PLAN REQUIREMENTS.—

(1) PHSA.—Part A of title XXVII of the Public Health Service Act (42 U.S.C. 300gg–11 et seq.), as amended by section 6(a), is further amended by inserting after section 2730 the following:

"SEC. 2731. PROVISION OF COST-SHARING INFORMATION.

"A group health plan or a health insurance issuer offering group or individual health insurance coverage shall provide a participant, beneficiary, or enrollee in the plan or coverage with a good faith estimate of the enrollee's cost-sharing (including deductibles, copayments, and coinsurance) for which the participant, beneficiary, or enrollee may be responsible for paying with respect to a specific health care service (including any service that is reasonably expected to be provided in conjunction with such specific service), as soon as practicable and not later than 2 business days after a request for such information by a participant, beneficiary, or enrollee."

(2) ERISA.—

(A) IN GENERAL.—Subpart B of part 7 of subtitle B of title I of the Employee Retirement Income Security Act of 1974 (29 U.S.C. 1185 et seq.), as amended by section 6(b), is further amended by adding at the end the following:

"SEC. 718. PROVISION OF COST-SHARING INFORMATION.

"A group health plan (or health insurance coverage offered in connection with such a plan) shall provide a participant or beneficiary in the plan or coverage with a good faith estimate of the participant's or beneficiary's cost-sharing (including deductibles, copayments, and coinsurance) for which the participant or beneficiary may be responsible for paying with respect to a specific health care service (including any service that is reasonably expected to be provided in conjunction with such specific service), as soon as practicable and not later than 2 business days after a request for such information by a participant or beneficiary. For purposes of the previous sentence, the Secretary shall develop and make available in multiple languages (as specified by the Secretary) a model form that is in easily understandable language and format."

(B) APPLICATION.—The amendment made by subparagraph (A) shall apply regardless of whether the model form described in the section 718 proposed to be added by such subparagraph has been developed or made available.

(3) IRC.—Subchapter B of chapter 100 of the Internal Revenue Code of 1986, as amended by section 6(c), is further amended by adding at the end the following:

"SEC. 9818. PROVISION OF COST-SHARING INFORMATION.

"A group health plan shall provide a participant or beneficiary in the plan with a good faith estimate of the participant's or beneficiary's cost-sharing (including deductibles, copayments, and coinsurance) for which the participant or beneficiary may be responsible for paying with respect to a specific health care service (including any service that is reasonably expected to be provided in conjunction with such specific service), as soon as practicable and not later than 2 business days after a request for such information by a participant or beneficiary."

(4) CLERICAL AMENDMENTS.—

(A) ERISA.—The table of contents in section 1 of the Employee Retirement Income Security Act of 1974 (29 U.S.C. 1001 et seq.), as amended by section 8(b)(4), is further amended by inserting after the item relating to section 717 the following new item:

"Sec. 718. Provision of cost-sharing information."

(B) IRC.—The table of sections for subchapter B of chapter 100 of the Internal Revenue Code of 1986, as amended by section 8(b)(4), is further amended by adding at the end the following new item:

"Sec. 9818. Provision of cost-sharing information."

(b) PROVIDER REQUIREMENTS.—Part D of title XXVII of the Public Health Service Act, as added by section 3 and amended by section 6, is further amended by inserting before section 2799A–7 the following new section:

"SEC. 2799A–6. PROVISION OF COST-SHARING INFORMATION.

"A provider that is in-network with respect to a group health plan or a health insurance issuer offering group or individual health insurance coverage shall, upon request by a participant, beneficiary, or enrollee, provide to a participant, beneficiary, or enrollee in the plan or coverage the following information, together with accurate and complete information about the participant's, beneficiary's, or enrollee's coverage under the applicable plan or coverage:

"(1) As soon as practicable and not later than 2 business days after the participant, beneficiary, or enrollee requests such information, a good faith estimate of the expected participant, beneficiary, or enrollee cost-sharing for the provision of a particular health care service (including any service that is reasonably expected to be provided in conjunction with such specific service).

"(2) As soon as practicable and not later than 2 business days after a participant, beneficiary, or enrollee requests such information, the contact information for any ancillary providers for a scheduled health care service."

(c) EFFECTIVE DATE.—The amendments made by subsections (a) and (b) shall apply with respect to plan years beginning on or after the date that is 18 months after the date of enactment of this Act.

SECTION 9. TRANSPARENCY REGARDING IN-NETWORK AND OUT-OF-NETWORK DEDUCTIBLES AND OUT-OF-POCKET LIMITATIONS.

(a) PHSA.—Section 2719A of the Public Health Service Act, as amended by section 2, is further amended by adding at the end the following new subsection:

"(g) TRANSPARENCY REGARDING IN-NETWORK AND OUT-OF-NETWORK DEDUCTIBLES AND OUT-OF-POCKET LIMITATIONS.—

"(1) IN GENERAL.—A group health plan or a health insurance issuer offering group or individual health insurance coverage and providing or covering any benefit with respect to items or services shall include, in clear writing, on any plan or insurance identification card issued to enrollees in the plan or coverage the amount of the in-network and out-of-network deductibles and the in-network and out-of-network out-of-pocket maximum limitation that apply to such plan or coverage.

"(2) GUIDANCE.—The Secretary, in consultation with the Secretary of Labor and Secretary of the Treasury, shall issue guidance to implement paragraph (1)."

(b) ERISA.—Section 716 of the Employee Retirement Income Security Act of 1974, as added by section 2 and as amended by sections 3(c) and 7(b), is further amended by adding at the end the following new subsection:

"(j) TRANSPARENCY REGARDING IN-NETWORK AND OUT-OF-NETWORK DEDUCTIBLES AND OUT-OF-POCKET LIMITATIONS.—

"(1) IN GENERAL.—A group health plan or a health insurance issuer offering group health insurance coverage and providing or covering any benefit with respect to items or services shall include, in clear writing, on any plan or insurance identification card issued to participants or beneficiaries in the plan or coverage the amount of the in-network and out-of-network deductibles and the in-network and out-of-network out-of-pocket maximum limitation that apply to such plan or coverage.

"(2) GUIDANCE.—The Secretary, in consultation with the Secretary of Health and Human Services and Secretary of the Treasury, shall issue guidance to implement paragraph (1)."

(c) IRC.—Section 9816 of the Internal Revenue Code of 1986, as added by section 2, is further amended by adding at the end the following new subsection:

"(h) TRANSPARENCY REGARDING IN-NETWORK AND OUT-OF-NETWORK DEDUCTIBLES AND OUT-OF-POCKET LIMITATIONS.—

"(1) IN GENERAL.—A group health plan providing or covering any benefit with respect to items or services shall include, in clear writing, on any plan or insurance identification card issued to participants or beneficiaries in the plan the amount of the in-network and out-of-network deductibles and the in-network and out-of-network out-of-pocket maximum limitation that apply to such plan. "(2) GUIDANCE.—The Secretary, in consultation with the Secretary of Health and Human Services and Secretary of Labor, shall issue guidance to implement paragraph (1)."

(d) EFFECTIVE DATE.—The amendments made by this subsection shall apply with respect to plan years beginning on or after January 1, 2022.

SECTION 10. CONTINUITY OF CARE.

(a) IN GENERAL.—Subpart B of part 7 of subtitle B of title I of the Employee Retirement Income Security Act of 1974 (29 U.S.C. 1185 et seq.), as amended by sections 2, 6, and 8, is further amended by adding at the end the following:

"SEC. 719. CONTINUITY OF CARE.

"(a) ENSURING CONTINUITY OF CARE WITH RESPECT TO TERMINATIONS OF CERTAIN CONTRACTUAL RELATIONSHIPS RESULTING IN CHANGES IN PROVIDER NETWORK STATUS.—

"(1) IN GENERAL.—In the case of an individual with benefits under a group health plan or health insurance coverage offered by a health insurance issuer in connection with a group health plan and with respect to a health care provider or facility that has a contractual relationship with such plan or such issuer (as applicable) for furnishing items and services under such plan or such coverage, if, while such individual is a continuing care patient (as defined in subsection (b)) with respect to such provider or facility—

"(A) such contractual relationship is terminated (as defined in paragraph (b));

"(B) benefits provided under such plan or such health insurance coverage with respect to such provider or facility are terminated because of a change in the terms of the participation of the provider or facility in such plan or coverage; or

"(C) a contract between such group health plan and a health insurance issuer offering health insurance coverage in connection with such plan is terminated, resulting in a loss of benefits provided under such plan with respect to such provider or facility; the plan or issuer, respectively, shall meet the requirements of paragraph (2) with respect to such individual.

"(2) REQUIREMENTS.—The requirements of this paragraph are that the plan or issuer—

"(A) notify each individual enrolled under such plan or coverage who is a continuing care patient with respect to a provider or facility at the time of a termination described in paragraph (1) affecting such provider or facility on a timely basis of such termination and such individual's right to elect continued transitional care from such provider or facility under this section;

"(B) provide such individual with an opportunity to notify the plan or issuer of the individual's need for transitional care; and

"(C) permit the patient to elect to continue to have benefits provided under such plan or such coverage, under the same terms and conditions as would have applied and with respect to such items and services as would have been covered under such plan or coverage had such termination not occurred, with respect to the course of treatment furnished by such provider or facility relating to such individual's status as a continuing care patient during the period beginning on the date on which the notice under subparagraph (A) is provided and ending on the earlier of—

"(i) the 90-day period beginning on such date; or

"(ii) the date on which such individual is no longer a continuing care patient with respect to such provider or facility.

"(b) DEFINITIONS.—In this section:

"(1) CONTINUING CARE PATIENT.—The term 'continuing care patient' means an individual who, with respect to a provider or facility—

"(A) is undergoing a course of treatment for a serious and complex condition from the provider or facility;

"(B) is undergoing a course of institutional or inpatient care from the provider or facility;

"(C) is scheduled to undergo nonelective surgery from the provide or facility, including receipt of postoperative care from such provider or facility with respect to such a surgery;

"(D) is pregnant and undergoing a course of treatment for the pregnancy from the provider or facility; or

"(E) is or was determined to be terminally ill (as determined under section 1861(dd)(3)(A) of the Social Security Act) and is receiving treatment for such illness from such provider or facility.

"(2) SERIOUS AND COMPLEX CONDITION.—The term 'serious and complex condition' means, with respect to a participant, beneficiary, or enrollee under a group health plan or health insurance coverage—

"(A) in the case of an acute illness, a condition that is serious enough to require specialized medical treatment to avoid the reasonable possibility of death or permanent harm; or

"(B) in the case of a chronic illness or condition, a condition that—

"(i) is life-threatening, degenerative, potentially disabling, or congenital; and

"(ii) requires specialized medical care over a prolonged period of time.

"(3) TERMINATED.—The term 'terminated' includes, with respect to a contract, the expiration or nonrenewal of the contract, but does not include a termination of the contract for failure to meet applicable quality standards or for fraud."

(b) CLERICAL AMENDMENT.—The table of contents in section 1 of the Employee Retirement Income Security Act of 1974 (29 U.S.C. 1001), as amended by sections 2, 6, and 8, is further amended by inserting after the item relating to section 718 the following new item:

"Sec. 719. Continuity of care."

(c) EFFECTIVE DATE.—The amendment made by subsection (a) shall apply with respect to plan years beginning on or after January 1, 2021.

SECTION 11. REPORT BY COMPTROLLER GENERAL ON ACCESS TO HEALTH CARE PROVIDERS.

Not later than January 1, 2023, the Comptroller General of the United States shall submit to Congress, and make publicly available, a report—

(1) on the effect of the provisions of, including amendments made by, this Act on access to health care providers, including in rural and underserved communities and health professional shortage areas (as defined in section 332 of the Public Health Service Act (42 U.S.C. 254e)); and

(2) including—

(A) an analysis of access to health care in the communities and areas described in paragraph (1) and the extent of provider shortages in such communities and areas; and

(B) legislative and regulatory recommendations to address any such shortage.

SECTION 12. REPORT BY COMPTROLLER GENERAL ON ADEQUACY OF PROVIDER NETWORKS.

Not later than January 1, 2023, the Comptroller General of the United States shall submit to Congress, and make publicly available, a report on the adequacy of provider networks in group health plans and group and individual health insurance coverage, including legislative recommendations to improve the adequacy of such networks.

SECTION 13. IMPLEMENTING PROTECTIONS AGAINST PROVIDER NONDISCRIMINATION.

Not later than 180 days after the date of the enactment of this Act, the Secretary of Health and Human Services, the Secretary of Labor, and the Secretary of the Treasury shall issue interim final rules implementing the protections of section 2706(a) of the Public Health Service Act

(42 U.S.C. 300gg–5(a)). The Secretaries shall accept and consider public comments on any interim final rule issued pursuant to this subsection for a period of 60 days after the date of such issuance.

Purpose and Summary

The Ban Surprise Billing Act is comprehensive, bipartisan legislation that makes several major reforms to protect consumers from surprise medical bills and improve transparency in health coverage. Surprise medical bills arise when a consumer covered by a health plan is unexpectedly treated by an out-of-network provider and is required to pay the difference between what the plan pays and the provider's charge. The issue of surprise bills, which can often expose a consumer to thousands of dollars of unforeseen medical costs, is widespread. In 2017, one in six Americans covered by an employer-sponsored plan received a surprise medical bill for out-of-network care despite having health insurance.[1] One in ten elective hospital admissions and one in five admissions from emergency departments result in surprise bills.[2]

First, the *Ban Surprise Billing Act* protects participants, bene-ficiaries, and enrollees in group health plans and coverage in the group or individual markets from surprise medical bills. To ensure that consumers are held harmless under the terms of their plan or coverage, it limits cost-sharing to the in-network rate: (1) in emergency situations, whenever a participant, beneficiary, or enrollee receives out-of-network emergency care without having a choice of provider; and (2) in non-emergency settings, when out-of-network care from certain ancillary providers is chosen without the individual's knowledge. It also extends these protections to patients who receive services from air ambulance providers.

Second, the *Ban Surprise Billing Act* includes strong prohibitions on balance billing by providers. Balance billing occurs when a patient is held financially liable for the difference between a provider's billed charge and the allowed amount under a health plan. The legislation prohibits out-of-network providers or facilities from balance billing patients in all emergency situations and in non-emergency situations by ancillary providers. It limits balance billing for elective out-of-network care at in-network facilities to situations in which a patient has a choice of an in-network provider at the facility and if the out-of-network provider complies with strong notice-and-consent requirements. Violations of these prohibitions on balance billing by providers will be enforced primarily by the states, who retain authority to regulate insurance coverage, and secondarily by the Secretary of Health and Human Services, subject to oversight by the Secretary of Labor regarding violations impacting participants and beneficiaries under group health plans or coverage.

Third, in order to resolve payment disputes between providers and health plans, the *Ban Surprise Billing Act* employs a hybrid approach that relies upon both a market-based benchmark payment and an Independent Dispute Resolution (IDR) process. For claims under $750 (under $25,000 for air ambulance claims), payment for out-of-network care will be based on the median contracted rate for similar services in the geographic area. For claims of at least $750

---

[1] Rachel Bluth, 1 In 6 Insured Hospital Patients Get a Surprise Bill for Out-Of-Network Care, *Kaiser Health News* (June 20, 2019), https://khn.org/news/1-in-6-insured-hospital-patients-get-a-surprise-bill-for-out-of-network-care/.

[2] Christopher Garmon & Benjamin Chartock, One in Five Inpatient Emergency Department Cases May Lead To Surprise Bills, 36 *Health Affairs* 177 (2017), https://www.healthaffairs.org/doi/pdf/10.1377/hlthaff.2016.0970.

($25,000 for air ambulance claims), the benchmark rate may serve as the payment amount or, alternatively, either the provider or plan may elect to utilize the binding IDR process to determine a fair payment amount. Importantly, guardrails—including a prohibition on consideration of provider billed charges by IDR entities—are put into effect to reduce costs for patients and prevent inflationary effects on health care costs.

Fourth, the *Ban Surprise Billing Act* takes additional steps to improve transparency in health coverage. For example, it requires group health plans and issuers offering coverage in the group or individual markets to establish business processes to verify and update provider directories and protect consumers from using inaccurate or out-of-date directory information. It improves the availability of information regarding cost-sharing on insurance cards. It requires brokers and consultants to disclose to group health plan sponsors and individual market consumers whether they have received any direct or indirect compensation for referrals. The *Ban Surprise Billing Act* also requires the Secretary of Labor to develop a standardized form to facilitate group health plans' information reporting to state All-Payer Claims Databases. These and other reforms will meaningfully improve the quality and affordability of care while increasing transparency in coverage and empowering patients to make informed decisions about their care.

Finally, the bill is drafted in a legally sound manner that will ensure its requirements are enforceable and fully protect participants, beneficiaries, and enrollees in group health plans and coverage in the group and individual markets from surprise medical bills. All provisions of the *Ban Surprise Billing Act* that are intended to apply to plans covered by the *Employee Retirement Income Security Act of 1974* (ERISA) are drafted as explicit amendments to ERISA, resolving any question as to their applicability and enforceability by the Secretary of Labor.

Committee Action

116th Congress

On April 2, 2019, the Committee on Education and Labor's (the Committee) Subcommittee on Health, Employment, Labor, and Pensions held the first ever Congressional hearing on surprise billing entitled "Examining Surprise Billing: Protecting Patients from Financial Pain" (April 2nd Subcommittee Hearing). The hearing explored the causes of surprise billing, the impact of surprise medical bills on consumers, and the policies needed to both protect consumers and improve transparency in health coverage. The Committee heard testimony from Ms. Christen Linke Young, Fellow, USC Brookings Schaeffer Initiative on Health Policy, Washington, DC; Ms. Ilyse Schuman, Senior Vice President, Health Policy, American Benefits Council, Washington, DC; Mr. Frederick Isasi, Executive Director, Families USA, Washington, DC; and Dr. Jack Hoadley, Research Professor Emeritus, Georgetown University Health Policy Institute, McCourt School of Public Policy, McLean, VA.

On February 7, 2020, Congressman Robert C. "Bobby" Scott (D– VA–3), Chairman of the Committee on Education and Labor, introduced H.R. 5800, the *Ban Surprise Billing Act*, with Congresswoman Virginia Foxx (R–NC–5), Ranking Member of the Committee on Education and Labor, as an original cosponsor.

On February 11, 2020, the Committee marked up H.R. 5800 and ordered it to be reported favorably, as amended, to the House of Representatives by a vote of 32 Yeas and 13 Nays.

At the markup, the Committee considered the following amendments to H.R. 5800:

- Congressman Scott offered an Amendment in the Nature of a Substitute (ANS) that made minor technical corrections to the bill. The ANS also requires the Comptroller General to conduct a study of the IDR process established by the bill and analyze potential financial relationships between providers or facilities that utilize the IDR process and private equity firms. The ANS, as amended with further amendments described below, was adopted by voice vote.
- Congresswoman Donna Shalala (D–FL–27) offered an amendment allowing for care begun with an in-network provider to continue at the in-network rate for 90 days if the provider leaves the network. The amendment was adopted by voice vote.
- Congressman Greg Murphy (R–NC–3) offered an amendment requiring certain provider directory documents to be retained by health plans for five years. The amendment was adopted by voice vote.
- Congresswoman Shalala offered an amendment requiring a rulemaking on provider nondiscrimination requirements. The amendment was adopted by voice vote.
- Congressman Murphy offered an amendment providing that the IDR process established under the bill must require public disclosure of the average response time following a billing discrepancy and the average time to resolve a billing discrepancy. The amendment was adopted by voice vote.
- Congresswoman Ilhan Omar (D–MN–5) offered an amendment requiring the Secretary of Labor to submit a template for disseminating cost-sharing information. The amendment was adopted by voice vote.
- Congressman Phil Roe (R–TN–1) offered an amendment striking the air ambulance provisions of the bill. The amendment was defeated by a vote of 8 Yeas and 37 Nays.
- Congresswoman Kim Schrier (D–WA–8) offered an amendment requiring the Comptroller General to conduct a study of network adequacy in health plans and coverage. The amendment was adopted by voice vote.
- Congressman Roe offered an amendment striking the median contracted rate benchmark and substituting "commercially reasonable" rates. The amendment was defeated by a vote of 15 Yeas and 30 Nays.
- Congresswoman Susie Lee (D–NV–3) offered an amendment requiring the Comptroller General to conduct a study of provider access in underserved areas. The amendment was adopted by voice vote.
- Congressman Roe offered an amendment striking the median contracted rate benchmark and substituting "previously contracted" rates. The amendment was defeated by a vote of 16 Yeas and 29 Nays.
- Congresswoman Schrier offered an amendment adding good faith efforts to contract as a consideration for IDR entities. The amendment was adopted by voice vote.
- Congressman Lloyd Smucker (R–PA–11) offered an amendment allowing for the continuation of certain contracting practices, notwithstanding the enactment of the *Ban Surprise Billing Act*. The amendment was withdrawn.

- Congressman Joe Morelle (D–NY–25) offered an ANS substituting the text of H.R. 5826, the *Consumer Protections against Surprise Medical Bills Act of 2020,* in place of the text of H.R. 5800. The amendment was withdrawn.
- Congressman Morelle offered an amendment to strike the threshold for claims to be eligible for the IDR process. The amendment was defeated by a vote of 15 Yeas and 30 Nays.

Committee Views

Introduction

As the Committee of jurisdiction over employer-sponsored health coverage, a central goal in developing and advancing the Ban Surprise Billing Act is to ensure that reforms apply throughout the health care system—not only in the individual market, but also to the approximately 157 million Americans who are covered through a workplace health plan.[3] In addition, while meaningfully improving the affordability of care for millions, the bill was carefully crafted to strike a balance between the various concerns of stakeholders—including providers, hospitals, labor unions, health insurers, and employers—many of whom have divergent views on how to effectively address the issue of surprise billing.

While striking a careful balance between the concerns of stakeholders, the *Ban Surprise Billing Act* puts consumers and patients first, and has been commended by dozens of advocacy groups. A coalition of twenty-three patient organizations, including the American Heart Association, American Lung Association, and American Cancer Society, applauded the bill for its "robust protections for all patients in all health settings. . . . Importantly, these protections extend to patients covered by employer-sponsored plans."[4] Similarly, the No Surprises coalition, a group of thirteen consumer organizations, including Families USA, National Consumers League, and Consumer Reports, highlighted the bill's strong protections against growth in health care premiums: "With health care costs a primary concern for America's families, we strongly prefer the benchmark approach taken by the Education and Labor [Committee] as the most effective cost control mechanism available."[5]

Background on Surprise Medical Bills

Surprise medical bills occur when consumers covered by health insurance are subject to higher-than-expected out-of-pocket costs when they receive care from a provider who is outside their plan's network. These costs can include cost-sharing at out-of-network rates under their health plan as well as balance bills from a provider requiring the consumer to pay the difference between the provider's out-of-network charge and the amount, if any, that the plan will pay for the item or service. The rise of managed care plans, such as Health Maintenance Organizations

---

[3] Kaiser Family Foundation, *Health Insurance Coverage of the Total Population*, https:// www.kff.org/other/state-indicator/total-population/ (last visited Feb. 23, 2020) (Covering the 2018 timeframe).

[4] Press Release, ALS Association, et al. (Feb. 11, 2020), https://rarediseases.org/wp-content/ uploads/2020/ 02/NORD-2020-EdLabor-SMB-Markup-STMT-FINAL.pdf.

[5] Letter from *No Surprises: People against Surprise Medical Bills* to the Honorable Robert C. "Bobby" Scott, Chairman, Committee on Education and Labor, et al. (Feb. 11, 2020) (on file with Committee).

(HMOs), Preferred Provider Organizations (PPOs), and Point of Service (POS) plans, in which the insurer contracts with a network of doctors, hospitals, or other health care providers, has placed an increasing number of consumers at risk of receiving surprise bills.[6]

Situations in which patients have little or no control over whether a provider is in- or out-of-network can arise in both emergency and non-emergency situations. Patients in emergency settings often receive care at a hospital that is not in their plan's network or are transported by an out-of-network ambulance. Non-emergency situations can also lead to surprise bills when patients receive care at a facility that is in-network but unknowingly receive services by out-of-network providers. Among the most common non-emergency services that result in surprise out-of-network bills are pathology, radiology, anesthesiology, and other ancillary health services for which the patient did not have an opportunity to choose the provider or was unaware the care was being provided at all.[7]

The Prevalence and Financial Impact of Surprise Medical Bills

Surprise medical bills are widespread in private health coverage, impacting consumers in both the group and individual markets. In 2017, one in six Americans covered by an employer-sponsored plan received a surprise medical bill for out-of-network care despite having health insurance.[8] One in ten elective hospital admissions and one in five admissions to emergency departments result in surprise bills.[9] Services particularly likely to be out-of-network include ambulance transportation, including more than half of all emergency ground ambulance transports[10] and nearly 70 percent of air ambulance transports.[11]

The financial liability imposed on patients by surprise medical bills can be staggering. A series of articles published by Vox in 2019 drew substantial public attention to the devastating stories of patients who have received surprise bills; among the most shocking was a spinal surgery patient who received a bill of $101,000 despite having confirmed that her surgeon was in-network.[12] These unexpected medical bills can result in financial ruin, as nearly four in ten American adults are unable to cover a $400 emergency expense,[13] yet the average surprise balance bill by emergency physicians in 2014 and 2015 was an estimated $620 greater than the

---

[6] Over the past three decades, the number of individuals enrolled in a conventional health insurance arrangement through their employer has declined from 73 percent of workers to approximately ten percent. By 2018, approximately 49 percent of individuals with employer-sponsored coverage were enrolled in a PPO, 16 percent in an HMO, and six percent in a POS plan. Kaiser Family Foundation, *2018 Employer Health Benefits Survey*, https://www.kff.org/report-section/2018-employer-health-benefits-survey-section-5-market-shares-of-health-plans/ (last visited May 20, 2020).

[7] Loren Adler et al., Stopping Surprise Medical Bills: Federal Action Is Needed, *Health Affairs* (Feb. 1, 2017), https://www.healthaffairs.org/do/10.1377/hblog20170201.058570/full/.

[8] Rachel Bluth, *supra* note 1.

[9] Christopher Garmon & Benjamin Chartock, *supra* note 2.

[10] *Id.*

[11] U.S. Gov't Accountability Off., GAO–19–292, *Air Ambulances: Available Data Show Privately-Insured Patients Are at Financial Risk* 16 (2019), https://www.gao.gov/assets/700/ 697684.pdf.

[12] Sarah Kliff, A Spinal Surgery, a $101,000 Bill, and a New Law to Prevent More Surprises, *Vox* (Mar. 19, 2019 8:00AM), https://www.vox.com/health-care/2019/3/19/18233051/surprise-medical-bills-arbitration-new-york.

[13] Board of Governors of the Federal Reserve System, *Economic Well-Being of U.S. Households in 2018* 21 (2019), https://www.federalreserve.gov/publications/files/2018-report-economic-well-being-us-households-201905.pdf.

Medicare rate for the same service.[14] The ever-present threat of out-of-pocket medical expenses contributes to the fact that approximately two-thirds of consumers have expressed a fear that they will not be able to afford an unanticipated medical expense for themselves or a family member.[15] These costs have further negative impacts on when and how patients receive needed care, often resulting in care delays and negatively affecting patient choices.[16] Surprise medical bills have devastating financial impacts on Americans and on their ability to afford needed health care. Consumers, who are subject to these bills through no fault of their own, should not be liable for unexpected and unreasonable out-of-pocket costs. There is substantial bipartisan interest in reducing the burden of surprise medical bills on consumers. In addition, there has been a growing sentiment among health care stakeholders that surprise billing must be addressed at the federal level, although opinions differ regarding the appropriate approach to do so.

Surprise Billing Represents a Market Failure

Economists generally regard the practice of surprise medical billing as arising from a failure in the health care market, which causes providers—particularly in certain specialties—to have little or no incentive to contract to join a health plan's network due to a number of unique circumstances. These providers face highly inelastic demands for their services because patients lack the ability to meaningfully choose or refuse care, such as during an emergency or when ancillary services are provided of which a patient may not even be aware. They also often hold substantial market power, resulting in one or only very few providers available to provide critical items or services in a geographic area. These circumstances enable some providers to charge amounts for their services that exceed the marginal cost of producing those services and resulting in compensation far above what is needed to sustain their practice.

The presence of this market failure in certain provider specialties is strongly supported by evidence reflecting the highly inflated payment rates for these services. For example, in comparison to the amount paid by Medicare for similar items or services, the median billed charge for emergency medicine is 465 percent of the Medicare rate; similar disparities are present for pathology (343 percent), diagnostic radiology (402 percent), and anesthesiology (551 percent).[17] These inflated payment rates are, in turn, reflected in the cost of in-network care. While the average in-network physician is paid at 128 percent of Medicare rates, in-network payments for emergency medicine (306 percent), radiology (200 percent), and

---

[14] Zack Cooper & Fiona Scott Morton, Out-of-Network Emergency-Physician Bills—An Unwelcome Surprise, 375 *New England Journal of Medicine* 1915 (2016), http://zackcooper.com/sites/default/files/paper-files/NEJM/surprise/billing.pdf.

[15] Jordan Rau, Surprise Medical Bills Are What Americans Fear Most in Paying for Health Care, *Kaiser Health News* (Sept. 5, 2018), https://khn.org/news/surprise-medical-bills-are-what-americans-fear-most-in-paying-for-health-care/.

[16] According to one survey, 45 percent of individuals, the majority of whom are covered by health insurance, report that they have delayed or avoided receiving health care due to high out-of-pocket costs. Kyle T. Smith et al., Access Is Necessary but Not Sufficient: Factors Influencing Delay and Avoidance of Health Care Services, 3 *Medical Decision Making Policy & Practice* 1 (2018). *See also* Benjamin Chartock et al., Consumers' Responses to Surprise Medical Bills in Elective Situations, 38 *Health Affairs* 425 (2019).

[17] *Examining Surprise Billing: Protecting Patients from Financial Pain before the Subcomm. on Health, Employment, Labor, and Pensions of the H. Comm. on Educ. & Labor*, 116th Cong. (2019) (written testimony of Christen Linke Young, Fellow, USC–Brookings Schaeffer Initiative on Health Policy at 17) [hereinafter Young Testimony].

anesthesiology (344 percent) far exceed Medicare rates.[18] These costs are directly felt through higher out-of-pocket expenses and exorbitant surprise bills for out-of-network care, as well as by all consumers who share in rising overall health care costs through higher premiums.

The financial opportunity from inflated out-of-network prices has made health care an attractive market for private equity firms, hedge funds, and venture capital firms.[19] For example, private equity deals related to health care more than doubled between 2008 and 2018,[20] and private equity firms now own the two largest physician staffing companies, which together account for 30 percent of the physician-staffing market.[21] Research on one large private equity-owned firm showed that when it entered a hospital network, out-of-network billing rates increased by more than 81 percentage points.[22]

Existing State Laws and the Need for Federal Action

A number of states have taken significant steps to address surprise medical bills through consumer protection laws that shield patients from surprise billing in the individual, small group, and fully-insured group markets. In total, about half of the states in the U.S. have enacted at least some form of surprise billing legislation; however, most Americans live in states that have not enacted laws that are considered comprehensive by experts.[23] Federal action is necessary to ensure that patients throughout the country are protected from unexpected costs arising from surprise billing practices. Moreover, states are unable to protect consumers fully in employer-sponsored plans from surprise bills because ERISA prohibits states from regulating self-insured group health plans, which cover more than 60 percent of people enrolled in employer-sponsored health plans.[24] ERISA contains a broad preemption clause providing that federal law "shall supersede any and all State laws insofar as they may now or hereafter relate to any employee benefit plan."[25] States are therefore unable to apply their surprise medical bill laws to millions of their residents, and as a result, a federal legislative response is necessary.

The Central Role of ERISA in Ensuring Surprise Billing Protections Apply

The *Patient Protection and Affordable Care Act* (ACA)[26] made a number of major changes to the private health insurance market through amendments to Part A of title XXVII of the *Public*

---

[18] Young Testimony at 9.

[19] Rachel Bluth & Emmarie Huetteman, Investors' Deep-Pocket Push to Defend Surprise Medical Bills, *Kaiser Health News* (Sept. 11, 2019), https://khn.org/news/investors-deep-pocket-push-to-defend-surprise-medical-bills/.

[20] Samantha Liss, Private Equity Sees Ripe Opportunity in Healthcare this Year, *Health Care Dive* (Mar. 25, 2019), https://www.healthcaredive.com/news/private-equity-sees-ripe-opportunity-in-healthcare-this-year/548831/.

[21] *Id.*

[22] Zack Cooper et al., Surprise! Out-of-Network Billing for Emergency Care in the United States 2018, 23 *National Bureau of Economic Research*, (2019) https://www.nber.org/papers/w23623.pdf.

[23] Jack Hoadley et al., State Efforts to Protect Consumers from Balance Billing, *Commonwealth Fund* (Jan. 18, 2019), https://www.commonwealthfund.org/blog/2019/state-efforts-protect-consumers-balance-billing.

[24] 2018 Employer Health Benefits Survey, Section 10: Plan Funding, *Kaiser Family Foundation* (Oct. 3, 2018), https://www.kff.org/report-section/2018-employer-health-benefits-survey-section-10-plan-funding/ (last visited June 5, 2020).

[25] 29 U.S.C. § 1144.

[26] 42 U.S.C. § 18001 et seq.

Health Service Act (PHSA).[27] These provisions, insofar as they impact group health plans and health insurance issuers providing health insurance coverage in connection with group health plans, are incorporated by reference into ERISA through Section 715 of ERISA.[28]

However, serious questions exist as to whether amendments to Part A of title XXVII of the PHSA enacted subsequent to the ACA are automatically incorporated into ERISA. A recent decision by the Supreme Court of the United States, *Jam v. International Finance Corp.*,[29] articulated an approach to statutory interpretation that would suggest that subsequent amendments are not automatically incorporated. In that decision, Chief Justice Roberts distinguished between two scenarios in which a statute incorporates external law by reference. In situations in which "a statute refers to a general subject, the statute adopts the law on that subject as it exists whenever a question under the statute arises."[30] However, the Court drew a clear distinction "when a statute [] refers to another statute by specific title or section number."[31] In such situations, the referring statute "in effect cuts and pastes the referenced statute as it existed when the referring statute was enacted, without any subsequent amendments."[32]

Although the statute at issue in *Jam* was the *International Organizations Immunities Act*, the principle of statutory interpretation articulated by the Court is directly applicable to title XXVII of the PHSA and the incorporation by reference provision of ERISA. Because Section 715 of ERISA *specifically* references "the provisions of part A of title XXVII of the Public Health Service Act," the Court's reasoning in *Jam* suggests that ERISA only incorporates the law in Part A of title XXVII of the PHSA as it stood on the date of enactment of the ACA on March 23, 2010. Therefore, in order for subsequent amendments to Part A of title XXVII of the PHSA to apply to ERISA, the amendments must be drafted directly to ERISA. Therefore, the *Ban Surprise Billing Act* is drafted in this manner in order to protect consumers comprehensively and unequivocally from surprise bills.

Comprehensive Protections Are Needed to Protect Consumers Fully

There is widespread agreement that any surprise billing solution must comprehensively protect consumers by "taking the consumer out of the middle" of surprise billing disputes. Since a large share of American consumers have very little financial cushion—as noted above, about 40 percent could not afford an unexpected $400 emergency expense in 2018—surprise medical bills can lead to financial stress, debt, damaged credit, and bankruptcy.[33] The fact that individual consumers are ill-equipped to bear the risk of large, unpredictable costs underpins the notion of insurance in the market for health care. Consumers do not need to receive an exorbitant bill themselves to be negatively affected by surprise billing practices; when plans

---

[27] 42 U.S.C. § § 300gg et seq.

[28] 29 U.S.C § 1185d. Note that a similar provision incorporates Part A of title XXVII of the *Public Health Service Act* into the Internal Revenue Code. 26 U.S.C. § 9815.

[29] 139 S. Ct. 759 (2019).

[30] *Id.* at 769.

[31] *Id.*

[32] *Id.*

[33] Federal Reserve Board, *supra note* 13.

pay high out-of-network bills, these costs are passed on to all consumers in the form of higher premiums.[34]

At the April 2nd Subcommittee Hearing, witnesses discussed several critical issues Congress must address to provide comprehensive protections for consumers from surprise medical billing. First, in order to hold a consumer truly harmless from the financial devastation of surprise bills, health plans must provide that cost-sharing be limited to in-network amounts in surprise billing situations to ensure that the patient is treated as if they were seeing an in-network provider.[35] Second, a surprise billing solution must prohibit providers from sending balance bills to patients for amounts in excess of their in-network cost-sharing under the plan.[36] Third, in order to resolve disputes between providers and plans over payments, legislation must establish a fair payment amount.[37]

In addition, witnesses and Members noted that measures to improve transparency in health coverage could serve as important complements to surprise billing legislation. Specifically, improvements to provider directories—described as "notoriously inaccurate" by Dr. Jack Hoadley during his testimony—were mentioned as potentially beneficial for consumers.[38] Further measures to improve transparency, such as including additional information regarding coverage on insurance cards, were also raised by Members such as Congressman Roe in his written questions for the hearing record.[39] However, witnesses emphasized that improvements to transparency, though helpful, are not substitutes for a comprehensive solution to the underlying issue of surprise medical billing.[40]

Resolving Payment Disputes between Providers and Health Plans

A key element of any solution to address surprise billing comprehensively is the payment rate, which is the amount that payers must remit to providers for out-of-network items and services. Two payment rate options have emerged as the predominant contenders to correct the market failure associated with surprise billing: (1) the benchmark rate model, and (2) the IDR process, also referred to as arbitration. Under a benchmark rate model, payments to providers for out-of-network items and services default to a pre-determined amount, such as a percentage of the Medicare rate (typically 125 percent of Medicare) or the median contracted (in-network) rate

---

[34] Young Testimony at 2.

[35] *Examining Surprise Billing: Protecting Patients from Financial Pain, Hearing Before the Subcomm. on Health, Employment, Labor, and Pensions of the H. Comm. on Educ. & Labor*, 116th Cong. (2019) (written testimony of Frederick Isasi, Executive Director, Families USA, Washington, DC at 6).

[36] *Id.*

[37] *Id.*

[38] H. Comm. on Educ. & Labor, *Examining Surprise Billing: Protecting Patients from Financial Pain*, YouTube (Apr. 7, 2019), https://www.youtube.com/watch?v=HyUd2-/YPN0 (see 46:33).

[39] *Examining Surprise Billing: Protecting Patients from Financial Pain, Hearing Before the Subcomm. on Health, Employment, Labor, and Pensions of the H. Comm. on Educ. & Labor*, 116th Cong 194–95 (response to Committee Member questions by Ilyse Schuman, Senior Vice President, Health Policy, American Benefits Council).

[40] *Examining Surprise Billing: Protecting Patients from Financial Pain, Hearing Before the Subcomm. on Health, Employment, Labor, and Pensions of the H. Comm. on Educ. & Labor*, 116th Cong. (2019) 202 (response to Committee Member questions by Christen Linke Young, Fellow, USC-Brookings Schaeffer Initiative on Health Policy) ("Enhanced transparency about cost-sharing can be useful, but I do not believe it will provide a meaningful tool to address surprise out-of-network billing").

in the geographic area where the service took place.[41] In contrast, the IDR process is mediated by a third-party arbitrator, and legislation typically specifies guidance or criteria for the arbitrator to consider. A common approach is to use "baseball-style" arbitration, under which each side submits a price, and the arbitrator chooses one, with both sides bound by the decision.[42]

Both approaches "take the consumer out of the middle" of surprise billing disputes. Both also offer the opportunity to tether payment rates for surprise out-of-network bills directly to market-based prices, curbing cost growth relative to the status quo. For example, the commonly considered median in-network benchmark rate is a market-based price; it reflects negotiations between providers and insurers in a local health care market. An IDR process may also partially reflect market-based prices if the arbitrator is instructed under the legislation to consider a market-derived price such as the median in-network rate, although the IDR process entails some additional administrative costs. However, some IDR process proposals would have the arbitrator consider non-market-based rates such as providers' billed charges,[43] which may drive up consumer costs.[44]

Of the two options, evidence indicates that benchmark rates will generally slow the rapid growth of health care costs, both by lowering costs in the near term relative to the status quo and by slowing the rate of health care cost inflation in future years.[45] Benchmark rates achieve this primarily by removing providers' incentives and ability to charge very high out-of-network

---

[41] When the benchmark is set at a negotiated rate such as the median in-network rate, it is typically linked to previously agreed-upon rates (such as 2019 rates) and linked to inflation thereafter, which prevents providers from influencing their own pay. Examples of recent federal legislation that rely exclusively on benchmark rates are the *Lower Health Care Costs Act* (S. 1895), which passed the Senate Health, Education, Labor, and Pensions (HELP) Committee on June 26, 2019, by a vote of 20–3, and the *No Surprises Act* (H.R. 3630), as introduced in the U.S. House of Representatives on June 9, 2019. Both bills set benchmark rates at the median contracted (in-network) rate, although H.R. 3630 was amended in the Committee on Energy and Commerce to allow for limited arbitration for disputed bills for which the median in-network rate is at least $1,250.

[42] An example of federal legislation that relies on the arbitration approach is the *Consumer Protections Against Surprise Medical Bills Act of 2020* (H.R. 5826) which was reported by the House Ways and Means Committee on February 12, 2020, by voice vote. The bill allows arbitration to take place if the payer and provider fail to negotiate a solution within 30 days; it instructs the arbitrator to consider the median in-network rate for the item or service, among other criteria.

[43] For example, under New York's surprise billing law, arbitration entities are instructed to consider several factors in baseball-style arbitration, including the 80th percentile of billed charges. Loren Adler, *Experience with New York's Arbitration Process for Surprise Out-of-network Bills*, Brookings Institution (Oct. 24, 2019), https://www.brookings.edu/blog/usc-brookings-schaeffer-on-health-policy/2019/10/24/experience-with-new-yorks-arbitration-process-for-surprise-out-of-network-bills/.

[44] Loren Adler et al., *Rep. Ruiz's Arbitration Proposal for Surprise Billing (H.R. 3502) Would Lead to Much Higher Costs And Deficits*," Health Affairs Blog (July 16, 2019), https:// www.healthaffairs.org/do/10.1377/hblog 20190716.355260/full/; *see also* David Hyman & Benedic Ippolito, Arbitration not the Answer to Fix Surprise Medical Billing, *Real Clear Policy* (Feb. 12, 2019), https://www.realclearpolicy.com/articles/2019/02/12/ arbitration/not/the/answer/to/fix/surprise/medical/billing/111042.html.

[45] For example, the Congressional Budget Office (CBO) estimates that the surprise billing provisions of the Senate HELP Committee bill, which sets the benchmark rate at the relevant median in-network payment rate, would reduce commercial insurance premiums by an average of one percent nationwide and decrease deficits by $25 billion over 10 years relative to the status quo. Of this $25 billion, approximately $24 billion stems from increased tax revenue due to lower premiums for tax-privileged employment-based insurance, while over $1 billion stems from reduced federal spending. Congressional Budget Office, S.1895, *Lower Health Care Costs Act* 3 (2019), https://www.cbo.gov/system/files/2019–07/s1895/0.pdf. By contrast, while CBO has not published a formal assessment of an IDR process model, CBO reportedly has stated that establishing a system similar to New York's at the national level would increase the federal deficit by "double digit billions" over a ten-year period. Rachana Pradhan, More States Crack Down on Vaping, *Politico* (Sep. 25, 2019), https://www.politico.com/newsletters/ politico-pulse/2019/09/25/more-states-crack-down-on-vaping-757620.

prices,[46] thus reducing providers' bargaining power to negotiate or demand higher prices of health plans,[47] the costs of which insurers typically pass on to consumers.[48] Slower growth in health care costs will, in turn, reduce growth in consumers' premiums and government spending on health care.

The IDR process, on the other hand, has the potential advantage of allowing payment rates "to vary more for specific circumstances and potentially adjust more easily over time."[49] This added flexibility may be particularly merited in high-stakes and complex situations in which a market-based benchmark such as the median in-network rate is less likely to reflect or be monetarily close to the cost of furnishing the item or service.

There is a wide range of opinions among various stakeholders about which approach to payment rates is optimal. To bridge this divide, the *Ban Surprise Billing Act* incorporates a hybrid approach that will ensure that an efficient, market-based payment benchmark is employed, while providing for a noninflationary IDR mechanism for cases in which claims of at least $750 (or $25,000 for air ambulance services). This strikes an appropriate balance between the views of various stakeholders and is designed to reduce premiums and the deficit.

Conclusion

H.R. 5800, the *Ban Surprise Billing Act*, protects consumers from the financial devastation of surprise medical billing through a targeted and balanced approach that carefully weighs the needs of all stakeholders with divergent views on the issue. Most importantly, the legislation provides robust protections from surprise medical bills for workers and families across the country.

Section-by-Section Analysis

Sec. 1. Short Title

This section states that the Act may be cited as the *Ban Surprise Billing Act*.

Sec. 2. Preventing Surprise Medical Bills

This section establishes consumer protections in the group and individual markets to protect participants, beneficiaries, and enrollees from surprise medical bills. It limits cost-sharing owed

---

[46] Michelle Andrews, California Surprise-Billing Law Protects Patients but Aggravates Many Doctors, *California Healthline* (Dec. 4, 2019), https://californiahealthline.org/news/california-surprise-billing-law-protects-patients-but-aggravates-many-doctors/.

[47] Loren Adler et al., Brookings, *State Approaches to Mitigating Surprise Out-of-Network Billing* at 9 (2019), https://www.brookings.edu/wp-content/uploads/2019/02/Adler/et-al/State-Approaches-to-Mitigating-Surprise-Billing-2019.pdf.

[48] *See* Glenn Melnick, Blame Emergency Rooms for the Out-of-Control Cost of Health Care, *New York Times* (Sept. 5, 2018), https://www.nytimes.com/2018/09/05/opinion/emergency-rooms-cost-insurance.html. Furthermore, ben chmarking obviates the additional administrative costs insurers face under an arbitration model which, if high enough, could "undermine the effectiveness of the policy by leading insurers to simply accede to providers' demands rather than pursue arbitration," causing insurers to pass increased costs on to consumers, again leading to health care cost inflation. Loren Adler et al., *supra* note 47.

[49] Loren Adler et al., *supra* note 47.

under a health plan or coverage to the in-network rate whenever a participant, beneficiary, or enrollee receives out-of-network emergency care, including air ambulance services and non-emergency care provided by out-of-network ancillary providers. It also requires that the costs of out-of-network care received in a situation where a surprise bill would have occurred in either emergency or non-emergency settings be counted toward the in-network deductible or out-of-pocket limit under the plan or coverage.

This section provides that the recognized amount under the plan or coverage for certain out-of-network items or services will be determined based on a market-based benchmark of the median contracted rate for similar services in the geographic area. The methodology for determining the benchmark will be established by the Secretaries of Health and Human Services, Labor, and the Treasury ("Secretaries") and the Secretaries shall establish a process whereby plans or providers may file complaints of violations of the requirements for determining the benchmark payment. Plans and issuers will be subject to audit by the Secretaries to ensure compliance with these requirements. The audit process specified in the bill is not intended to limit, restrict, or otherwise interfere with the Secretary of Labor's existing investigative and enforcement authority under Part 5 of ERISA, including the Secretary's authority to conduct additional audits regarding the median contracted rate and any other provisions of the bill.

This section also provides that in determining the allowed amount under the plan or coverage, state laws for determining the payment amount may remain in effect with respect to plans and coverage within the jurisdiction of states, including amounts determined under an All-Payer Model Agreement under Section 1115A of the *Social Security Act*. In cases in which no applicable state law is in effect, the allowed amount will be the median of the in-network rate recognized by the plan or issuer for a similar item or service provided in the same geographic region.

Sec. 3. Preventing Certain Cases of Balance Billing

This section prohibits out-of-network facilities and providers, including air ambulance providers, from engaging in balance billing of a participant, beneficiary, or enrollee in a group or individual health plan or coverage. In emergency situations, providers are prohibited from holding a participant, beneficiary, or enrollee liable for an amount greater than the cost-sharing owed under the plan or coverage. In non-emergency situations, ancillary providers are prohibited from holding a participant, beneficiary, or enrollee liable for an amount greater than the cost-sharing owed under the plan or coverage. This section further specifies that such ancillary services include emergency medicine, anesthesiology, pathology, radiology, neonatology, and certain diagnostic services. In addition, in cases in which no in-network provider can furnish the item or service at the facility, such out-of-network services will be treated as ancillary services.

In cases in which elective out-of-network care is sought, this section requires that out-of-network providers and facilities provide notice to a participant, beneficiary, or enrollee of their network status and a good faith estimate of charges that may be applied for the out-of-network care. In order for the item or service to be treated as out-of-network, this information must be provided at the time an appointment is scheduled and the consent of the patient must be obtained at least 72 hours in advance of when the items or services are furnished.

This section also provides for state enforcement under the Act of provider requirements and the prohibition on balance billing. In cases in which states fail to implement the requirements and do not substantially enforce the prohibitions, this section provides that the Secretary of Health and Human Services shall have the authority to apply, with respect to a facility or provider, a civil monetary penalty of up to $10,000 per violation. In addition, this section requires states and the Secretary of Health and Human Services to inform the Secretary of Labor of violations of requirements impacting individuals in group health plans or coverage and any enforcement actions, including the disposition of such actions.

Sec. 4. Independent Dispute Resolution

This section requires the Secretaries of Health and Human Services, the Treasury, and Labor to jointly establish an Independent Dispute Resolution (IDR) process to determine payment amounts. The Secretaries shall jointly certify such IDR entities, subject to standards to prevent conflicts of interest and financial relationships between certified entities and either providers or plans. This section permits providers and payers to elect to utilize the IDR process for any amounts for which the median contracted rate is at least $750 ($25,000 for air ambulance services).

This section authorizes certified IDR entities to consider several factors in determining payment amounts, including the median contracted rate for a similar item or service furnished in the same geographic area, the level of training and experience of the provider, and extenuating circumstances such as the complexity of the specific case or the acuity of the patient. It prohibits IDR entities from considering the billed charges of the provider for the item or service.

Sec. 5. Advisory Committee on Ground Ambulance and Patient Billing

This section requires the Secretaries of Health and Human Services, Labor, and the Treasury to establish an advisory committee to develop recommendations to protect consumers from ground ambulance balance bills.

Sec. 6. Improving Provider Directories

This section requires group health plans and issuers offering coverage in the group or individual markets to establish business processes to verify and update provider directories and to respond to inquiries with respect to the network status of a provider within one business day of a request. It limits cost-sharing to the in-network rate when a participant, beneficiary, or enrollee relied in good faith on out-of-date provider directories under the plan or coverage.

Sec. 7. Improving Transparency in Health Coverage

This section requires brokers and consultants to disclose to group health plan sponsors and consumers enrolled in coverage in the individual market whether they have received any direct or indirect compensation for referrals.

This section also requires the Secretary of Labor to develop a standardized form to allow group health plans and issuers to report information to state All-Payer Claims Databases.

Sec. 8. Access to Cost-Sharing Information

This section requires providers, group health plans, and issuers offering coverage in the group or individual markets to provide to a participant, beneficiary, or enrollee a good faith estimate of cost-sharing owed for a health care service within two business days of a request.

Sec. 9. Transparency Regarding in-Network and Out-of-Network Deductibles and Out-of-Pocket Limitations

This section requires group health plans and issuers offering coverage in the group or individual markets to include on insurance identification cards the amount of the in-network and out-of-network deductibles and out-of-pocket limitations under the plan or coverage.

Explanation of Amendments

The amendments, including the amendment in the nature of a substitute, are explained in the descriptive portions of this report.

Application of Law to the Legislative Branch

Pursuant to section 102(b)(3) of the *Congressional Accountability Act*, Pub. L. No. 104–1, H.R. 5800, as amended, does not apply to terms and conditions of employment or to access to public services or accommodations within the legislative branch.

Unfunded Mandate Statement

Pursuant to Section 423 of the *Congressional Budget and Impoundment Control Act* (as amended by Section 101(a)(2) of the *Unfunded Mandates Reform Act*, Pub. L. No. 104 4), the Committee adopts as its own the estimate of and statement regarding federal mandates in H.R. 5800, as amended, prepared by the Director of the Congressional Budget Office.

Earmark Statement

In accordance with clause 9 of rule XXI of the Rules of the House of Representatives, H.R. 5800 does not contain any congressional earmarks, limited tax benefits, or limited tariff benefits as described in clauses 9(e), 9(f), and 9(g) of rule XXI.

Roll Call Votes

In compliance with clause 3(b) of rule XIII of the Rules of the House of Representatives, the Committee advises that the following roll call votes occurred during the Committee's consideration of H.R. 5800:

Date: 2/11/2020

COMMITTEE ON EDUCATION AND LABOR RECORD OF COMMITTEE VOTE

Roll Call: 1 Bill: H.R. 5800 Amendment Number: 7

Disposition: defeated by a vote of 8-37

Sponsor/Amendment: Roe/ Strikes air ambulance provision

Name & State	Aye	No	Not Voting	Name & State	Aye	No	Not Voting
Mr. SCOTT (VA) (Chairman)		X		Mrs. FOXX (NC) (Ranking)		X	
Mrs. DAVIS (CA)		X		Mr. ROE (TN)	X		
Mr. GRIJALVA (AZ)		X		Mr. THOMPSON (PA)		X	
Mr. COURNTEY (CT)		X		Mr. WALBERG (MI)		X	
Ms. FUDGE (OH)			X	Mr. GUTHRIE (KY)		X	
Mr. SABLAN (MP)		X		Mr. BYRNE (AL)			X
Ms. WILSON (FL)		X		Mr. GROTHMAN (WI)	X		
Ms. BONAMICI (OR)		X		Ms. STEFANIK (NY)		X	
Mr. TAKANO (CA)		X		Mr. ALLEN (GA)	X		
Ms. ADAMS (NC)			X	Mr. SMUCKER (PA)	X		
Mr. DESAULNIER (CA)		X		Mr. BANKS (IN)	X		
Mr. NORCROSS (NJ)		X		Mr. WALKER (NC)			X
Ms. JAYAPAL (WA)		X		Mr. COMER (KY)		X	
Mr. MORELLE (NY)		X		Mr. CLINE (VA)		X	
Ms. WILD (PA)		X		Mr. FULCHER (ID)		X	
Mr. HARDER (CA)		X		Mr. WATKINS (KS)	X		
Mrs. MCBATH (GA)		X		Mr. WRIGHT (TX)			X
Ms. SCHRIER (WA)		X		Mr. MEUSER (PA)		X	
Ms. UNDERWOOD (IL)		X		Mr. JOHNSON (SD)	X		
Mrs. HAYES (CT)		X		Mr. KELLER (PA)		X	
Ms. SHALALA (FL)		X		Mr. MURPHY (NC)	X		
Mr. LEVIN (MI)		X		Mr. VAN DREW (NJ)		X	
Ms. OMAR (MN)		X					
Mr. TRONE (MD)		X					
Ms. STEVENS (MI)		X					
Mrs. LEE (NV)		X					
Mrs. TRAHAN (MA)		X					
Mr. CASTRO (TX)		X					

TOTALS: Ayes: 8 Nos: 37 Not Voting: 5

Total: 50 / Quorum: / Report:

(28 D - 22 R)

^Although not present for the recorded vote, Member expressed he/she would have voted AYE if present at time of vote.

*Although not present for the recorded vote, Member expressed he/she would have voted NO if present at time of vote.

Date: 2/11/2020

COMMITTEE ON EDUCATION AND LABOR RECORD OF COMMITTEE VOTE

Roll Call: 2 Bill: H.R. 5800 Amendment Number: 9

Disposition: defeated by a vote of 15-30

Sponsor/Amendment: Roe /Changes median in-network to "commercially reasonable" rates

Name & State	Aye	No	Not Voting	Name & State	Aye	No	Not Voting
Mr. SCOTT (VA) (Chairman)		X		Mrs. FOXX (NC) (Ranking)		X	
Mrs. DAVIS (CA)		X		Mr. ROE (TN)	X		
Mr. GRIJALVA (AZ)		X		Mr. THOMPSON (PA)	X		
Mr. COURNTEY (CT)		X		Mr. WALBERG (MI)		X	
Ms. FUDGE (OH)			X	Mr. GUTHRIE (KY)		X	
Mr. SABLAN (MP)		X		Mr. BYRNE (AL)			X
Ms. WILSON (FL)		X		Mr. GROTHMAN (WI)	X		
Ms. BONAMICI (OR)		X		Ms. STEFANIK (NY)		X	
Mr. TAKANO (CA)		X		Mr. ALLEN (GA)	X		
Ms. ADAMS (NC)			X	Mr. SMUCKER (PA)	X		
Mr. DESAULNIER (CA)		X		Mr. BANKS (IN)	X		
Mr. NORCROSS (NJ)		X		Mr. WALKER (NC)			X
Ms. JAYAPAL (WA)		X		Mr. COMER (KY)		X	
Mr. MORELLE (NY)	X			Mr. CLINE (VA)		X	
Ms. WILD (PA)	X			Mr. FULCHER (ID)	X		
Mr. HARDER (CA)		X		Mr. WATKINS (KS)	X		
Mrs. MCBATH (GA)		X		Mr. WRIGHT (TX)			X
Ms. SCHRIER (WA)	X			Mr. MEUSER (PA)		X	
Ms. UNDERWOOD (IL)		X		Mr. JOHNSON (SD)		X	
Mrs. HAYES (CT)		X		Mr. KELLER (PA)		X	
Ms. SHALALA (FL)	X			Mr. MURPHY (NC)	X		
Mr. LEVIN (MI)		X		Mr. VAN DREW (NJ)	X		
Ms. OMAR (MN)		X					
Mr. TRONE (MD)		X					
Ms. STEVENS (MI)		X					
Mrs. LEE (NV)	X						
Mrs. TRAHAN (MA)		X					
Mr. CASTRO (TX)		X					

TOTALS: Ayes: 15 Nos: 30 Not Voting: 5

Total: 50 / Quorum: / Report:

(28 D - 22 R)

^Although not present for the recorded vote, Member expressed he/she would have voted AYE if present at time of vote.

*Although not present for the recorded vote, Member expressed he/she would have voted NO if present at time of vote.

Date: 2/11/2020

COMMITTEE ON EDUCATION AND LABOR RECORD OF COMMITTEE VOTE

Roll Call: 3 Bill: H.R. 5800 Amendment Number: 11

Disposition: defeated by a vote of 16-29

Sponsor/Amendment: Roe /Changes median in-network to "previously contracted" rates

Name & State	Aye	No	Not Voting	Name & State	Aye	No	Not Voting
Mr. SCOTT (VA) (Chairman)		X		Mrs. FOXX (NC) (Ranking)		X	
Mrs. DAVIS (CA)		X		Mr. ROE (TN)	X		
Mr. GRIJALVA (AZ)		X		Mr. THOMPSON (PA)	X		
Mr. COURNTEY (CT)		X		Mr. WALBERG (MI)		X	
Ms. FUDGE (OH)			X	Mr. GUTHRIE (KY)		X	
Mr. SABLAN (MP)		X		Mr. BYRNE (AL)			X
Ms. WILSON (FL)		X		Mr. GROTHMAN (WI)	X		
Ms. BONAMICI (OR)		X		Ms. STEFANIK (NY)		X	
Mr. TAKANO (CA)		X		Mr. ALLEN (GA)	X		
Ms. ADAMS (NC)			X	Mr. SMUCKER (PA)	X		
Mr. DESAULNIER (CA)		X		Mr. BANKS (IN)	X		
Mr. NORCROSS (NJ)		X		Mr. WALKER (NC)			X
Ms. JAYAPAL (WA)		X		Mr. COMER (KY)		X	
Mr. MORELLE (NY)	X			Mr. CLINE (VA)		X	
Ms. WILD (PA)	X			Mr. FULCHER (ID)	X		
Mr. HARDER (CA)		X		Mr. WATKINS (KS)	X		
Mrs. MCBATH (GA)		X		Mr. WRIGHT (TX)			X
Ms. SCHRIER (WA)	X			Mr. MEUSER (PA)		X	
Ms. UNDERWOOD (IL)		X		Mr. JOHNSON (SD)		X	
Mrs. HAYES (CT)		X		Mr. KELLER (PA)		X	
Ms. SHALALA (FL)	X			Mr. MURPHY (NC)	X		
Mr. LEVIN (MI)		X		Mr. VAN DREW (NJ)	X		
Ms. OMAR (MN)		X					
Mr. TRONE (MD)		X					
Ms. STEVENS (MI)	X						
Mrs. LEE (NV)	X						
Mrs. TRAHAN (MA)		X					
Mr. CASTRO (TX)		X					

TOTALS: Ayes: 16 Nos: 29 Not Voting: 5

Total: 50 / Quorum: / Report:

(28 D - 22 R)

^Although not present for the recorded vote, Member expressed he/she would have voted AYE if present at time of vote.

*Although not present for the recorded vote, Member expressed he/she would have voted NO if present at time of vote.

Date: 2/11/2020

COMMITTEE ON EDUCATION AND LABOR RECORD OF COMMITTEE VOTE

Roll Call: 4 Bill: H.R. 5800 Amendment Number: 15

Disposition: defeated by a vote of 15-30

Sponsor/Amendment: Morelle/ Deletes the threshold for arbitration

Name & State	Aye	No	Not Voting	Name & State	Aye	No	Not Voting
Mr. SCOTT (VA) (Chairman)		X		Mrs. FOXX (NC) (Ranking)		X	
Mrs. DAVIS (CA)		X		Mr. ROE (TN)	X		
Mr. GRIJALVA (AZ)		X		Mr. THOMPSON (PA)	X		
Mr. COURNTEY (CT)		X		Mr. WALBERG (MI)		X	
Ms. FUDGE (OH)			X	Mr. GUTHRIE (KY)		X	
Mr. SABLAN (MP)		X		Mr. BYRNE (AL)			X
Ms. WILSON (FL)		X		Mr. GROTHMAN (WI)	X		
Ms. BONAMICI (OR)		X		Ms. STEFANIK (NY)	X		
Mr. TAKANO (CA)		X		Mr. ALLEN (GA)	X		
Ms. ADAMS (NC)			X	Mr. SMUCKER (PA)	X		
Mr. DESAULNIER (CA)		X		Mr. BANKS (IN)		X	
Mr. NORCROSS (NJ)		X		Mr. WALKER (NC)			X
Ms. JAYAPAL (WA)		X		Mr. COMER (KY)		X	
Mr. MORELLE (NY)	X			Mr. CLINE (VA)		X	
Ms. WILD (PA)		X		Mr. FULCHER (ID)	X		
Mr. HARDER (CA)		X		Mr. WATKINS (KS)	X		
Mrs. MCBATH (GA)		X		Mr. WRIGHT (TX)			X
Ms. SCHRIER (WA)	X			Mr. MEUSER (PA)		X	
Ms. UNDERWOOD (IL)		X		Mr. JOHNSON (SD)	X		
Mrs. HAYES (CT)		X		Mr. KELLER (PA)		X	
Ms. SHALALA (FL)	X			Mr. MURPHY (NC)	X		
Mr. LEVIN (MI)		X		Mr. VAN DREW (NJ)	X		
Ms. OMAR (MN)		X					
Mr. TRONE (MD)		X					
Ms. STEVENS (MI)		X					
Mrs. LEE (NV)	X						
Mrs. TRAHAN (MA)		X					
Mr. CASTRO (TX)		X					

TOTALS: Ayes: 15 Nos: 30 Not Voting: 5

Total: 50 / Quorum: / Report:

(28 D - 22 R)

^Although not present for the recorded vote, Member expressed he/she would have voted AYE if present at time of vote.

*Although not present for the recorded vote, Member expressed he/she would have voted NO if present at time of vote.

Date: 2/11/2020

COMMITTEE ON EDUCATION AND LABOR RECORD OF COMMITTEE VOTE

Roll Call: 5 Bill: H.R. 5800 Amendment Number: Motion

Disposition: adopted by a vote of 32-13

Sponsor/Amendment: Takano/ to report to the House with an amendment and with the recommendation that the amendment be agreed to, and the bill as amended, do pass

Name & State	Aye	No	Not Voting	Name & State	Aye	No	Not Voting
Mr. SCOTT (VA) (Chairman)	X			Mrs. FOXX (NC) (Ranking)	X		
Mrs. DAVIS (CA)	X			Mr. ROE (TN)		X	
Mr. GRIJALVA (AZ)	X			Mr. THOMPSON (PA)		X	
Mr. COURNTEY (CT)	X			Mr. WALBERG (MI)	X		
Ms. FUDGE (OH)			X	Mr. GUTHRIE (KY)	X		
Mr. SABLAN (MP)	X			Mr. BYRNE (AL)			X
Ms. WILSON (FL)	X			Mr. GROTHMAN (WI)		X	
Ms. BONAMICI (OR)	X			Ms. STEFANIK (NY)	X		
Mr. TAKANO (CA)	X			Mr. ALLEN (GA)		X	
Ms. ADAMS (NC)			X	Mr. SMUCKER (PA)		X	
Mr. DESAULNIER (CA)	X			Mr. BANKS (IN)	X		
Mr. NORCROSS (NJ)	X			Mr. WALKER (NC)			X
Ms. JAYAPAL (WA)	X			Mr. COMER (KY)	X		
Mr. MORELLE (NY)		X		Mr. CLINE (VA)		X	
Ms. WILD (PA)	X			Mr. FULCHER (ID)		X	
Mr. HARDER (CA)	X			Mr. WATKINS (KS)		X	
Mrs. MCBATH (GA)	X			Mr. WRIGHT (TX)			X
Ms. SCHRIER (WA)	X			Mr. MEUSER (PA)	X		
Ms. UNDERWOOD (IL)	X			Mr. JOHNSON (SD)		X	
Mrs. HAYES (CT)	X			Mr. KELLER (PA)	X		
Ms. SHALALA (FL)		X		Mr. MURPHY (NC)		X	
Mr. LEVIN (MI)	X			Mr. VAN DREW (NJ)		X	
Ms. OMAR (MN)	X						
Mr. TRONE (MD)	X						
Ms. STEVENS (MI)	X						
Mrs. LEE (NV)	X						
Mrs. TRAHAN (MA)	X						
Mr. CASTRO (TX)	X						

TOTALS: Ayes: 32 Nos: 13 Not Voting: 5

Total: 50 / Quorum: / Report:

(28 D - 22 R)

^Although not present for the recorded vote, Member expressed he/she would have voted AYE if present at time of vote.

*Although not present for the recorded vote, Member expressed he/she would have voted NO if present at time of vote.

Statement of Performance Goals and Objectives

Pursuant to clause (3)(c) of rule XIII of the Rules of the House of Representatives, the goals of H.R. 5800 are to end surprise medical billing and increase transparency in health coverage.

Duplication of Federal Programs

Pursuant to clause 3(c)(5) of rule XIII of the Rules of the House of Representatives, the Committee states that no provision of H.R. 5800 establishes or reauthorizes a program of the Federal Government known to be duplicative of another federal program, a program that was included in any report from the Government Accountability Office to Congress pursuant to section 21 of Pub. L. No. 111–139, or a program related to a program identified in the most recent Catalog of Federal Domestic Assistance.

Hearings

Pursuant to section 103(i) of H. Res. 6 for the 116th Congress, on April 2, 2019, the Committee on Education and Labor's Subcommittee on Health, Employment, Labor, and Pensions held a hearing entitled "Examining Surprise Billing: Protecting Patients from Financial Pain," which was used to develop H.R. 5800. The hearing explored the causes of surprise billing, the impact of surprise medical bills on patients, and policies to both protect consumers and improve transparency in health coverage. The Committee heard testimony from: Ms. Christen Linke Young, Fellow, USC-Brookings Schaeffer Initiative on Health Policy, Washington, DC; Ms. Ilyse Schuman Senior Vice President, Health Policy, American Benefits Council Washington, DC; Mr. Frederick Isasi, Executive Director, Families USA, Washington, DC; and Dr. Jack Hoadley, Research Professor Emeritus, Georgetown University Health Policy Institute, McCourt School of Public Policy, McLean, VA.

Statement of Oversight Findings and Recommendations of the Committee

In compliance with clause 3(c)(1) of rule XIII and clause 2(b)(1) of rule X of the Rules of the House of Representatives, the Committee's oversight findings and recommendations are reflected in the descriptive portions of this report.

New Budget Authority and CBO Cost Estimate

Pursuant to clause 3(c)(2) of rule XIII of the Rules of the House of Representatives and section 308(a) of the *Congressional Budget Act of 1974*, and pursuant to clause 3(c)(3) of rule XIII of the Rules of the House of Representatives and section 402 of the *Congressional Budget Act of 1974,* the Committee has received the following estimate for H.R. 5800 from the Director of the Congressional Budget Office:

H.R. 5800, The Ban Surprise Billing Act, as ordered reported by the House Committee on Education and Labor on February 11, 2020 estimated budgetary effects

	By fiscal year, millions of dollars—												
	2020	2021	2022	2023	2024	2025	2026	2027	2028	2029	2030	2020–2025	2020–2030
Increases or Decreases (−) in Direct Spending													
Protections Against Surprise Medical Bills:													
Estimated Budget Authority	0	0	*	−44	−89	−103	−111	−119	−123	−128	−134	−236	−851
Estimated Outlays	0	0	*	−44	−89	−103	−111	−119	−123	−128	−134	−236	−851
Increases in Revenues													
Protections Against Surprise Medical Bills:	0	0	872	1,809	2,170	2,335	2,689	2,944	3,153	3,387	3,642	7,186	23,002
On-budget revenues	0	0	619	1,284	1,544	1,664	1,970	2,176	2,335	2,511	2,701	5,112	16,804
Off-budget revenues	0	0	253	525	625	671	720	768	819	877	940	2,074	6,198
Increases or Decreases (−) in the Deficit from Direct Spending and Revenues													
Estimated Effect on the Deficit:	0	0	−872	−1,853	−2,259	−2,438	−2,801	−3,063	−3,276	−3,515	−3,776	−7,423	−23,853
Estimated Changes in On-Budget Deficits	0	0	−619	−1,328	−1,633	−1,767	−2,081	−2,295	−2,458	−2,638	−2,835	−5,348	−17,656
Estimated Changes in Off-Budget Deficits	0	0	−253	−525	−625	−671	−720	−768	−819	−877	−940	−2,074	−6,198

Sources: Congressional Budget Office; staff of the Joint Committee on Taxation. Components may not sum to totals because of rounding; * = between zero and $500,000.

H.R. 5800 would establish patient protections from surprise medical billing, and in certain circumstances would require insurers to reimburse out-of-network providers on the basis of the median payment rate for in-network care. The bill also would establish a process for health care providers and insurers to settle disputes over out-of-network bills greater than $750.

CBO and JCT expect that under the bill, in facilities where surprise bills are likely, the average of payment rates for both in- and out-of-network care would move toward the median in-network rate, which tends to be lower than average rates. CBO and JCT estimate that in most affected markets in most years, lower payments to some providers would reduce premiums by roughly 1 percent. Lower costs for health insurance would reduce federal deficits because the federal government subsidizes most private insurance through tax preferences for employment-based coverage and through the health insurance marketplaces established under the Affordable Care Act.

Committee Cost Estimate

Clause 3(d)(1) of rule XIII of the Rules of the House of Representatives requires an estimate and a comparison of the costs that would be incurred in carrying out H.R. 5800. However, clause 3(d)(2)(B) of that rule provides that this requirement does not apply when the committee has included in its report a timely submitted cost estimate of the bill prepared by the Director of the Congressional Budget Office under section 402 of the *Congressional Budget Act of 1974*. Pursuant to clause 3(d)(1) of rule XIII, the Committee adopts as its own the cost estimate prepared by the Director of the Congressional Budget Office pursuant to section 402 of the *Congressional Budget Act of 1974*.

Changes in Existing Law Made by the Bill, as Reported

In compliance with clause 3(e) of rule XIII of the Rules of the House of Representatives, changes in existing law made by the bill, H.R. 5800, as reported, are shown as follows:

Changes in Existing Law Made by The Bill, as Reported

In compliance with clause 3(e) of rule XIII of the Rules of the House of Representatives, changes in existing law made by the bill, as reported, are shown as follows (existing law proposed to be omitted is enclosed in black brackets, new matter is printed in italics, and existing law in which no change is proposed is shown in roman):

Public Health Service Act

Title XXVII—Requirements Relating to Health Insurance Coverage

Part A—Individual and Group Market Reforms

Subpart II—Improving Coverage

SEC. 2719A. PATIENT PROTECTIONS.

(a) CHOICE OF HEALTH CARE PROFESSIONAL.—If a group health plan, or a health insurance issuer offering group or individual health insurance coverage, requires or provides for designation by a participant, beneficiary, or enrollee of a participating primary care provider, then the plan or issuer shall permit each participant, beneficiary, and enrollee to designate any participating primary care provider who is available to accept such individual.

[(b) COVERAGE OF EMERGENCY SERVICES.—

[(1) IN GENERAL.—If a group health plan, or a health insurance issuer offering group or individual health insurance issuer, provides or covers any benefits with respect to services in an emergency department of a hospital, the plan or issuer shall cover emergency services (as defined in paragraph (2)(B))—

[(A) without the need for any prior authorization determination;

[(B) whether the health care provider furnishing such services is a participating provider with respect to such services;

[(C) in a manner so that, if such services are provided to a participant, beneficiary, or enrollee—

[(i) by a nonparticipating health care provider with or without prior authorization; or

[(ii)(I) such services will be provided without imposing any requirement under the plan for prior authorization of services or any limitation on coverage where the provider of services does not have a contractual relationship with the plan for the providing of services that is more restrictive than the requirements or limitations that apply to emergency department services received from providers who do have such a contractual relationship with the plan; and

[(II) if such services are provided out-of-network, the cost-sharing requirement (expressed as a copayment amount or coinsurance rate) is the same requirement that would apply if such services were provided in-network;

[(D) without regard to any other term or condition of such coverage (other than exclusion or coordination of benefits, or an affiliation or waiting period, permitted under section 2701 of this Act, section 701 of the Employee Retirement Income Security Act of 1974, or section 9801 of the Internal Revenue Code of 1986, and other than applicable cost-sharing).

[(2) DEFINITIONS.—In this subsection:

[(A) EMERGENCY MEDICAL CONDITION.—The term "emergency medical condition" means a medical condition manifesting itself by acute symptoms of sufficient severity (including severe pain) such that a prudent layperson, who possesses an average knowledge of health and medicine, could reasonably expect the absence of immediate medical attention to result in a condition described in clause (i), (ii), or (iii) of section 1867(e)(1)(A) of the Social Security Act.

[(B) EMERGENCY SERVICES.—The term "emergency services" means, with respect to an emergency medical condition—

[(i) a medical screening examination (as required under section 1867 of the Social Security Act) that is within the capability of the emergency department of a hospital, including ancillary services routinely available to the emergency department to evaluate such emergency medical condition, and

[(ii) within the capabilities of the staff and facilities available at the hospital, such further medical examination and treatment as are required under section 1867 of such Act to stabilize the patient.

[(C)STABILIZE.—The term "to stabilize," with respect to an emergency medical condition (as defined in subparagraph (A)), has the meaning give in section 1867(e)(3) of the Social Security Act (42 U.S.C. 1395dd(e)(3)).

(b) COVERAGE OF EMERGENCY SERVICES.—

(1) IN GENERAL.—If a group health plan, or a health insurance issuer offering group or individual health insurance coverage, provides or covers any benefits with respect to services in an emergency department of a hospital or with respect to emergency services in an independent freestanding emergency department (as defined in paragraph (3)(D)), the plan or issuer shall cover emergency services (as defined in paragraph (3)(C))—

(A) without the need for any prior authorization determination;

(B) whether the health care provider furnishing such services is a participating provider or a participating emergency facility, as applicable, with respect to such services;

(C) in a manner so that, if such services are provided to a participant, beneficiary, or enrollee by a nonparticipating provider or a nonparticipating emergency facility—

(i) such services will be provided without imposing any requirement under the plan or coverage for prior authorization of services or any limitation on coverage that is more restrictive than the requirements or limitations that apply to emergency services received from participating providers and participating emergency facilities with respect to such plan or coverage, respectively;

(ii) the cost-sharing requirement (expressed as a copayment amount or coinsurance rate) is not greater than the requirement that would apply if such services were provided by a participating provider or a participating emergency facility;

(iii) such cost-sharing requirement is calculated as if the total amount that would have been charged for such services by such participating provider or participating emergency facility were equal to the recognized amount (as defined in paragraph (3)(H)) for such services, plan or coverage, and year;

(iv) the group health plan or health insurance issuer, respectively, pays to such provider or facility, respectively the amount by which the recognized amount for such services and year involved exceeds the cost-sharing amount for such services (as determined in accordance with clauses (ii) and (iii)) and year; and

(v) any cost-sharing payments made by the participant, beneficiary, or enrollee with respect to such emergency services so furnished shall be counted toward any in-network deductible or out-of-pocket maximums applied under the plan or coverage, respectively (and such in-network deductible and out-of-pocket maximums shall be applied) in the same manner as if such cost-sharing payments were made with respect to emergency services furnished by a participating provider or a participating emergency facility; and

(D) *without regard to any other term or condition of such coverage (other than exclusion or coordination of benefits, or an affiliation or waiting period, permitted under section 2704 of this Act, including as incorporated pursuant to section 715 of the Employee Retirement Income Security Act of 1974 and section 9815 of the Internal Revenue Code of 1986, and other than applicable cost-sharing).*

(2) AUDIT PROCESS AND REGULATIONS FOR MEDIAN CONTRACTED RATES.—

(A) AUDIT PROCESS.—

(i) IN GENERAL.—Not later than July 1, 2021, the Secretary, in consultation with appropriate State agencies and the Secretary of Labor and the Secretary of the Treasury, shall establish through rulemaking a process, in accordance with clause (ii), under which group health plans and health insurance issuers offering health insurance coverage in the group or individual market are audited by the Secretary or applicable State authority to ensure that—

(I) such plans and coverage are in compliance with the requirement of applying a median contracted rate under this section; and

(II) such median contracted rate so applied satisfies the definition under paragraph (3)(E) with respect to the year involved, including with respect to a group health plan or health insurance issuer described in clause (ii) of such paragraph (3)(E).

(ii) AUDIT SAMPLES.—Under the process established pursuant to clause (i), the Secretary—

(I) shall conduct audits described in such clause, with respect to a year (beginning with 2022), of a sample with respect to such year of claims data from not more than 25 group health plans and health insurance issuers offering health insurance coverage in the group or individual market; and

(II) may audit any group health plan or health insurance issuer offering health insurance coverage in the group or individual market if the Secretary has received any complaint about such plan or coverage, respectively, that involves the compliance of the plan or coverage, respectively, with either of the requirements described in subclauses (I) and (II) of such clause.

(iii) REPORTS.—Beginning for 2022, the Secretary shall annually submit to Congress a report on the number of plans and issuers with respect to which audits were conducted during such year pursuant to this subparagraph.

(B) RULEMAKING.—Not later than July 1, 2021, the Secretary, in consultation with the Secretary of Labor and the Secretary of the Treasury, shall establish through rulemaking—

(i) the methodology the group health plan or health insurance issuer offering health insurance coverage in the group or individual market shall use to determine the median contracted rate, differentiating by line of business;

(ii) the information such plan or issuer, respectively, shall share with the nonparticipating provider or nonparticipating facility, as applicable, when making such a determination;

(iii) the geographic regions applied for purposes of this subparagraph, taking into account access to items and services in rural and underserved areas, including health professional shortage areas, as defined in section 332; and

(iv) a process to receive complaints of violations of the requirements described in subclauses (I) and (II) of subparagraph (A)(i) by group health plans and health insurance issuers offering health insurance coverage in the group or individual market.

Such rulemaking shall take into account payments that are made by such plan or issuer, respectively, that are not on a fee-for-service basis. Such methodology may account for relevant payment adjustments that take into account quality or facility type (including higher acuity settings and the case-mix of various facility types) that are otherwise taken into account for purposes of determining payment amounts with respect to participating facilities. In carrying out clause (iii), the Secretary shall consult with the National Association of Insurance Commissioners to establish the geographic regions under such clause and shall periodically update such regions, as appropriate.

(3) DEFINITIONS.—In this part:

(A) EMERGENCY DEPARTMENT OF A HOSPITAL.—The term "emergency department of a hospital" includes a hospital outpatient department that provides emergency services.

(B) EMERGENCY MEDICAL CONDITION.—The term "emergency medical condition" means a medical condition manifesting itself by acute symptoms of sufficient severity (including severe pain) such that a prudent layperson, who possesses an average knowledge of health and medicine, could reasonably expect the absence of immediate medical attention to result in a condition described in clause (i), (ii), or (iii) of section 1867(e)(1)(A) of the Social Security Act.

(C) EMERGENCY SERVICES.—

(i) IN GENERAL.—The term "emergency services," with respect to an emergency medical condition, means—

(I) a medical screening examination (as required under section 1867 of the Social Security Act, or as would be required under such section if such section applied to an independent freestanding emergency department) that is within the capability of the emergency department of a hospital or of an independent freestanding emergency department, as applicable, including ancillary services routinely available to the emergency department to evaluate such emergency medical condition; and

(II) within the capabilities of the staff and facilities available at the hospital or the independent freestanding emergency department, as applicable, such further medical examination and treatment as are required under section 1867 of such Act, or as would be required under such section if such section applied to an independent freestanding emergency department, to stabilize the patient.

(ii) INCLUSION OF CERTAIN SERVICES OUTSIDE OF EMERGENCY DEPARTMENT.—

(I) IN GENERAL.—For purposes of this subsection and section 2799A–1, in the case of an individual enrolled in a group health plan or health insurance coverage offered by a health insurance issuer in the group or individual market who is furnished services described in clause (i) by a participating or nonparticipating provider or a participating or nonparticipating emergency facility to stabilize such individual with respect to an emergency medical condition, the term "emergency services" shall include, unless each of the conditions described in subclause (II) are met, in addition to the items and services described in clause (i), items and services for which benefits are provided or covered under the plan or coverage, respectively, furnished by a nonparticipating provider or nonparticipating facility, regardless of the department of the hospital in which such individual is furnished such items or services, if, after such stabilization but during such visit in which such individual is so stabilized, the provider or facility determines that such items or services are needed.

(II) CONDITIONS.—For purposes of subclause (I), the conditions described in this subclause, with respect to an individual who is stabilized and furnished additional items and services described in subclause (I) after such stabilization by a provider or facility described in subclause (I), are the following:

(aa) Such a provider or facility determines such individual is able to travel using nonmedical transportation or nonemergency medical transportation.

(bb) Such provider furnishing such additional items and services satisfies the notice and consent criteria of section 2799A–2(d) with respect to such items and services.

(cc) Such an individual is in a condition to receive (as determined in accordance with guidance issued by the Secretary) the information described in section 2799A–2 and to provide informed consent under such section, in accordance with applicable State law.

(D) INDEPENDENT FREESTANDING EMERGENCY DEPARTMENT.—The term "independent freestanding emergency department" means a facility that—

(i) is geographically separate and distinct and licensed separately from a hospital under applicable State law; and

(ii) provides any emergency services (as defined in subparagraph (C)).

(E) MEDIAN CONTRACTED RATE.—

(i) IN GENERAL.—The term "median contracted rate" means, subject to clauses (ii) and (iii), with respect to a sponsor of a group health plan and health insurance issuer offering health insurance coverage in the group or individual market—

(I) *for an item or service furnished during 2022, the median of the contracted rates recognized by the plan or issuer, respectively (determined with respect to all such plans of such sponsor or all such coverage offered by such issuer that are offered within the same line of business as the plan or coverage) as the total maximum payment (including the cost-sharing amount imposed for such item or service and the amount to be paid by the plan or issuer, respectively) under such plans or coverage, respectively, on January 31, 2019, for the same or a similar item or service that is provided by a provider in the same or similar specialty and provided in the geographic region in which the item or service is furnished, consistent with the methodology established by the Secretary under paragraph (2)(B), increased by the percentage increase in the consumer price index for all urban consumers (United States city average) over 2019, such percentage increase over 2020, and such percentage increase over 2021; and*

(II) *for an item or service furnished during 2023 or a subsequent year, the median contracted rate determined under this clause for such an item or service furnished in the previous year, increased by the percentage increase in the consumer price index for all urban consumers (United States city average) over such previous year.*

(ii) *NEW PLANS AND COVERAGE.—The term "median contracted rate" means, with respect to a sponsor of a group health plan or health insurance issuer offering health insurance coverage in the group or individual market in a geographic region in which such sponsor or issuer, respectively, did not offer any group health plan or health insurance coverage during 2019—*

(I) *for the first year in which such group health plan or health insurance coverage, respectively, is offered in such region, a rate (determined in accordance with a methodology established by the Secretary) for items and services that are covered by such plan and furnished during such first year; and*

(II) *for each subsequent year such group health plan or health insurance coverage, respectively, is offered in such region, the median contracted rate determined under this clause for such items and services furnished in the previous year, increased by the percentage increase in the consumer price index for all urban consumers (United States city average) over such previous year.*

(iii) *INSUFFICIENT INFORMATION; NEWLY COVERED ITEMS AND SERVICES.—In the case of a sponsor of a group health plan or health insurance issuer offering health insurance coverage in the group or individual market that does not have sufficient information to calculate the median of the contracted rates described in clause (i)(I) in 2019 (or, in the case of a newly covered item or service (as defined in clause (iv)(III)), in the first coverage year (as defined in clause (iv)(I)) for such item or service with respect to such plan or coverage) for an item or service (including with respect to provider type, or amount, of claims for items or services (as determined by the Secretary) provided in a particular geographic region (other than in a case with respect to which clause (ii) applies)) the term "median contracted rate"—*

(I) for an item or service furnished during 2022 (or, in the case of a newly covered item or service, during the first coverage year for such item or service with respect to such plan or coverage), means such rate for such item or service determined by the sponsor or issuer, respectively, through use of any database that is determined, in accordance with rulemaking described in paragraph (2)(B), to not have any conflicts of interest and to have sufficient information reflecting allowed amounts paid to a health care provider or facility for relevant services furnished in the applicable geographic region (such as a State all-payer claims database);

(II) for an item or service furnished in a subsequent year (before the first sufficient information year (as defined in clause (iv)(II)) for such item or service with respect to such plan or coverage), means the rate determined under subclause (I) or this subclause, as applicable, for such item or service for the year previous to such subsequent year, increased by the percentage increase in the consumer price index for all urban consumers (United States city average) over such previous year;

(III) for an item or service furnished in the first sufficient information year for such item or service with respect to such plan or coverage, has the meaning given the term median contracted rate in clause (i)(I), except that in applying such clause to such item or service, the reference to "furnished during 2022" shall be treated as a reference to furnished during such first sufficient information year, the reference to "in 2019" shall be treated as a reference to such sufficient information year, and the increase described in such clause shall not be applied; and

(IV) for an item or service furnished in any year subsequent to the first sufficient information year for such item or service with respect to such plan or coverage, has the meaning given such term in clause (i)(II), except that in applying such clause to such item or service, the reference to "furnished during 2023 or a subsequent year" shall be treated as a reference to furnished during the year after such first sufficient information year or a subsequent year.

(iv) DEFINITIONS.—For purposes of this subparagraph:

(I) FIRST COVERAGE YEAR.—The term "first coverage year" means, with respect to a group health plan or health insurance coverage offered by a health insurance issuer in the group or individual market and an item or service for which coverage is not offered in 2019 under such plan or coverage, the first year after 2019 for which coverage for such item or service is offered under such plan or health insurance coverage.

(II) FIRST SUFFICIENT INFORMATION YEAR.—The term "first sufficient information year" means, with respect to a group health plan or health insurance coverage offered by a health insurance issuer in the group or individual market—

(aa) in the case of an item or service for which the plan or coverage does not have sufficient information to calculate the median of the contracted rates described in clause (i)(I) in 2019, the first year subsequent to 2022 for which the sponsor or issuer has such sufficient information to calculate the median of such contracted rates in the year previous to such first subsequent year; and

(bb) in the case of a newly covered item or service, the first year subsequent to the first coverage year for such item or service with respect to such plan or coverage for which the sponsor or issuer has sufficient information to calculate the median of the contracted rates described in clause (i)(I) in the year previous to such first subsequent year.

(III) NEWLY COVERED ITEM OR SERVICE.—The term "newly covered item or service" means, with respect to a group health plan or health insurance issuer offering health insurance coverage in the group or individual market, an item or service for which coverage was not offered in 2019 under such plan or coverage, but is offered under such plan or coverage in a year after 2019.

(F) NONPARTICIPATING EMERGENCY FACILITY; PARTICIPATING EMERGENCY FACILITY.—

(i) NONPARTICIPATING EMERGENCY FACILITY.—The term "nonparticipating emergency facility" means, with respect to an item or service and a group health plan or health insurance coverage offered by a health insurance issuer in the group or individual market, an emergency department of a hospital, or an independent freestanding emergency department, that does not have a contractual relationship directly or indirectly with the plan or issuer, respectively, for furnishing such item or service under the plan or coverage, respectively.

(ii) PARTICIPATING EMERGENCY FACILITY.—The term "participating emergency facility" means, with respect to an item or service and a group health plan or health insurance coverage offered by a health insurance issuer in the group or individual market, an emergency department of a hospital, or an independent freestanding emergency department, that has a contractual relationship directly or indirectly with the plan or issuer, respectively, with respect to the furnishing of such an item or service at such facility.

(G) NONPARTICIPATING PROVIDERS; PARTICIPATING PROVIDERS.—

(i) NONPARTICIPATING PROVIDER.—The term "nonparticipating provider" means, with respect to an item or service and a group health plan or health insurance coverage offered by a health insurance issuer in the group or individual market, a physician or other health care provider who is acting within the scope of practice of that provider's license or

certification under applicable State law and who does not have a contractual relationship with the plan or issuer, respectively, for furnishing such item or service under the plan or coverage, respectively.

(ii) PARTICIPATING PROVIDER.—The term "participating provider" means, with respect to an item or service and a group health plan or health insurance coverage offered by a health insurance issuer in the group or individual market, a physician or other health care provider who is acting within the scope of practice of that provider's license or certification under applicable State law and who has a contractual relationship with the plan or issuer, respectively, for furnishing such item or service under the plan or coverage, respectively.

(H) RECOGNIZED AMOUNT.—The term "recognized amount" means, with respect to an item or service furnished by a nonparticipating provider or emergency facility during a year and a group health plan or health insurance coverage offered by a health insurance issuer in the group or individual market—

(i) subject to clause (iii), in the case of such item or service furnished in a State that has in effect a specified State law with respect to such plan, coverage, or issuer, respectively, such a nonparticipating provider or emergency facility, and such an item or service, the amount determined in accordance with such law;

(ii) subject to clause (iii), in the case of such item or service furnished in a State that does not have in effect a specified State law, with respect to such plan, coverage, or issuer, respectively, such a nonparticipating provider or emergency facility, and such an item or service, an amount that is the median contracted rate (as defined in subparagraph (E)) for such year and determined in accordance with rulemaking described in paragraph (2)(B)) for such item or service; or

(iii) in the case of such item or service furnished in a State with an All-Payer Model Agreement under section 1115A of the Social Security Act, the amount that the State approves under such system for such item or service so furnished.

(I) SPECIFIED STATE LAW.—The term "specified State law" means, with respect to a State, an item or service furnished by a nonparticipating provider or emergency facility during a year and a group health plan or health insurance coverage offered by a health insurance issuer in the group or individual market, a State law that provides for a method for determining the amount of payment that is required to be covered by such a plan, coverage, or issuer, respectively (to the extent such State law applies to such plan, coverage, or issuer, subject to section 514 of the Employee Retirement Income Security Act of 1974) in the case of a participant, beneficiary, or enrollee covered under such plan or coverage and receiving such item or service from such a nonparticipating provider or emergency facility.

(J) STABILIZE.—The term "to stabilize," with respect to an emergency medical condition (as defined in subparagraph (B)), has the meaning give in section 1867(e)(3) of the Social Security Act (42 U.S.C. 1395dd(e)(3)).

(c) ACCESS TO PEDIATRIC CARE.—

(1) PEDIATRIC CARE.—In the case of a person who has a child who is a participant, beneficiary, or enrollee under a group health plan, or health insurance coverage offered by a health insurance issuer in the group or individual market, if the plan or issuer requires or provides for the designation of a participating primary care provider for the child, the plan or issuer shall permit such person to designate a physician (allopathic or osteopathic) who specializes in pediatrics as the child's primary care provider if such provider participates in the network of the plan or issuer.

(2) CONSTRUCTION.—Nothing in paragraph (1) shall be construed to waive any exclusions of coverage under the terms and conditions of the plan or health insurance coverage with respect to coverage of pediatric care.

(d) PATIENT ACCESS TO OBSTETRICAL AND GYNECOLOGICAL CARE.—

(1) GENERAL RIGHTS.—

(A) DIRECT ACCESS.—A group health plan, or health insurance issuer offering group or individual health insurance coverage, described in paragraph (2) may not require authorization or referral by the plan, issuer, or any person (including a primary care provider described in paragraph (2)(B)) in the case of a female participant, beneficiary, or enrollee who seeks coverage for obstetrical or gynecological care provided by a participating health care professional who specializes in obstetrics or gynecology. Such professional shall agree to otherwise adhere to such plan's or issuer's policies and procedures, including procedures regarding referrals and obtaining prior authorization and providing services pursuant to a treatment plan (if any) approved by the plan or issuer.

(B) OBSTETRICAL AND GYNECOLOGICAL CARE.—A group health plan or health insurance issuer described in paragraph (2) shall treat the provision of obstetrical and gynecological care, and the ordering of related obstetrical and gynecological items and services, pursuant to the direct access described under subparagraph (A), by a participating health care professional who specializes in obstetrics or gynecology as the authorization of the primary care provider.

(2) APPLICATION OF PARAGRAPH.—A group health plan, or health insurance issuer offering group or individual health insurance coverage, described in this paragraph is a group health plan or coverage that—

(A) provides coverage for obstetric or gynecologic care; and

(B) requires the designation by a participant, beneficiary, or enrollee of a participating primary care provider.

(3) CONSTRUCTION.—Nothing in paragraph (1) shall be construed to—

(A) waive any exclusions of coverage under the terms and conditions of the plan or health insurance coverage with respect to coverage of obstetrical or gynecological care; or

(B) preclude the group health plan or health insurance issuer involved from requiring that the obstetrical or gynecological provider notify the primary care health care professional or the plan or issuer of treatment decisions.

(e) COVERAGE OF NON-EMERGENCY SERVICES PERFORMED BY NON-PARTICIPATING PROVIDERS AT CERTAIN PARTICIPATING FACILITIES.—

(1) IN GENERAL.—In the case of items or services (other than emergency services to which subsection (b) applies) for which any benefits are provided or covered by a group health plan or health insurance issuer offering health insurance coverage in the group or individual market furnished to a participant, beneficiary, or enrollee of such plan or coverage by a nonparticipating provider (as defined in subsection (b)(3)(G)(i)) (and who, with respect to such items and services, has not satisfied the notice and consent criteria of section 2799A–2(d)) with respect to a visit (as defined by the Secretary in accordance with paragraph (2)(B)) at a participating health care facility (as defined in paragraph (2)(A)), with respect to such plan or coverage, respectively, the plan or coverage, respectively—

(A) shall not impose on such participant, beneficiary, or enrollee a cost-sharing amount (expressed as a copayment amount or coinsurance rate) for such items and services so furnished that is greater than the cost-sharing amount that would apply under such plan or coverage, respectively, had such items or services been furnished by a participating provider (as defined in subsection (b)(3)(G)(ii));

(B) shall calculate such cost-sharing amount as if the total amount that would have been charged for such items and services by such participating provider were equal to the recognized amount (as defined in subsection (b)(3)(H)) for such items and services, plan or coverage, and year;

(C) shall pay to such provider furnishing such items and services to such participant, beneficiary, or enrollee the amount by which the recognized amount (as defined in subsection (b)(3)(H)) for such items and services and year involved exceeds the cost-sharing amount imposed under the plan or coverage, respectively, for such items and services (as determined in accordance with subparagraphs (A) and (B)); and

(D) shall count toward any in-network deductible and in-network out-of-pocket maximums (as applicable) applied under the plan or coverage, respectively, any cost-sharing payments made by the participant, beneficiary, or enrollee (and such in-network deductible and out-of-pocket maximums shall be applied) with respect to such items and services so furnished in the same manner as if such cost-sharing payments were with respect to items and services furnished by a participating provider.

(2) DEFINITIONS.—In this section:

(A) PARTICIPATING HEALTH CARE FACILITY.—

(i) IN GENERAL.—The term "participating health care facility" means, with respect to an item or service and a group health plan or health insurance issuer offering health insurance coverage in the group or individual market, a health care facility described in clause (ii) that has a contractual relationship with the plan or issuer, respectively, with respect to the furnishing of such an item or service at the facility.

(ii) HEALTH CARE FACILITY DESCRIBED.—A health care facility described in this clause, with respect to a group health plan or health

insurance coverage offered in the group or individual market, is each of the following:

(I) A hospital (as defined in 1861(e) of the Social Security Act).

(II) A hospital outpatient department.

(III)A critical access hospital (as defined in section 1861(mm) of such Act).

(IV)An ambulatory surgical center (as defined in section 1833(i)(1)(A) of such Act).

(V) Any other facility that provides items or services for which coverage is provided under the plan or coverage, respectively.

(B) VISIT.—The term "visit" shall, with respect to items and services furnished to an individual at a participating health care facility, include equipment and devices, telemedicine services, imaging services, laboratory services, and such other items and services as the Secretary may specify, regardless of whether or not the provider furnishing such items or services is at the facility.

(f) AIR AMBULANCE SERVICES.—

(1) IN GENERAL.—In the case of a participant, beneficiary, or enrollee in a group health plan or health insurance coverage offered in the group or individual market who receives air ambulance services from a nonparticipating provider (as defined in subsection (b)(3)(G)) with respect to such plan or coverage, if such services would be covered if provided by a participating provider (as defined in such section) with respect to such plan or coverage—

(A) the cost-sharing requirement (expressed as a copayment amount, coinsurance rate, or deductible) with respect to such services shall be the same requirement that would apply if such services were provided by such a participating provider, and any coinsurance or deductible shall be based on rates that would apply for such services if they were furnished by such a participating provider;

(B) such cost-sharing amounts shall be counted toward the in-network deductible and in-network out-of-pocket maximum amount under the plan or coverage for the plan year (and such in-network deductible shall be applied) with respect to such items and services so furnished in the same manner as if such cost-sharing payments were with respect to items and services furnished by a participating provider; and

(C) the plan or coverage shall pay to such provider furnishing such services to such participant, beneficiary, or enrollee the amount by which the recognized amount (as defined in and determined pursuant to subsection (b)(3)(H)(ii)) for such services and year involved exceeds the cost-sharing amount imposed under the plan or coverage, respectively, for such services (as determined in accordance with subparagraphs (A) and (B)).

(2) AIR AMBULANCE SERVICE DEFINED.—For purposes of this section, the term "air ambulance service" means medical transport by helicopter or airplane for patients.

(g) CERTAIN ACCESS FEES TO CERTAIN DATABASES.—In the case of a sponsor of a group health plan or health insurance issuer offering health insurance coverage in the group or individual market that, pursuant to subsection (b)(3)(E)(iii), uses a database

described in such subsection to determine a rate to apply under such subsection for an item or service by reason of having insufficient information described in such subsection with respect to such item or service, such sponsor or issuer shall cover the cost for access to such database.

(g) TRANSPARENCY REGARDING IN-NETWORK AND OUT-OF-NETWORK DEDUCTIBLES AND OUT-OF-POCKET LIMITATIONS.—

(1) IN GENERAL.—A group health plan or a health insurance issuer offering group or individual health insurance coverage and providing or covering any benefit with respect to items or services shall include, in clear writing, on any plan or insurance identification card issued to enrollees in the plan or coverage the amount of the in-network and out-of-network deductibles and the in-network and out-of-network out-of-pocket maximum limitation that apply to such plan or coverage.

(2) GUIDANCE.—The Secretary, in consultation with the Secretary of Labor and Secretary of the Treasury, shall issue guidance to implement paragraph (1).

SEC. 2730. PROTECTING PATIENTS AND IMPROVING THE ACCURACY OF PROVIDER DIRECTORY INFORMATION.

(a) NETWORK STATUS OF PROVIDERS.—

(1) IN GENERAL.—Beginning on the date that is one year after the date of enactment of this section, a group health plan or a health insurance issuer offering group or individual health insurance coverage shall—

(A) establish business processes to ensure that all enrollees in such plan or coverage receive proof of a health care provider's network status, based on what a plan or issuer knows or should know—

(i) upon a telephone inquiry by an enrollee—

(I) through a written electronic communication from the plan or issuer to the enrollee, as soon as practicable and not later than 1 business day after such inquiry is made by such participant, beneficiary, or enrollee for such information;

(II) through an oral communication from the plan or issuer to the enrollee, as soon as practicable and not later than 1 business day after such inquiry is made by such enrollee for such information, which communication shall be documented by such plan or issuer, and such documentation shall be kept in the enrollee's file for a minimum of 2 years; and

(ii) in real-time through an online health care provider directory search tool maintained by the plan or issuer; and

(B) include in any print directory—

(i) a disclosure that the information included in the directory is accurate as of the date of the last data update and that enrollees or prospective enrollees should consult the group health plan's or issuer's electronic provider directory on its website or call a specified customer service telephone number to obtain the most current provider directory information; and

(ii) a list of the categories of providers of ancillary services for which the plan or coverage has no in-network providers.

(2) GROUP HEALTH PLAN AND HEALTH INSURANCE ISSUER BUSINESS PROCESSES.—Beginning on the date that is one year after the date of the enactment of this section, a group health plan or a health insurance issuer offering group or individual health insurance coverage shall establish business processes to—

(A) verify and update, at least once every 90 days, the provider directory information for all providers included in the online health care provider directory search tool described in paragraph (1)(A)(ii); and

(B) remove any provider from such online directory search tool if such provider has not verified the directory information within the previous 6 months or the plan or issuer has been unable to verify the provider's network participation.

(b) COST-SHARING LIMITATIONS.—A group health plan or a health insurance issuer offering group or individual health insurance coverage shall not apply, and shall ensure that no provider applies, cost-sharing to an enrollee for treatment or services provided by a health care provider in excess of the normal cost-sharing applied for such treatment or services provided in-network (including any balance bill issued by the health care provider involved), if such enrollee, or health care provider referring such enrollee, demonstrates (based on the electronic, written information described in subsection (a)(1)(A)(i)(I), the oral confirmation described in subsection (a)(1)(A)(i)(II) received by the enrollee not more than 30 days before the date the treatment or services were received, or a copy of the online provider directory described in subsection (a)(1)(A)(ii) on a date not more than 30 days before the date the treatment or services were received), that the enrollee relied on the information described in subsection (a)(1) for which such enrollee provides such documentation, that indicated that the provider is an in-network provider, if the provider was out-of-network at the time the treatment or service involved was received.

(c) DEFINITION.—For purposes of this section, the term "provider directory information" includes the names, addresses, specialty, and telephone numbers of individual health care providers, and the names, addresses, and telephone numbers of each medical group, clinic, or facility contracted to participate in any of the networks of the group health plan or health insurance coverage involved.

(d) RULE OF CONSTRUCTION.—Nothing in this section shall be construed to preempt any provision of State law relating to health care provider directories.

SEC. 2731. PROVISION OF COST-SHARING INFORMATION.

A group health plan or a health insurance issuer offering group or individual health insurance coverage shall provide a participant, beneficiary, or enrollee in the plan or coverage with a good faith estimate of the enrollee's cost-sharing (including deductibles, copayments, and coinsurance) for which the participant, beneficiary, or enrollee may be responsible for paying with respect to a specific health care service (including any service that is reasonably expected to be provided in conjunction with such specific service), as soon as practicable and not later than 2 business days after a request for such information by a participant, beneficiary, or enrollee.

Part B—Individual Market Rules

Subpart I—Portability, Access, and Renewability Requirements

SEC. 2746. DISCLOSURE TO ENROLLEES OF INDIVIDUAL MARKET COVERAGE.

(a) IN GENERAL.—A health insurance issuer offering individual health insurance coverage shall make disclosures to enrollees in such coverage, as described in subsection (b), and reports to the Secretary, as described in subsection (c), regarding direct or indirect compensation provided to an agent or broker associated with enrolling individuals in such coverage.

(b) DISCLOSURE.—A health insurance issuer described in subsection (a) shall disclose to an enrollee the amount of direct or indirect compensation provided to an agent or broker for services provided by such agent or broker associated with plan selection and enrollment. Such disclosure shall be—

(1) made prior to the individual finalizing plan selection; and

(2) included on any documentation confirming the individual's enrollment.

(c) REPORTING.—A health insurance issuer described in subsection (a) shall annually report to the Secretary, prior to the beginning of open enrollment, any direct or indirect compensation provided to an agent or broker associated with enrolling individuals in such coverage.

(d) RULEMAKING.—Not later than 1 year after the date of enactment of the Ban Surprise Billing Act, the Secretary shall finalize, through notice-and-comment rulemaking, the form and manner in which issuers described in subsection (a) are required to make the disclosures described in subsection (b) and the reports described in subsection (c). Such rulemaking may also include adjustments to notice requirements to reflect the different processes for plan renewals, in order to provide enrollees with full, timely information.

Part D—Health Care Provider Requirements

SEC. 2799A–1. BALANCE BILLING IN CASES OF EMERGENCY SERVICES.

(a) IN GENERAL.—In the case of a participant, beneficiary, or enrollee with benefits under a group health plan or health insurance coverage offered by a health insurance issuer in the group or individual market who is furnished during a plan year beginning on or after January 1, 2022, emergency services for which any benefit is provided under such plan or coverage with respect to an emergency medical condition with respect to a visit at an emergency department of a hospital or an independent freestanding emergency department—

(1) in the case that the hospital or independent freestanding emergency department is a nonparticipating emergency facility, the emergency department of a hospital or independent free-standing emergency department shall not hold the participant,

beneficiary, or enrollee liable for a payment amount for such emergency services so furnished that is more than the cost-sharing amount for such services (as determined in accordance with clauses (ii) and (iii) of section 2719A(b)(1)(C), section 716(b)(1)(C) of the Employee Retirement Income Security Act of 1974, and section 9816(b)(1)(C) of the Internal Revenue Code of 1986, as applicable); and

(2) in the case that such services are furnished by a nonparticipating provider, the health care provider shall not hold such participant, beneficiary, or enrollee liable for a payment amount for an emergency service furnished to such individual by such provider with respect to such emergency medical condition and visit for which the individual receives emergency services at the hospital or emergency department that is more than the cost-sharing amount for such services furnished by the provider (as determined in accordance with clauses (ii) and (iii) of section 2719A(b)(1)(C), section 716(b)(1)(C) of the Employee Retirement Income Security Act of 1974, and section 9816(b)(1)(C) of the Internal Revenue Code of 1986, as applicable).

(b) DEFINITION.—In this section, the term "visit" shall have such meaning as applied to such term for purposes of section 2719A(e).

SEC. 2799A–2. BALANCE BILLING IN CASES OF NON-EMERGENCY SERVICES PERFORMED BY NONPARTICIPATING PROVIDERS AT CERTAIN PARTICIPATING FACILITIES.

(a) IN GENERAL.—Subject to subsection (b), in the case of a participant, beneficiary, or enrollee with benefits under a group health plan or health insurance coverage offered by a health insurance issuer in the group or individual market who is furnished during a plan year beginning on or after January 1, 2022, items or services (other than emergency services to which section 2799A–1 applies) for which any benefit is provided under such plan or coverage at a participating health care facility by a nonparticipating provider, such provider shall not bill, and shall not hold liable, such participant, beneficiary, or enrollee for a payment amount for such an item or service furnished by such provider with respect to a visit at such facility that is more than the cost-sharing amount for such item or service (as determined in accordance with subparagraphs (A) and (B) of section 2719A(e)(1), section 716(e)(1) of the Employee Retirement Income Security Act of 1974, and section 9816(e)(1) of the Internal Revenue Code of 1986, as applicable).

(b) EXCEPTION.—

(1) IN GENERAL.—Subsection (a) shall not apply with respect to items or services (other than ancillary services described in paragraph (2)) furnished by a nonparticipating provider to a participant, beneficiary, or enrollee of a group health plan or health insurance coverage offered by a health insurance issuer in the group or individual market, if the provider satisfies the notice and consent criteria of subsection (d).

(2) ANCILLARY SERVICES DESCRIBED.—For purposes of paragraph (1), ancillary services described in this paragraph are, with respect to a participating health care facility—

(A) subject to paragraph (3), items and services related to emergency medicine, anesthesiology, pathology, radiology, and neonatology, whether or not provided by a physician or non-physician practitioner, and items and services provided by assistant surgeons, hospitalists, and intensivists;

(B) subject to paragraph (3), diagnostic services (including radiology and laboratory services);

(C) items and services provided by such other specialty practitioners, as the Secretary specifies through rulemaking; and

(D) items and services provided by a nonparticipating provider if there is no participating provider who can furnish such item or service at such facility.

(3) EXCEPTION.—The Secretary may, through rulemaking, establish a list (and update such list) of advanced diagnostic laboratory tests, which shall not be included as an ancillary service described in paragraph (2) and with respect to which subsection (a) would apply.

(c) CLARIFICATION.—In the case of a nonparticipating provider that satisfies the notice and consent criteria of subsection (d) with respect to an item or service (referred to in this subsection as a "covered item or service"), such notice and consent criteria may not be construed as applying with respect to any item or service that is furnished as a result of unforeseen, urgent medical needs that arise at the time such covered item or service is furnished. For purposes of the previous sentence, a covered item or service shall not include an ancillary service described in subsection (b)(2).

(d) NOTICE AND CONSENT TO BE TREATED BY A NONPARTICIPATING PROVIDER OR NONPARTICIPATING FACILITY.—

(1) IN GENERAL.—A nonparticipating provider or nonparticipating facility satisfies the notice and consent criteria of this subsection, with respect to items or services furnished by the provider or facility to a participant, beneficiary, or enrollee of a group health plan or health insurance coverage offered by a health insurance issuer in the group or individual market, if the provider (or, if applicable, the participating health care facility on behalf of such provider) or nonparticipating facility—

(A) provides to the participant, beneficiary, or enrollee (or to an authorized representative of the participant, beneficiary, or enrollee) on the date on which the individual is furnished such items or services and, in the case that the participant, beneficiary, or enrollee makes an appointment to be furnished such items or services, on such date the appointment is made—

(i) an oral explanation of the written notice described in clause (ii); and

(ii) a written notice in paper or electronic form (and including electronic notification, as practicable) specified by the Secretary, not later than July 1, 2021, through guidance (which shall be updated as determined necessary by the Secretary) that—

(I) contains the information required under paragraph (2);

(II) clearly states that consent to receive such items and services from such nonparticipating provider or nonparticipating facility is optional and that the participant, beneficiary, or enrollee may instead seek care from a participating provider or at a participating facility, with respect to such plan or coverage, as applicable, in which

case the cost-sharing responsibility of the participant, beneficiary, or enrollee would not exceed such responsibility that would apply with respect to such an item or service that is furnished by a participating provider or participating facility, as applicable with respect to such plan;

(III) is available in the 15 most common languages in the geographic region of the applicable facility and, in the case the primary language of the beneficiary, participant, or enrollee, respectively, is not one of such 15 language, makes a good faith effort to also provide such notice orally in such primary language of the beneficiary, participant, or enrollee; and

(IV) is signed and dated by the participant, beneficiary, or enrollee (or by an authorized representative of the participant, beneficiary, or enrollee) and, with respect to items or services to be furnished by such a provider that are not poststabilization services described in section 2719A(b)(3)(C)(ii), is so signed and dated not less than 72 hours prior to the participant, beneficiary, or enrollee being furnished such items or services by such provider; and

(B) obtains from the participant, beneficiary, or enrollee (or from such an authorized representative) the consent described in paragraph (3) to be treated by a nonparticipating provider or nonparticipating facility.

(2) INFORMATION REQUIRED UNDER WRITTEN NOTICE.—For purposes of paragraph (1)(A)(ii)(I), the information described in this paragraph, with respect to a nonparticipating provider or nonparticipating facility and a participant, beneficiary, or enrollee of a group health plan or health insurance coverage offered by a health insurance issuer in the group or individual market, is each of the following:

(A) Notification, as applicable, that the health care provider is a nonparticipating provider with respect to the health plan or the health care facility is a nonparticipating facility with respect to the health plan.

(B) Notification of the good faith estimated amount that such provider or facility may charge the participant, beneficiary, or enrollee for such items and services involved, including a notification that the provision of such estimate or consent to be treated under paragraph (3) does not constitute a contract with respect to the charges estimated for such items and services.

(C) In the case of a participating facility and a nonparticipating provider, a list of any participating providers at the facility who are able to furnish such items and services involved and notification that the participant, beneficiary, or enrollee may be referred, at their option, to such a participating provider.

(D) Information about whether prior authorization or other care management limitations may be required in advance of receiving such items or services at the facility.

(3) CONSENT DESCRIBED TO BE TREATED BY A NONPARTICIPATING PROVIDER OR NONPARTICIPATING FACILITY.—For purposes of paragraph (1)(B), the consent described in this paragraph, with respect to a participant, beneficiary, or enrollee of a group health plan or health insurance coverage

offered by a health insurance issuer in the group or individual market who is to be furnished items or services by a nonparticipating provider or nonparticipating facility, is a document specified by the Secretary through rulemaking, in consultation with the Secretary of Labor, that—

(A) acknowledges that the participant, beneficiary, or enrollee has been—

(i) provided with a written good faith estimate and an oral explanation of the charge that may be applied for the items or services anticipated to be furnished by such provider or facility; and

(ii) informed that the payment of such charge by the participant, beneficiary, or enrollee may not accrue toward meeting any limitation that the plan or coverage places on cost-sharing, including an explanation that such payment may not apply to an in-network deductible applied under the plan or coverage; and

(B) documents the consent of the participant, beneficiary, or enrollee to be furnished such item or services by such provider or facility.

(4) RULE OF CONSTRUCTION.—The consent described in paragraph (3), with respect to a participant, beneficiary, or enrollee of a group health plan or health insurance coverage offered by a health insurance issuer in the group or individual market, shall constitute only consent to the receipt of the information provided pursuant to this subsection and shall not constitute a contractual agreement of the participant, beneficiary, or enrollee to any estimated charge or amount included in such information.

(e) RETENTION OF CERTAIN DOCUMENTS.—A nonparticipating facility (with respect to such facility or any nonparticipating provider at such facility) or a participating facility (with respect to nonparticipating providers at such facility) that obtains from a participant, beneficiary, or enrollee of a group health plan or health insurance coverage offered by a health insurance issuer in the group or individual market (or an authorized representative of such participant, beneficiary, or enrollee) a written notice in accordance with subsection (d)(1)(A)(ii), with respect to furnishing an item or service to such participant, beneficiary, or enrollee, shall retain such notice for at least a 2-year period after the date on which such item or service is so furnished.

(f) DEFINITIONS.—In this section:

(1) The terms "nonparticipating provider" and "participating provider" have the meanings given such terms, respectively, in subsection (b)(3) of section 2719A.

(2) The term "participating health care facility" has the meaning given such term in subsection (e)(2) of section 2719A.

(3) The term "nonparticipating facility" means—

(A) with respect to emergency services (as defined in section 2719A(b)(3)(C)(i)) and a group health plan or health insurance coverage offered by a health insurance issuer in the group or individual market, an emergency department of a hospital, or an independent freestanding emergency department, that does not have a contractual relationship with the plan or issuer, respectively, with respect to the furnishing of such services under the plan or coverage, respectively; and

(B) with respect to services described in section 2719A(b)(3)(C)(ii) and a group health plan or health insurance coverage offered by a health insurance issuer

in the group or individual market, a hospital or an independent freestanding emergency department, that does not have a contractual relationship with the plan or issuer, respectively, with respect to the furnishing of such services under the plan or coverage, respectively.

(4) The term "participating facility" means—

(A) with respect to emergency services (as defined in clause (i) of section 2719A(b)(3)(C)) that are not described in clause (ii) of such section and a group health plan or health insurance coverage offered by a health insurance issuer in the group or individual market, an emergency department of a hospital, or an independent freestanding emergency department, that has a contractual relationship with the plan or issuer, respectively, with respect to the furnishing of such services under the plan or coverage, respectively; and

(B) with respect to services that pursuant to clause (ii) of section 2719A(b)(3)(C) are included as emergency services (as defined in clause (i) of such section) and a group health plan or health insurance coverage offered by a health insurance issuer in the group or individual market, a hospital or an independent freestanding emergency department, that has a contractual relationship with the plan or coverage, respectively, with respect to the furnishing of such services under the plan or coverage, respectively.

SEC. 2799A–3. PROVIDER REQUIREMENT WITH RESPECT TO PUBLIC PROVISION OF INFORMATION.

(a) IN GENERAL.—Each health care provider and health care facility shall make publicly available, and (if applicable) post on a public website of such provider or facility and provide to individuals who are participants, beneficiaries, or enrollees of a group health plan or health insurance coverage offered by a health insurance issuer in the group or individual market a one-page notice in plain language containing information on—

(1) the requirements and prohibitions of such provider or facility under sections 2799A–1, 2799A–2, and 2799A–4 (relating to prohibitions on balance billing in certain circumstances);

(2) if provided for under applicable State law, any other requirements on such provider or facility regarding the amounts such provider or facility may, with respect to an item or service, charge a participant, beneficiary, or enrollee of a group health plan or health insurance coverage offered by a health insurance issuer in the group or individual market with respect to which such provider or facility does not have a contractual relationship for furnishing such item or service under the plan or coverage, respectively, after receiving payment from the plan or coverage, respectively, for such item or service and any applicable cost-sharing payment from such participant, beneficiary, or enrollee; and

(3) information on contacting appropriate State and Federal agencies in the case that an individual believes that such provider or facility has violated any requirement described in paragraph (1) or (2) with respect to such individual.

(b) GUIDANCE.—Not later than 6 months after the date of the enactment of this section, the Secretary, in consultation with the Secretary of Labor, shall issue guidance on the requirements for the notice under this section.

SEC. 2799A–4. AIR AMBULANCE SERVICES.

In the case of a participant, beneficiary, or enrollee with benefits under a group health plan or health insurance coverage offered by a health insurance issuer in the group or individual market who is furnished on or after January 1, 2022, air ambulance services from a nonparticipating provider (as defined in section 2719A(b)(3)(G)) with respect to such plan or coverage, such provider shall not bill, and shall not hold liable, such participant, beneficiary, or enrollee for a payment amount for such service furnished by such provider that is more than the cost-sharing amount for such service (as determined in accordance with paragraphs (1) and (2) of section 2719A(f), section 716(f) of the Employee Retirement Income Security Act of 1974, or section 9816(f) of the Internal Revenue Code of 1986, as applicable).

SEC. 2799A–5. PROVIDER REQUIREMENTS TO PROTECT PATIENTS AND IMPROVE THE ACCURACY OF PROVIDER DIRECTORY INFORMATION.

(a) PROVIDER BUSINESS PROCESSES.—A health care provider shall have in place business processes to ensure the timely provision of provider directory information to a group health plan or a health insurance issuer offering group or individual health insurance coverage to support compliance by such plans or issuers with section 2730(a)(1), section 717(a)(1) of the Employee Retirement Income Security Act of 1974, or section 9817(a)(1) of the Internal Revenue Code of 1986 (as applicable). Such providers shall submit provider directory information to a plan or issuers, at a minimum—

(1) when the provider begins a network agreement with a plan or with an issuer with respect to certain coverage;

(2) when the provider terminates a network agreement with a plan or with an issuer with respect to certain coverage;

(3) when there are material changes to the content of provider directory information described in section 2730(a)(1), section 717(a)(1) of the Employee Retirement Income Security Act of 1974, or section 9817(a)(1) of the Internal Revenue Code of 1986 (as applicable); and

(4) every 90 days throughout the duration of the network agreement with a plan or issuer.

(b) ENFORCEMENT.—

(1) CIVIL PENALTIES.—

(A) IN GENERAL.—Subject to paragraph (2), a health care provider that violates a requirement under subsection (a) or takes actions that prevent a group health plan or health insurance issuer from complying with subsection (a)(1) or (b) of sections 2730, 717 of the Employee Retirement Income Security Act of 1974, or 9817 of the Internal Revenue Code of 1986 (as applicable) shall be subject to a civil monetary penalty of not more than $10,000 for each act constituting such violation.

(B) *SAFE HARBOR.—The Secretary may waive the penalty described under paragraph (1) with respect to a health care provider that unknowingly violates section 2730(b)(1), section 717(b)(1) of the Employee Retirement Income Security Act of 1974, or section 9817(b)(1) of the Internal Revenue Code of 1986 (as applicable) with respect to an enrollee if such provider rescinds the bill involved and, if applicable, reimburses the enrollee within 30 days of the date on which the provider billed the enrollee in violation of such subsection.*

(C) *PROCEDURE.—The provisions of section 1128A of the Social Security Act, other than subsections (a) and (b) and the first sentence of subsection (c)(1) of such section, shall apply to civil money penalties under this subsection in the same manner as such provisions apply to a penalty or proceeding under section 1128A of the Social Security Act.*

(2) *REFUNDS TO ENROLLEES.—If a health care provider submits a bill to an enrollee based on cost-sharing for treatment or services provided by the health care provider that is in excess of the normal cost-sharing applied for such treatment or services provided in-network, as prohibited under section 2730(b), section 717(b) of the Employee Retirement Income Security Act of 1974, or section 9817(b) of the Internal Revenue Code of 1986 (as applicable) and the enrollee pays such bill, the provider shall reimburse the enrollee for the full amount paid by the enrollee in excess of the in-network cost-sharing amount for the treatment or services involved, plus interest, at an interest rate determined by the Secretary.*

(c) *LIMITATION.—Nothing in this section shall prohibit a provider from requiring in the terms of a contract, or contract termination, with a group health plan or health insurance issuer—*

(1) *that the plan or issuer remove, at the time of termination of such contract, the provider from a directory of the plan or issuer described in section 2730(a)(1), section 717(a)(1) of the Employee Retirement Income Security Act of 1974, or section 9817(a)(1) of the Internal Revenue Code of 1986 (as applicable); or*

(2) *that the plan or issuer bear financial responsibility, including under section 2730(b), section 717(b) of the Employee Retirement Income Security Act of 1974, or section 9817(b) of the Internal Revenue Code of 1986 (as applicable) for providing inaccurate network status information to an enrollee.*

(d) *DEFINITION.—For purposes of this section, the term "provider directory information" includes the names, addresses, specialty, and telephone numbers of individual health care providers, and the names, addresses, and telephone numbers of each medical group, clinic, or facility contracted to participate in any of the networks of the group health plan or health insurance coverage involved.*

(e) *RULE OF CONSTRUCTION.—Nothing in this section shall be construed to preempt any provision of State law relating to health care provider directories.*

SEC. 2799A–6. PROVISION OF COST-SHARING INFORMATION.

A provider that is in-network with respect to a group health plan or a health insurance issuer offering group or individual health insurance coverage shall, upon request by a participant, beneficiary, or enrollee, provide to a participant, beneficiary, or enrollee in the plan or coverage the following information, together with accurate and complete information about the participant's, beneficiary's, or enrollee's coverage under the applicable plan or coverage:

(1) As soon as practicable and not later than 2 business days after the participant, beneficiary, or enrollee requests such information, a good faith estimate of the expected participant, beneficiary, or enrollee cost-sharing for the provision of a particular health care service (including any service that is reasonably expected to be provided in conjunction with such specific service).

(2) As soon as practicable and not later than 2 business days after a participant, beneficiary, or enrollee requests such information, the contact information for any ancillary providers for a scheduled health care service.

SEC. 2799A–7. ENFORCEMENT.

(a) STATE ENFORCEMENT.—

(1) STATE AUTHORITY.—Each State may require a provider or health care facility (including a provider of air ambulance services) subject to the requirements of this part (except section 2799A–5) to satisfy such requirements applicable to the provider or facility.

(2) FAILURE TO IMPLEMENT REQUIREMENTS.—In the case of a determination by the Secretary that a State has failed to substantially enforce the requirements specified in paragraph (1) with respect to applicable providers and facilities in the State, the Secretary shall enforce such requirements under subsection (b) insofar as they relate to violations of such requirements occurring in such State.

(3) NOTIFICATION OF SECRETARY OF LABOR.—A State may notify the Secretary of Labor of instances of violations of sections 2799A–1, 2799A–2, or 2799A–4 with respect to participants or beneficiaries under a group health plan or health insurance coverage offered by a health insurance issuer in the group market and any enforcement actions taken against providers or facilities as a result of such violations, including the disposition of any such enforcement actions.

(b) SECRETARIAL ENFORCEMENT AUTHORITY.—

(1) IN GENERAL.—If a provider or facility is found to be in violation of a requirement specified in subsection (a)(1) by the Secretary, the Secretary may apply a civil monetary penalty with respect to such provider or facility (including, as applicable, a provider of air ambulance services) in an amount not to exceed $10,000 per violation. The provisions of subsections (c) (with the exception of the first sentence of paragraph (1) of such subsection), (d), (e), (g), (h), (k), and (l) of section 1128A of the Social Security Act shall apply to a civil monetary penalty or assessment under this subsection in the same manner as such provisions apply to a penalty, assessment, or proceeding under subsection (a) of such section.

(2) LIMITATION.—The provisions of paragraph (1) shall apply to enforcement of a provision (or provisions) specified in subsection (a)(1) only as provided under subsection (a)(2).

(3) COMPLAINT PROCESS.—The Secretary shall, through rulemaking conducted in consultation with the Secretary of Labor, establish a process to receive consumer complaints of violations of such provisions and resolve such complaints within 60

days of receipt of such complaints. Such process shall provide that the Secretary of Labor be informed of complaints by participants or beneficiaries under a group health plan or health insurance coverage offered by a health insurance issuer in the group market and any enforcement actions against providers resulting from such complaints, including the disposition of any such enforcement actions.

(4) *EXCEPTION.—The Secretary may waive the penalties described under paragraph (1) with respect to a facility or provider (including a provider of air ambulance services) who does not knowingly violate, and should not have reasonably known it violated, sections 2799A–1, 2799A–2, or 2799A–4 with respect to a participant, beneficiary, or enrollee, if such facility or provider, within 30 days of the violation, withdraws the bill that was in violation of such provision and reimburses the health plan or participant, beneficiary, or enrollee, as applicable, in an amount equal to the difference between the amount billed and the amount allowed to be billed under the provision, plus interest, at an interest rate determined by the Secretary.*

(5) *HARDSHIP EXEMPTION.—The Secretary may establish a hardship exemption to the penalties under this subsection.*

(c) *CONTINUED APPLICABILITY OF STATE LAW.—The sections specified in subsection (a)(1) shall not be construed to supersede any provision of State law which establishes, implements, or continues in effect any requirement or prohibition except to the extent that such requirement or prohibition prevents the application of a requirement or prohibition of such a section.*

Employee Retirement Income Security Act of 1974

Short Title and Table of Contents

SECTION 1. This Act may be cited as the "Employee Retirement Income Security Act of 1974."

Title I—Protection of Employee Benefit Rights

Subtitle B—Regulatory Provisions

Part 4—Fiduciary Responsibility

Exemptions from Prohibited Transactions
SEC. 408.

(a) The Secretary shall establish an exemption procedure for purposes of this subsection. Pursuant to such procedure, he may grant a conditional or unconditional exemption of any fiduciary or transaction, or class of fiduciaries or transactions, from all or part of the restrictions imposed by sections 406 and 407(a). Action under this subsection may be taken only after consultation and coordination with the Secretary of the Treasury. An exemption granted under this section shall not relieve a fiduciary from any other applicable provision of this Act. The Secretary may not grant an exemption under this subsection unless he finds that such exemption is—
(1) administratively feasible,
(2) in the interests of the plan and of its participants and beneficiaries, and
(3) protective of the rights of participants and beneficiaries of such plan.

Before granting an exemption under this subsection from section 406(a) or 407(a), the Secretary shall publish notice in the Federal Register of the pendency of the exemption, shall require that adequate notice be given to interested persons, and shall afford interested persons opportunity to present views. The Secretary may not grant an exemption under this subsection from section 406(b) unless he affords an opportunity for a hearing and makes a determination on the record with respect to the findings required by paragraphs (1), (2), and (3) of this subsection.

(b) The prohibitions provided in section 406 shall not apply to any of the following transactions:
(1) Any loans made by the plan to parties in interest who are participants or beneficiaries of the plan if such loans (A) are available to all such participants and beneficiaries on a reasonably equivalent basis, (B) are not made available to highly compensated employees (within the meaning of section 414(q) of the Internal Revenue Code of 1986) in an amount greater than the amount made available to other employees, (C) are made in accordance with specific provisions regarding such loans set forth in the plan, (D) bear a reasonable rate of interest, and (E) are adequately secured. A loan made by a plan shall not fail to meet the requirements of the preceding sentence by reason of a loan repayment suspension described under section 414(u)(4) of the Internal Revenue Code of 1986. [(2) Contracting or making
[(2) (A) Contracting or making] reasonable arrangements with a party in interest for office space, or legal, accounting, or other services necessary for the establishment or operation of the plan, if no more than reasonable compensation is paid therefor.

(B)(i) No contract or arrangement for services between a covered plan and a covered service provider, and no extension or renewal of such a contract or arrangement, is reasonable within the meaning of this paragraph unless the requirements of this subparagraph are met.

(ii)(I) For purposes of this subparagraph:

(aa) The term "covered plan" means a group health plan as defined section 733(a).

(bb) The term "covered service provider" means a service provider that enters into a contract or arrangement with the covered plan and reasonably expects $1,000 (or such amount as the Secretary may establish in regulations to account for inflation since the date of the enactment of the Ban Surprise Billing Act, as appropriate) or more in compensation, direct or indirect, to be received in connection with providing one or more of the following services, pursuant to the contract or arrangement, regardless of whether such services will be performed, or such compensation received, by the covered service provider, an affiliate, or a subcontractor:

(AA) Brokerage services, for which the covered service provider, an affiliate, or a subcontractor reasonably expects to receive indirect compensation or direct compensation described in item (dd), provided to a covered plan with respect to selection of insurance products (including vision and dental), recordkeeping services, medical management vendor, benefits administration (including vision and dental), stop-loss insurance, pharmacy benefit management services, wellness services, transparency tools and vendors, group purchasing organization preferred vendor panels, disease management vendors and products, compliance services, employee assistance programs, or third party administration services.

(BB) Consulting, for which the covered service provider, an affiliate, or a subcontractor reasonably expects to receive indirect compensation or direct compensation described in item (dd), related to the development or implementation of plan design, insurance or insurance product selection (including vision and dental), recordkeeping, medical management, benefits administration selection (including vision and dental), stop-loss insurance, pharmacy benefit management services, wellness design and management services, transparency tools, group purchasing organization agreements and services, participation in and services from preferred vendor panels, disease management, compliance services, employee assistance programs, or third party administration services.

(cc) The term "affiliate," with respect to a covered service provider, means an entity that directly or indirectly (through one or more intermediaries) controls, is controlled by, or is under common control with, such provider, or is an officer, director, or employee of, or partner in, such provider.

(dd)(AA) The term "compensation" means anything of monetary value, but does not include non-monetary compensation valued at $250 (or such amount as the Secretary may establish in regulations to account for inflation since the date of enactment of the Ban Surprise Billing Act, as appropriate) or less, in the aggregate, during the term of the contract or arrangement.

(BB) The term "direct compensation" means compensation received directly from a covered plan.

(CC) The term "indirect compensation" means compensation received from any source other than the covered plan, the plan sponsor, the covered service provider, or an affiliate. Compensation received from a subcontractor is indirect compensation, unless it is received in connection with services performed under a contract or arrangement with a subcontractor.

(ee) The term "responsible plan fiduciary" means a fiduciary with authority to cause the covered plan to enter into, or extend or renew, the contract or arrangement.

(ff) The term "subcontractor" means any person or entity (or an affiliate of such person or entity) that is not an affiliate of the covered service provider and that, pursuant to a contract or arrangement with the covered service provider or an affiliate, reasonably expects to receive $1,000 (or such amount as the Secretary may establish in regulations to account for inflation since the date of enactment of the Ban Surprise Billing Act, as appropriate) or more in compensation for performing one or more services described in item (bb) under a contract or arrangement with the covered plan.

(II) For purposes of this subparagraph, a description of compensation or cost may be expressed as a monetary amount, formula, or a per capita charge for each enrollee or, if the compensation or cost cannot reasonably be expressed in such terms, by any other reasonable method, including a disclosure that additional compensation may be earned but may not be calculated at the time of contract if such a disclosure includes a description of the circumstances under which the additional compensation may be earned and a reasonable and good faith estimate if the covered service provider cannot otherwise readily describe compensation or cost and explains the methodology and assumptions used to prepare such estimate. Any such description shall contain sufficient information to permit evaluation of the reasonableness of the compensation or cost.

(III) No person or entity is a "covered service provider" within the meaning of subclause (I)(bb) solely on the basis of providing services as an affiliate or a subcontractor that is performing one or more of the services described in subitem (AA) or (BB) of such subclause under the contract or arrangement with the covered plan.

(i) A covered service provider shall disclose to a responsible plan fiduciary, in writing, the following:

(I) A description of the services to be provided to the covered plan pursuant to the contract or arrangement.

(II) If applicable, a statement that the covered service provider, an affiliate, or a subcontractor will provide, or reasonably expects to provide, services pursuant to the contract or arrangement directly to the covered plan as a fiduciary (within the meaning of section 3(21)).

(III) A description of all direct compensation, either in the aggregate or by service, that the covered service provider, an affiliate, or a subcontractor reasonably expects to receive in connection with the services described in subclause (I).

(IV)(aa) A description of all indirect compensation that the covered service provider, an affiliate, or a subcontractor reasonably expects to receive in connection with the services described in subclause (I)—

(AA) including compensation from a vendor to a brokerage firm based on a structure of incentives not solely related to the contract with the covered plan; and

(BB) not including compensation received by an employee from an employer on account of work performed by the employee.

(bb) A description of the arrangement between the payer and the covered service provider, an affiliate, or a subcontractor, as applicable, pursuant to which such indirect compensation is paid.

(cc) Identification of the services for which the indirect compensation will be received, if applicable.

(dd) Identification of the payer of the indirect compensation.

(V) A description of any compensation that will be paid among the covered service provider, an affiliate, or a subcontractor, in connection with the services described in subclause (I) if such compensation is set on a transaction basis (such as commissions, finder's fees, or other similar incentive compensation based on business placed or retained), including identification of the services for which such compensation will be paid and identification of the payers and recipients of such compensation (including the status of a payer or recipient as an affiliate or a subcontractor), regardless of whether such compensation also is disclosed pursuant to subclause (III) or (IV).

(VI) A description of any compensation that the covered service provider, an affiliate, or a subcontractor reasonably expects to receive in connection with termination of the contract or arrangement, and how any prepaid amounts will be calculated and refunded upon such termination.

(ii) A covered service provider shall disclose to a responsible plan fiduciary, in writing a description of the manner in which the compensation described in clause (iii), as applicable, will be received.

(v)(I) A covered service provider shall disclose the information required under clauses (iii) and (iv) to the responsible plan fiduciary not later than the date that is reasonably in advance of the date on which the contract or arrangement is entered into, and extended or renewed.

(II) A covered service provider shall disclose any change to the information required under clause (iii) and (iv) as soon as practicable, but not later than 60 days from the date on which the covered service provider is informed of such change, unless such disclosure is precluded due to extraordinary circumstances beyond the covered service provider's control, in which case the information shall be disclosed as soon as practicable.

(vi)(I) Upon the written request of the responsible plan fiduciary or covered plan administrator, a covered service provider shall furnish any other information relating to the compensation received in connection with the contract or arrangement that is required for the covered plan to comply with the reporting and disclosure requirements under this Act.

(II) The covered service provider shall disclose the information required under clause (iii)(I) reasonably in advance of the date upon which such responsible plan fiduciary or covered plan administrator states that it is required to comply with the applicable reporting or disclosure requirement, unless such disclosure is precluded due to extraordinary circumstances beyond the covered service provider's control, in which case the information shall be disclosed as soon as practicable.

(vii)No contract or arrangement will fail to be reasonable under this subparagraph solely because the covered service provider, acting in good faith and with reasonable diligence, makes an error or omission in disclosing the information required pursuant to clause (iii) (or a change to such information disclosed pursuant to clause (v)(II)) or clause (vi), provided that the covered service provider discloses the correct information to the responsible plan fiduciary as soon as practicable, but not later than 30 days from the date on which the covered service provider knows of such error or omission.

(viii)(I) Pursuant to subsection (a), subparagraphs (C) and (D) of section 406(a)(1) shall not apply to a responsible plan fiduciary, notwithstanding any failure by a covered service provider to disclose information required under clause (iii), if the following conditions are met:

(aa)The responsible plan fiduciary did not know that the covered service provider failed or would fail to make required disclosures and reasonably believed that the covered service provider disclosed the information required to be disclosed.

(bb)The responsible plan fiduciary, upon discovering that the covered service provider failed to disclose the required

information, requests in writing that the covered service provider furnish such information.

(cc) If the covered service provider fails to comply with a written request described in subclause (II) within 90 days of the request, the responsible plan fiduciary notifies the Secretary of the covered service provider's failure, in accordance with subclauses (II) and (III).

(II) A notice described in subclause (I)(cc) shall contain—

(aa) the name of the covered plan;

(bb) the plan number used for the annual report on the covered plan;

(cc) the plan sponsor's name, address, and employer identification number;

(dd) the name, address, and telephone number of the responsible plan fiduciary;

(ee) the name, address, phone number, and, if known, employer identification number of the covered service provider;

(ff) a description of the services provided to the covered plan;

(gg) a description of the information that the covered service provider failed to disclose;

(hh) the date on which such information was requested in writing from the covered service provider; and

(ii) a statement as to whether the covered service provider continues to provide services to the plan.

(III) A notice described in subclause (I)(cc) shall be filed with the Department not later than 30 days following the earlier of— (aa) The covered service provider's refusal to furnish the information requested by the written request described in subclause (I)(bb); or

(bb) 90 days after the written request referred to in subclause (I)(cc) is made.

(IV) If the covered service provider fails to comply with the written request under subclause (I)(bb) within 90 days of such request, the responsible plan fiduciary shall determine whether to terminate or continue the contract or arrangement under section 404. If the requested information relates to future services and is not disclosed promptly after the end of the 90-day period, the responsible plan fiduciary shall terminate the contract or arrangement as expeditiously as possible, consistent with such duty of prudence.

(ix) Nothing in this subparagraph shall be construed to supersede any provision of State law that governs disclosures by parties that provide the services described in this section, except to the extent that such law prevents the application of a requirement of this section.

(3) A loan to an employee stock ownership plan (as defined in section 407(d)(6)), if—

(A) such loan is primarily for the benefit of participants and beneficiaries of the plan, and

(B) such loan is at an interest rate which is not in excess of a reasonable rate.

If the plan gives collateral to a party in interest for such loan, such collateral may consist only of qualifying employer securities (as defined in section 407(d)(5)).

(4) The investment of all or part of a plan's assets in deposits which bear a reasonable interest rate in a bank or similar financial institution supervised by the United States or a State, if such bank or other institution is a fiduciary of such plan and if—

(A) the plan covers only employees of such bank or other institution and employees of affiliates of such bank or other institution, or

(B) such investment is expressly authorized by a provision of the plan or by a fiduciary (other than such bank or institution or affiliate thereof) who is expressly empowered by the plan to so instruct the trustee with respect to such investment.

(5) Any contract for life insurance, health insurance, or annuities with one or more insurers which are qualified to do business in a State, if the plan pays no more than adequate consideration, and if each such insurer or insurers is—

(A) the employer maintaining the plan, or

(B) a party in interest which is wholly owned (directly or indirectly) by the employer maintaining the plan, or by any person which is a party in interest with respect to the plan, but only if the total premiums and annuity considerations written by such insurers for life insurance, health insurance, or annuities for all plans (and their employers) with respect to which such insurers are parties in interest (not including premiums or annuity considerations written by the employer maintaining the plan) do not exceed 5 percent of the total premiums and annuity considerations written for all lines of insurance in that year by such insurers (not including premiums or annuity considerations written by the employer maintaining the plan).

(6) The providing of any ancillary service by a bank or similar financial institution supervised by the United States or a State, if such bank or other institution is a fiduciary of such plan, and if—

(A) such bank or similar financial institution has adopted adequate internal safeguards which assure that the providing of such ancillary service is consistent with sound banking and financial practice, as determined by Federal or State supervisory authority, and

(B) the extent to which such ancillary service is provided is subject to specific guidelines issued by such bank or similar financial institution (as determined by the Secretary after consultation with Federal and State supervisory authority), and adherence to such guidelines would reasonably preclude such bank or similar financial institution from providing such ancillary service (i) in an excessive or unreasonable manner, and (ii) in a manner that would be inconsistent with the best interests of participants and beneficiaries of employee benefit plans.

Such ancillary services shall not be provided at more than reasonable compensation.

(7) The exercise of a privilege to convert securities, to the extent provided in regulations of the Secretary, but only if the plan receives no less than adequate consideration pursuant to such conversion.

(8) Any transaction between a plan and (i) a common or collective trust fund or pooled investment fund maintained by a party in interest which is a bank or trust company supervised by a State or Federal agency or (ii) a pooled investment fund of an insurance company qualified to do business in a State, if—

(A) the transaction is a sale or purchase of an interest in the fund,

(B) the bank, trust company, or insurance company receives not more than reasonable compensation, and

(C) such transaction is expressly permitted by the instrument under which the plan is maintained, or by a fiduciary (other than the bank, trust company, or insurance company, or an affiliate thereof) who has authority to manage and control the assets of the plan.

(9) The making by a fiduciary of a distribution of the assets of the plan in accordance with the terms of the plan if such assets are distributed in the same manner as provided under section 4044 of this Act (relating to allocation of assets).

(10) Any transaction required or permitted under part 1 of subtitle E of title IV.

(11) A merger of multiemployer plans, or the transfer of assets or liabilities between multiemployer plans, determined by the Pension Benefit Guaranty Corporation to meet the requirements of section 4231.

(12) The sale by a plan to a party in interest on or after December 18, 1987, of any stock, if—

(A) the requirements of paragraphs (1) and (2) of subsection (e) are met with respect to such stock,

(B) on the later of the date on which the stock was acquired by the plan, or January 1, 1975, such stock constituted a qualifying employer security (as defined in section 407(d)(5) as then in effect), and

(C) such stock does not constitute a qualifying employer security (as defined in section 407(d)(5) as in effect at the time of the sale).

(13) Any transfer made before January 1, 2026, of excess pension assets from a defined benefit plan to a retiree health account in a qualified transfer permitted under section 420 of the Internal Revenue Code of 1986 (as in effect on the date of the enactment of the Surface Transportation and Veterans Health Care Choice Improvement Act of 2015).

(14) Any transaction in connection with the provision of investment advice described in section 3(21)(A)(ii) to a participant or beneficiary of an individual account plan that permits such participant or beneficiary to direct the investment of assets in their individual account, if—

(A) the transaction is—

(i) the provision of the investment advice to the participant or beneficiary of the plan with respect to a security or other property available as an investment under the plan,

(ii) the acquisition, holding, or sale of a security or other property available as an investment under the plan pursuant to the investment advice, or

(iii) the direct or indirect receipt of fees or other compensation by the fiduciary adviser or an affiliate thereof (or any employee, agent, or registered representative of the fiduciary adviser or affiliate) in connection with the provision of the advice or in connection with an acquisition, holding, or sale of a security or other property available as an investment under the plan pursuant to the investment advice; and

(B) the requirements of subsection (g) are met.

(15)(A) Any transaction involving the purchase or sale of securities, or other property (as determined by the Secretary), between a plan and a party in interest (other than a fiduciary described in section 3(21)(A)) with respect to a plan if—

(i) the transaction involves a block trade,

(ii) at the time of the transaction, the interest of the plan (together with the interests of any other plans maintained by the same plan sponsor), does not exceed 10 percent of the aggregate size of the block trade,

(iii) the terms of the transaction, including the price, are at least as favorable to the plan as an arm's length transaction, and

(iv) the compensation associated with the purchase and sale is not greater than the compensation associated with an arm's length transaction with an unrelated party.

(B) For purposes of this paragraph, the term "block trade" means any trade of at least 10,000 shares or with a market value of at least $200,000 which will be allocated across two or more unrelated client accounts of a fiduciary.

(16) Any transaction involving the purchase or sale of securities, or other property (as determined by the Secretary), between a plan and a party in interest if—

(A) the transaction is executed through an electronic communication network, alternative trading system, or similar execution system or trading venue subject to regulation and oversight by—

(i) the applicable Federal regulating entity, or

(ii) such foreign regulatory entity as the Secretary may determine by regulation,

(B) either—

(i) the transaction is effected pursuant to rules designed to match purchases and sales at the best price available through the execution system in accordance with applicable rules of the Securities and Exchange Commission or other relevant governmental authority, or

(ii) neither the execution system nor the parties to the transaction take into account the identity of the parties in the execution of trades,

(C) the price and compensation associated with the purchase and sale are not greater than the price and compensation associated with an arm's length transaction with an unrelated party,

(D) if the party in interest has an ownership interest in the system or venue described in subparagraph (A), the system or venue has been authorized by the plan sponsor or other independent fiduciary for transactions described in this paragraph, and

(E) not less than 30 days prior to the initial transaction described in this paragraph executed through any system or venue described in subparagraph (A), a plan fiduciary is provided written or electronic notice of the execution of such transaction through such system or venue.

(17)(A) Transactions described in subparagraphs (A), (B), and (D) of section 406(a)(1) between a plan and a person that is a party in interest other than a fiduciary (or an affiliate) who has or exercises any discretionary authority or control with respect to the investment of the plan assets involved in the transaction or renders investment advice (within the meaning of section 3(21)(A)(ii)) with respect to those assets, solely by reason of providing services to the plan or solely by reason of a relationship to such a service provider described in subparagraph (F), (G), (H), or (I) of section 3(14), or both, but only if in connection with such transaction the plan receives no less, nor pays no more, than adequate consideration.

(B) For purposes of this paragraph, the term "adequate consideration" means—

(i) in the case of a security for which there is a generally recognized market—

(II) the price of the security prevailing on a national securities exchange which is registered under section 6 of the Securities Exchange Act of 1934, taking into account factors such as the size of the transaction and marketability of the security, or

(II) if the security is not traded on such a national securities exchange, a price not less favorable to the plan than the offering price for the security as established by the current bid and asked prices quoted by persons independent of the issuer and of the party in interest, taking into account factors such as the size of the transaction and marketability of the security, and

(ii) in the case of an asset other than a security for which there is a generally recognized market, the fair market value of the asset as determined in good faith by a fiduciary or fiduciaries in accordance with regulations prescribed by the Secretary.

(18) FOREIGN EXCHANGE TRANSACTIONS.—Any foreign exchange transactions, between a bank or broker-dealer (or any affiliate of either), and a plan (as defined in section 3(3)) with respect to which such bank or broker-dealer (or affiliate) is a trustee, custodian, fiduciary, or other party in interest, if—

(A) the transaction is in connection with the purchase, holding, or sale of securities or other investment assets (other than a foreign exchange transaction unrelated to any other investment in securities or other investment assets),

(B) at the time the foreign exchange transaction is entered into, the terms of the transaction are not less favorable to the plan than the terms generally available in comparable arm's length foreign exchange transactions between unrelated parties, or the terms afforded by the bank or broker-dealer (or any affiliate of either) in comparable arm's-length foreign exchange transactions involving unrelated parties,

(C) the exchange rate used by such bank or broker-dealer (or affiliate) for a particular foreign exchange transaction does not deviate by more than 3 percent from the interbank bid and asked rates for transactions of comparable size and maturity at the time of the transaction as displayed on an independent service that reports rates of exchange in the foreign currency market for such currency, and

(D) the bank or broker-dealer (or any affiliate of either) does not have investment discretion, or provide investment advice, with respect to the transaction.

(19)CROSS TRADING.—Any transaction described in sections 406(a)(1)(A) and 406(b)(2) involving the purchase and sale of a security between a plan and any other account managed by the same investment manager, if—

(A) the transaction is a purchase or sale, for no consideration other than cash payment against prompt delivery of a security for which market quotations are readily available,

(B) the transaction is effected at the independent current market price of the security (within the meaning of section 270.17a–7(b) of title 17, Code of Federal Regulations),

(C) no brokerage commission, fee (except for customary transfer fees, the fact of which is disclosed pursuant to subparagraph (D)), or other remuneration is paid in connection with the transaction,

(D) a fiduciary (other than the investment manager engaging in the cross-trades or any affiliate) for each plan participating in the transaction authorizes in advance of any cross-trades (in a document that is separate from any other written agreement of the parties) the investment manager to engage in cross trades at the investment manager's discretion, after such fiduciary has received disclosure regarding the conditions under which cross trades may take place (but only if such disclosure is separate from any other agreement or disclosure involving the asset management relationship), including the written policies and procedures of the investment manager described in subparagraph (H),

(E) each plan participating in the transaction has assets of at least $100,000,000, except that if the assets of a plan are invested in a master trust containing the assets of plans maintained by employers in the same controlled group (as defined in section 407(d)(7)), the master trust has assets of at least $100,000,000,

(F) the investment manager provides to the plan fiduciary who authorized cross trading under subparagraph a quarterly report detailing all cross trades executed by the investment manager in which the plan participated during such quarter, including the following information, as applicable: (i) the identity of each security bought or sold; (ii) the number of shares or units traded; (iii) the parties involved in the cross-trade; and (iv) trade price and the method used to establish the trade price,

(G) the investment manager does not base its fee schedule on the plan's consent to cross trading, and no other service (other than the investment opportunities and cost savings available through a cross trade) is conditioned on the plan's consent to cross trading,

(H) the investment manager has adopted, and crosstrades are effected in accordance with, written cross-trading policies and procedures that are fair and equitable to all accounts participating in the cross-trading program, and that include a description of the manager's pricing policies and procedures, and the manager's policies and procedures for allocating cross trades in an objective manner among accounts participating in the cross-trading program, and

(I) the investment manager has designated an individual responsible for periodically reviewing such purchases and sales to ensure compliance with the written policies and procedures described in subparagraph (H), and following such review, the individual shall issue an annual written report no later than 90 days following the period to which it relates signed under penalty of perjury to the plan fiduciary who authorized cross trading under subparagraph (D) describing the steps performed during the course of the review, the level of compliance, and any specific instances of non-compliance.

The written report under subparagraph (I) shall also notify the plan fiduciary of the plan's right to terminate participation in the investment manager's cross-trading program at any time.

(20)(A) Except as provided in subparagraphs (B) and (C), a transaction described in section 406(a) in connection with the acquisition, holding, or disposition of any security or commodity, if the transaction is corrected before the end of the correction period.

(B) Subparagraph (A) does not apply to any transaction between a plan and a plan sponsor or its affiliates that involves the acquisition or sale of an employer security (as defined in section 407(d)(1)) or the acquisition, sale, or lease of employer real property (as defined in section 407(d)(2)).

(C) In the case of any fiduciary or other party in interest (or any other person knowingly participating in such transaction), subparagraph (A) does not apply to any transaction if, at the time the transaction occurs, such fiduciary or party in interest (or other person) knew (or reasonably should have known) that the transaction would (without regard to this paragraph) constitute a violation of section 406(a).

(D) For purposes of this paragraph, the term "correction period" means, in connection with a fiduciary or party in interest (or other person knowingly participating in the transaction), the 14-day period beginning on the date on which such fiduciary or party in interest (or other person) discovers, or reasonably should have discovered, that the transaction would (without regard to this paragraph) constitute a violation of section 406(a).

(E) For purposes of this paragraph—

(i) The term "security" has the meaning given such term by section 475(c)(2) of the Internal Revenue Code of 1986 (without regard to subparagraph (F)(iii) and the last sentence thereof).

(ii) The term "commodity" has the meaning given such term by section 475(e)(2) of such Code (without regard to subparagraph (D)(iii) thereof).

(iii) The term "correct" means, with respect to a transaction—

(I) to undo the transaction to the extent possible and in any case to make good to the plan or affected account any losses resulting from the transaction, and

(II) to restore to the plan or affected account any profits made through the use of assets of the plan.

(c) Nothing in section 406 shall be construed to prohibit any fiduciary from—

(1) receiving any benefit to which he may be entitled as a participant or beneficiary in the plan, so long as the benefit is computed and paid on a basis which is consistent with the terms of the plan as applied to all other participants and beneficiaries;

(2) receiving any reasonable compensation for services rendered, or for the reimbursement of expenses properly and actually incurred, in the performance of his duties with the plan; except that no person so serving who already receives full time pay from an employer or an association of employers, whose employees are participants in the plan, or from an employee organization whose members are participants in such plan shall receive compensation from such plan, except for reimbursement of expenses properly and actually incurred; or

(3) serving as a fiduciary in addition to being an officer, employee, agent, or other representative of a party in interest.

(d)(1) Section 407(b) and subsections (b), (c), and (e) of this section shall not apply to a transaction in which a plan directly or indirectly—

(A) lends any part of the corpus or income of the plan to,

(B) pays any compensation for personal services rendered to the plan to, or

(C) acquires for the plan any property from, or sells any property to, any person who is with respect to the plan an owner-employee (as defined in section 401(c)(3) of the Internal Revenue Code of 1986), a member of the family (as defined in section 267(c)(4) of such Code) of any such owner-employee, or any corporation in which any such owner-employee owns, directly or indirectly, 50 percent or more of the total combined voting power of all classes of stock entitled to vote or 50 percent or more of the total value of shares of all classes of stock of the corporation.

(2)(A) For purposes of paragraph (1), the following shall be treated as owner-employees:

(i) A shareholder-employee.

(ii) A participant or beneficiary of an individual retirement plan (as defined in section 7701(a)(37) of the Internal Revenue Code of 1986).

(iii) An employer or association of employees which establishes such an individual retirement plan under section 408(c) of such Code.

(B) Paragraph (1)(C) shall not apply to a transaction which consists of a sale of employer securities to an employee stock ownership plan (as defined in section 407(d)(6)) by a shareholder-employee, a member of the family (as defined in section 267(c)(4) of such Code) of any such owner-employee, or a corporation in which such a shareholder-employee owns stock representing a 50 percent or greater interest described in paragraph (1).

(C) For purposes of paragraph (1)(A), the term "owner-employee" shall only include a person described in clause (ii) or (iii) of subparagraph (A).

(3) For purposes of paragraph (2), the term "shareholder-employee" means an employee or officer of an S corporation (as defined in section 1361(a)(1) of such Code) who owns (or is considered as owning within the meaning of section

318(a)(1) of such Code) more than 5 percent of the outstanding stock of the corporation on any day during the taxable year of such corporation.

(e) Sections 406 and 407 shall not apply to the acquisition or sale by a plan of qualifying employer securities (as defined in section 407(d)(5)) or acquisition, sale or lease by a plan of qualifying employer real property (as defined in section 407(d)(4))—

(1) if such acquisition, sale, or lease is for adequate consideration (or in the case of a marketable obligation, at a price not less favorable to the plan than the price determined under section 407(e)(1)),

(2) if no commission is charged with respect thereto, and

(3) if—

(A) the plan is an eligible individual account plan (as defined in section 407(d)(3)), or

(B) in the case of an acquisition or lease of qualifying employer real property by a plan which is not an eligible individual account plan, or of an acquisition of qualifying employer securities by such a plan, the lease or acquisition is not prohibited by section 407(a).

(f) Section 406(b)(2) shall not apply to any merger or transfer described in subsection (b)(11).

(g) PROVISION OF INVESTMENT ADVICE TO PARTICIPANT AND BENEFICIARIES.—

(1) IN GENERAL.—The prohibitions provided in section 406 shall not apply to transactions described in subsection (b)(14) if the investment advice provided by a fiduciary adviser is provided under an eligible investment advice arrangement.

(2) ELIGIBLE INVESTMENT ADVICE ARRANGEMENT.—For purposes of this subsection, the term "eligible investment advice arrangement" means an arrangement—

(A) which either—

(i) provides that any fees (including any commission or other compensation) received by the fiduciary adviser for investment advice or with respect to the sale, holding, or acquisition of any security or other property for purposes of investment of plan assets do not vary depending on the basis of any investment option selected, or

(ii) uses a computer model under an investment advice program meeting the requirements of paragraph

(3) in connection with the provision of investment advice by a fiduciary adviser to a participant or beneficiary, and

(B) with respect to which the requirements of paragraph (4), (5), (6), (7), (8), and (9) are met.

(3) INVESTMENT ADVICE PROGRAM USING COMPUTER MODEL.—

(A) IN GENERAL.—An investment advice program meets the requirements of this paragraph if the requirements of subparagraphs (B), (C), and (D) are met.

(B) COMPUTER MODEL.—The requirements of this subparagraph are met if the investment advice provided under the investment advice program is provided pursuant to a computer model that—

(i) applies generally accepted investment theories that take into account the historic returns of different asset classes over defined periods of time,

(ii) utilizes relevant information about the participant, which may include age, life expectancy, retirement age, risk tolerance, other assets or sources of income, and preferences as to certain types of investments,

(iii) utilizes prescribed objective criteria to provide asset allocation portfolios comprised of investment options available under the plan,

(iv) operates in a manner that is not biased in favor of investments offered by the fiduciary adviser or a person with a material affiliation or contractual relationship with the fiduciary adviser, and

(v) takes into account all investment options under the plan in specifying how a participant's account balance should be invested and is not inappropriately weighted with respect to any investment option.

(C) CERTIFICATION.—

(i) IN GENERAL.—The requirements of this subparagraph are met with respect to any investment advice program if an eligible investment expert certifies, prior to the utilization of the computer model and in accordance with rules prescribed by the Secretary, that the computer model meets the requirements of subparagraph (B).

(ii) RENEWAL OF CERTIFICATIONS.—If, as determined under regulations prescribed by the Secretary, there are material modifications to a computer model, the requirements of this subparagraph are met only if a certification described in clause (i) is obtained with respect to the computer model as so modified.

(iii) ELIGIBLE INVESTMENT EXPERT.—The term "eligible investment expert" means any person—

(I) which meets such requirements as the Secretary may provide, and

(II) does not bear any material affiliation or contractual relationship with any investment adviser or a related person thereof (or any employee, agent, or registered representative of the investment adviser or related person).

(D) EXCLUSIVITY OF RECOMMENDATION.—The requirements of this subparagraph are met with respect to any investment advice program if—

(i) the only investment advice provided under the program is the advice generated by the computer model described in subparagraph (B), and

(ii) any transaction described in subsection (b)(14)(A)(ii) occurs solely at the direction of the participant or beneficiary.

Nothing in the preceding sentence shall preclude the participant or beneficiary from requesting investment advice other than that described in subparagraph (A), but only if such request has not been solicited by any person connected with carrying out the arrangement.

(4) EXPRESS AUTHORIZATION BY SEPARATE FIDUCIARY.—The requirements of this paragraph are met with respect to an arrangement if the arrangement is expressly authorized by a plan fiduciary other than the person offering the investment advice program, any person providing investment options under the plan, or any affiliate of either.

(5) ANNUAL AUDIT.—The requirements of this paragraph are met if an independent auditor, who has appropriate technical training or experience and proficiency and so represents in writing—
- (A) conducts an annual audit of the arrangement for compliance with the requirements of this subsection, and
- (B) following completion of the annual audit, issues a written report to the fiduciary who authorized use of the arrangement which presents its specific findings regarding compliance of the arrangement with the requirements of this subsection.

For purposes of this paragraph, an auditor is considered independent if it is not related to the person offering the arrangement to the plan and is not related to any person providing investment options under the plan.

(6) DISCLOSURE.—The requirements of this paragraph are met if—
- (A) the fiduciary adviser provides to a participant or a beneficiary before the initial provision of the investment advice with regard to any security or other property offered as an investment option, a written notification (which may consist of notification by means of electronic communication)—
  - (i) of the role of any party that has a material affiliation or contractual relationship with the fiduciary adviser in the development of the investment advice program and in the selection of investment options available under the plan,
  - (ii) of the past performance and historical rates of return of the investment options available under the plan,
  - (iii) of all fees or other compensation relating to the advice that the fiduciary adviser or any affiliate there- of is to receive (including compensation provided by any third party) in connection with the provision of the advice or in connection with the sale, acquisition, or holding of the security or other property,
  - (iv) of any material affiliation or contractual relationship of the fiduciary adviser or affiliates thereof in the security or other property,
  - (v) the manner, and under what circumstances, any participant or beneficiary information provided under the arrangement will be used or disclosed,
  - (vi) of the types of services provided by the fiduciary adviser in connection with the provision of investment advice by the fiduciary adviser,
  - (vii)that the adviser is acting as a fiduciary of the plan in connection with the provision of the advice, and
  - (viii)that a recipient of the advice may separately arrange for the provision of advice by another adviser, that could have no material affiliation with and receive no fees or other compensation in connection with the security or other property, and
- (B) at all times during the provision of advisory services to the participant or beneficiary, the fiduciary adviser—
  - (i) maintains the information described in subparagraph (A) in accurate form and in the manner described in paragraph (8),

(ii) provides, without charge, accurate information to the recipient of the advice no less frequently than annually,

(iii) provides, without charge, accurate information to the recipient of the advice upon request of the recipient, and

(iv) provides, without charge, accurate information to the recipient of the advice concerning any material change to the information required to be provided to the recipient of the advice at a time reasonably contemporaneous to the change in information.

(7) OTHER CONDITIONS.—The requirements of this paragraph are met if—

(A) the fiduciary adviser provides appropriate disclosure, in connection with the sale, acquisition, or holding of the security or other property, in accordance with all applicable securities laws,

(B) the sale, acquisition, or holding occurs solely at the direction of the recipient of the advice,

(C) the compensation received by the fiduciary adviser and affiliates thereof in connection with the sale, acquisition, or holding of the security or other property is reasonable, and

(D) the terms of the sale, acquisition, or holding of the security or other property are at least as favorable to the plan as an arm's length transaction would be.

(8) STANDARDS FOR PRESENTATION OF INFORMATION.—

(A) IN GENERAL.—The requirements of this paragraph are met if the notification required to be provided to participants and beneficiaries under paragraph (6)(A) is written in a clear and conspicuous manner and in a manner calculated to be understood by the average plan participant and is sufficiently accurate and comprehensive to reasonably apprise such participants and beneficiaries of the information required to be provided in the notification.

(B) MODEL FORM FOR DISCLOSURE OF FEES AND OTHER COMPENSATION.—The Secretary shall issue a model form for the disclosure of fees and other compensation required in paragraph (6)(A)(iii) which meets the requirements of subparagraph (A).

(9) MAINTENANCE FOR 6 YEARS OF EVIDENCE OF COMPLIANCE.—The requirements of this paragraph are met if a fiduciary adviser who has provided advice referred to in paragraph (1) maintains, for a period of not less than 6 years after the provision of the advice, any records necessary for determining whether the requirements of the preceding provisions of this subsection and of subsection (b)(14) have been met. A transaction prohibited under section 406 shall not be considered to have occurred solely because the records are lost or destroyed prior to the end of the 6-year period due to circumstances beyond the control of the fiduciary adviser.

(10) EXEMPTION FOR PLAN SPONSOR AND CERTAIN OTHER FIDUCIARIES.—

(A) IN GENERAL.—Subject to subparagraph (B), a plan sponsor or other person who is a fiduciary (other than a fiduciary adviser) shall not be treated as failing to meet the requirements of this part solely by reason of the provision of investment advice referred to in section 3(21)(A)(ii) (or solely by reason of contracting for or otherwise arranging for the provision of the advice), if—

(i) the advice is provided by a fiduciary adviser pursuant to an eligible investment advice arrangement between the plan sponsor or other fiduciary and the fiduciary adviser for the provision by the fiduciary adviser of investment advice referred to in such section,

(ii) the terms of the eligible investment advice arrangement require compliance by the fiduciary adviser with the requirements of this subsection, and

(iii) the terms of the eligible investment advice arrangement include a written acknowledgment by the fiduciary adviser that the fiduciary adviser is a fiduciary of the plan with respect to the provision of the advice.

(B) CONTINUED DUTY OF PRUDENT SELECTION OF ADVISER AND PERIODIC REVIEW.—Nothing in subparagraph (A) shall be construed to exempt a plan sponsor or other person who is a fiduciary from any requirement of this part for the prudent selection and periodic review of a fiduciary adviser with whom the plan sponsor or other person enters into an eligible investment advice arrangement for the provision of investment advice referred to in section 3(21)(A)(ii). The plan sponsor or other person who is a fiduciary has no duty under this part to monitor the specific investment advice given by the fiduciary adviser to any particular recipient of the advice.

(C) AVAILABILITY OF PLAN ASSETS FOR PAYMENT FOR ADVICE.—Nothing in this part shall be construed to preclude the use of plan assets to pay for reasonable expenses in providing investment advice referred to in section 3(21)(A)(ii).

(11) DEFINITIONS.—For purposes of this subsection and subsection (b)(14)—

(A) FIDUCIARY ADVISER.—The term "fiduciary adviser" means, with respect to a plan, a person who is a fiduciary of the plan by reason of the provision of investment advice referred to in section 3(21)(A)(ii) by the person to a participant or beneficiary of the plan and who is—

(i) registered as an investment adviser under the Investment Advisers Act of 1940 (15 U.S.C. 80b–1 et seq.) or under the laws of the State in which the fiduciary maintains its principal office and place of business,

(ii) a bank or similar financial institution referred to in subsection (b)(4) or a savings association (as defined in section 3(b)(1) of the Federal Deposit Insurance Act (12 U.S.C. 1813(b)(1)), but only if the advice is provided through a trust department of the bank or similar financial institution or savings association which is subject to periodic examination and review by Federal or State banking authorities,

(iii) an insurance company qualified to do business under the laws of a State,

(iv) a person registered as a broker or dealer under the Securities Exchange Act of 1934 (15 U.S.C. 78a et seq.),

(v) an affiliate of a person described in any of clauses (i) through (iv), or

(vi) an employee, agent, or registered representative of a person described in clauses (i) through (v) who satisfies the requirements of applicable insurance, banking, and securities laws relating to the provision of the advice.

For purposes of this part, a person who develops the computer model described in paragraph (3)(B) or markets the investment advice program or computer model shall be treated as a person who is a fiduciary of the plan by reason of the provision of investment advice referred to in section 3(21)(A)(ii) to a participant or beneficiary and shall be treated as a fiduciary adviser for purposes of this subsection and subsection (b)(14), except that the Secretary may prescribe rules under which only 1 fiduciary adviser may elect to be treated as a fiduciary with respect to the plan.

(B) AFFILIATE.—The term "affiliate" of another entity means an affiliated person of the entity (as defined in section 2(a)(3) of the Investment Company Act of 1940 (15 U.S.C. 80a–2(a)(3))).

(C) REGISTERED REPRESENTATIVE.—The term "registered representative" of another entity means a person described in section 3(a)(18) of the Securities Exchange Act of 1934 (15 U.S.C. 78c(a)(18)) (substituting the entity for the broker or dealer referred to in such section) or a person described in section 202(a)(17) of the Investment Advisers Act of 1940 (15 U.S.C. 80b-2(a)(17)) (substituting the entity for the investment adviser referred to in such section).

(h) PROVISION OF PHARMACY BENEFIT SERVICES.—

(1) IN GENERAL.—Provided that all of the conditions described in paragraph (2) are met, the restrictions imposed by subsections (a), (b)(1), and (b)(2) of section 406 shall not apply to—

(A) the offering of pharmacy benefit services to a group health plan that is sponsored by an entity described in section 3(37)(G)(vi) or to any other group health plan that is sponsored by a regional council, local union, or other labor organization affiliated with such entity;

(B) the purchase of pharmacy benefit services by plan participants and beneficiaries of a group health plan that is sponsored by an entity described in section 3(37)(G)(vi) or of any other group health plan that is sponsored by a regional council, local union, or other labor organization affiliated with such entity; or

(C) the operation or implementation of pharmacy benefit services by an entity described in section 3(37)(G)(vi) or by any other group health plan that is sponsored by a regional council, local union, or other labor organization affiliated with such entity, in any arrangement where such entity described in section 3(37)(G)(vi) or any related organization or subsidiary of such entity provides pharmacy benefit services that include prior authorization and appeals, a retail pharmacy network, pharmacy benefit administration, mail order fulfillment, formulary support, manufacturer payments, audits, and specialty pharmacy and goods, to any such group health plan.

(2) CONDITIONS.—The conditions described in this paragraph are the following:

(A) The terms of the arrangement are at least as favorable to the group health plan as such group health plan could obtain in a similar arm's length arrangement with an unrelated third party.

(B) At least 50 percent of the providers participating in the pharmacy benefit services offered by the arrangement are unrelated to the contributing employers or any other party in interest with respect to the group health plan.

(C) The group health plan retains an independent fiduciary who will be responsible for monitoring the group health plan's consultants, contractors, subcontractors, and other service providers for purposes of pharmacy benefit services described in paragraph (1) offered by such entity or any of its related organizations or subsidiaries and monitors the transactions of such entity and any of its related organizations or subsidiaries to ensure that all conditions of this exemption are satisfied during each plan year.

(D) Any decisions regarding the provision of pharmacy benefit services described in paragraph (1) are made by the group health plan's independent fiduciary, based on objective standards developed by the independent fiduciary in reliance on information provided by the arrangement.

(E) The independent fiduciary of the group health plan provides an annual report to the Secretary and the congressional committees of jurisdiction attesting that the conditions described in subparagraphs (C) and (D) have been met for the applicable plan year, together with a statement that use of the arrangement's services are in the best interest of the participants and beneficiaries in the aggregate for that plan year compared to other similar arrangements the group health plan could have obtained in transactions with an unrelated third party.

(F) The arrangement is not designed to benefit any party in interest with respect to the group health plan.

(3) VIOLATIONS.—In the event an entity described in section 3(37)(G)(vi) or any affiliate of such entity violates any of the conditions of such exemption, such exemption shall not apply with respect to such entity or affiliate and all enforcement and claims available under this Act shall apply with respect to such entity or affiliate.

(4) RULE OF CONSTRUCTION.—Nothing in this subsection shall be construed to modify any obligation of a group health plan otherwise set forth in this Act.

(5) GROUP HEALTH PLAN.—In this subsection, the term "group health plan" has the meaning given such term in section 733(a).

Part 5—Administration and Enforcement

SEC. 522. INVESTIGATIVE AUTHORITY REGARDING VIOLATIONS OF CERTAIN HEALTH CARE PROVIDER REQUIREMENTS; COMPLAINT PROCESS.

(a) INVESTIGATIVE AUTHORITY.—Upon receiving a notice from a State or the Secretary of Health and Human Services of violations of sections 2799A–1, 2799A–2, or 2799A–4 of the Public Health Service Act, the Secretary of Labor shall have the power to conduct an investigation to identify patterns of such violations with respect to participants or beneficiaries under a group health plan or health insurance coverage offered in connection with a group health plan by a health insurance issuer in the group market. The Secretary may assist States, the Secretary of Health and Human Services, plans, or issuers to ensure that appropriate measures have been taken to correct such violations retrospectively and prospectively with respect to participants or beneficiaries under a group health plan or health insurance coverage

offered in connection with a group health plan by a health insurance issuer in the group market.

(b) COMPLAINT PROCESS.—Not later than January 1, 2022, the Secretary shall establish a process under which the Secretary—

(1) may receive complaints from participants and beneficiaries of group health plans or health insurance coverage offered in connection with such plans relating to alleged violations of the sections specified in subsection (a); and

(2) transmits such complaints to States or the Secretary of Health and Human Services (as determined appropriate by the Secretary) for potential enforcement actions.

Part 7—Group Health Plan Requirements

Subpart B—Other Requirements

SEC. 716. CONSUMER PROTECTIONS.

(a) CHOICE OF HEALTH CARE PROFESSIONAL.—If a group health plan or health insurance issuer offering group health insurance coverage requires or provides for designation by a participant or beneficiary of a participating primary care provider, then the plan or issuer shall permit each participant or beneficiary to designate any participating primary care provider who is available to accept such individual.

(b) COVERAGE OF EMERGENCY SERVICES.—

(1) IN GENERAL.—If a group health plan, or a health insurance issuer offering group health insurance coverage, provides or covers any benefits with respect to services in an emergency department of a hospital or with respect to emergency services in an independent freestanding emergency department (as defined in paragraph (3)(D)), the plan or issuer shall cover emergency services (as defined in paragraph (3)(C))—

(A) without the need for any prior authorization determination;

(B) whether the health care provider furnishing such services is a participating provider or a participating emergency facility, as applicable, with respect to such services;

(C) in a manner so that, if such services are provided to a participant or beneficiary by a nonparticipating provider or a nonparticipating emergency facility—

(i) such services will be provided without imposing any requirement under the plan for prior authorization of services or any limitation on coverage that is more restrictive than the requirements or limitations that apply to emergency services received from participating providers and participating emergency facilities with respect to such plan or coverage, respectively;

(ii) the cost-sharing requirement (expressed as a copayment amount or coinsurance rate) is not greater than the requirement that would apply if

such services were provided by a participating provider or a participating emergency facility;

(iii) such cost-sharing requirement is calculated as if the total amount that would have been charged for such services by such participating provider or participating emergency facility were equal to the recognized amount (as defined in paragraph (3)(H)) for such services, plan or coverage, and year;

(iv) the group health plan or health insurance issuer, respectively, pays to such provider or facility, respectively, the amount by which the recognized amount for such services and year involved exceeds the cost-sharing amount for such services (as determined in accordance with clauses (ii) and (iii)) and year; and

(v) any cost-sharing payments made by the participant or beneficiary with respect to such emergency services so furnished shall be counted toward any in-network deductible or out-of-pocket maximums applied under the plan or coverage, respectively (and such in-network deductible and out-of-pocket maximums shall be applied) in the same manner as if such cost-sharing payments were made with respect to emergency services furnished by a participating provider or a participating emergency facility; and

(D) without regard to any other term or condition of such coverage (other than exclusion or coordination of benefits, or an affiliation or waiting period, permitted under section 2704 of the Public Health Service Act, including as incorporated pursuant to section 715 of this Act and section 9815 of the Internal Revenue Code of 1986, and other than applicable cost-sharing).

(2) AUDIT PROCESS AND REGULATIONS FOR MEDIAN CONTRACTED RATES.—

(A) AUDIT PROCESS.—

(i) IN GENERAL.—Not later than July 1, 2021, the Secretary, in consultation with appropriate State agencies and the Secretary of Health and Human Services and the Secretary of the Treasury, shall establish through rulemaking a process, in accordance with clause (ii), under which group health plans and health insurance issuers offering health insurance coverage in the group market are audited by the Secretary or applicable State authority to ensure that—

(I) such plans and coverage are in compliance with the requirement of applying a median contracted rate under this section; and

(II) such median contracted rate so applied satisfies the definition under paragraph (3)(E) with respect to the year involved, including with respect to a group health plan or health insurance issuer described in clause (ii) of such paragraph (3)(E).

(ii) AUDIT SAMPLES.—Under the process established pursuant to clause (i), the Secretary—

(I) shall conduct audits described in such clause, with respect to a year (beginning with 2022), of a sample with respect to such year of claims

data from not more than 25 group health plans and health insurance issuers offering health insurance coverage in the group market; and

(II) may audit any group health plan or health insurance issuer offering health insurance coverage in the group market if the Secretary has received any complaint about such plan or coverage, respectively, that involves the compliance of the plan or coverage, respectively, with either of the requirements described in subclauses (I) and (II) of such clause.

(iii) REPORTS.—Beginning for 2022, the Secretary shall annually submit to Congress information on the number of plans and issuers with respect to which audits were conducted during such year pursuant to this subparagraph.

(B) RULEMAKING.—Not later than July 1, 2021, the Secretary, in consultation with the Secretary of the Treasury and the Secretary of Health and Human Services, shall establish through rulemaking—

(i) the methodology the group health plan or health insurance issuer offering health insurance coverage in the group market shall use to determine the median contracted rate, differentiating by line of business;

(ii) the information such plan or issuer, respectively, shall share with the nonparticipating provider or nonparticipating facility, as applicable, when making such a determination;

(iii) the geographic regions applied for purposes of this subparagraph, taking into account access to items and services in rural and underserved areas, including health professional shortage areas, as defined in section 332 of the Public Health Service Act; and

(iv) a process to receive complaints of violations of the requirements described in subclauses (I) and (II) of paragraph (2)(A)(i) by group health plans and health insurance issuers offering health insurance coverage in the group market.

Such rulemaking shall take into account payments that are made by such plan or issuer, respectively, that are not on a fee-for-service basis. Such methodology may account for relevant payment adjustments that take into account quality or facility type (including higher acuity settings and the case-mix of various facility types) that are otherwise taken into account for purposes of determining payment amounts with respect to participating facilities. In carrying out clause (iii), the Secretary shall consult with the National Association of Insurance Commissioners to establish the geographic regions under such clause and shall periodically update such regions, as appropriate.

(3) DEFINITIONS.—In this section:

(A) EMERGENCY DEPARTMENT OF A HOSPITAL.—The term "emergency department of a hospital" includes a hospital outpatient department that provides emergency services.

(B) EMERGENCY MEDICAL CONDITION.—The term "emergency medical condition" means a medical condition manifesting itself by acute symptoms of sufficient severity (including severe pain) such that a prudent layperson,

who possesses an average knowledge of health and medicine, could reasonably expect the absence of immediate medical attention to result in a condition described in clause (i), (ii), or (iii) of section 1867(e)(1)(A) of the Social Security Act.

(C) EMERGENCY SERVICES.—

(i) IN GENERAL.—The term "emergency services," with respect to an emergency medical condition, means—

(I) a medical screening examination (as required under section 1867 of the Social Security Act, or as would be required under such section if such section applied to an independent freestanding emergency department) that is within the capability of the emergency department of a hospital or of an independent freestanding emergency department, as applicable, including ancillary services routinely available to the emergency department to evaluate such emergency medical condition; and

(II) within the capabilities of the staff and facilities available at the hospital or the independent freestanding emergency department, as applicable, such further medical examination and treatment as are required under section 1867 of such Act, or as would be required under such section if such section applied to an independent freestanding emergency department, to stabilize the patient.

(ii) INCLUSION OF CERTAIN SERVICES OUTSIDE OF EMERGENCY DEPARTMENT.—

(I) IN GENERAL.—For purposes of this subsection and section 2799A–1, in the case of an individual enrolled in a group health plan or health insurance coverage offered by a health insurance issuer in the group or individual market who is furnished services described in clause (i) by a participating or nonparticipating provider or a participating or nonparticipating emergency facility to stabilize such individual with respect to an emergency medical condition, the term "emergency services" shall include, unless each of the conditions described in subclause (II) are met, in addition to the items and services described in clause (i), items and services for which benefits are provided or covered under the plan or coverage, respectively, furnished by a nonparticipating provider or nonparticipating facility, regardless of the department of the hospital in which such individual is furnished such items or services, if, after such stabilization but during such visit in which such individual is so stabilized, the provider or facility determines that such items or services are needed.

(II) CONDITIONS.—For purposes of subclause (I), the conditions described in this subclause, with respect to an individual who is stabilized and furnished additional items and services described in subclause (I) after such stabilization by a provider or facility described in subclause (I), are the following:

(aa) Such a provider or facility determines such individual is able to travel using nonmedical transportation or nonemergency medical transportation.

(bb) Such provider furnishing such additional items and services satisfies the notice and consent criteria of section 2799A–2(d) of the Public Health Service Act with respect to such items and services.

(cc) Such an individual is in a condition to receive (as determined in accordance with guidance issued by the Secretary) the information described in section 2799A–2 of the Public Health Service Act and to provide informed consent under such section, in accordance with applicable State law.

(D) INDEPENDENT FREESTANDING EMERGENCY DEPARTMENT.—The term "independent freestanding emergency department" means a facility that—

(i) is geographically separate and distinct and licensed separately from a hospital under applicable State law; and

(ii) provides any emergency services (as defined in subparagraph (C)).

(E) MEDIAN CONTRACTED RATE.—

(i) IN GENERAL.—The term "median contracted rate" means, subject to clauses (ii) and (iii), with respect to a sponsor of a group health plan and health insurance issuer offering health insurance coverage in the group market—

(I) for an item or service furnished during 2022, the median of the contracted rates recognized by the plan or issuer, respectively (determined with respect to all such plans of such sponsor or all such coverage offered by such issuer that are offered within the same line of business as the plan or coverage) as the total maximum payment (including the cost-sharing amount imposed for such item or service and the amount to be paid by such plan or such issuer, respectively) under such plans or coverage, respectively, on January 31, 2019, for the same or a similar item or service that is provided by a provider in the same or similar specialty and provided in the geographic region in which the item or service is furnished, consistent with the methodology established by the Secretary under paragraph (2)(B), increased by the percentage increase in the consumer price index for all urban consumers (United States city average) over 2019, such percentage increase over 2020, and such percentage increase over 2021; and

(II) for an item or service furnished during 2023 or a subsequent year, the median contracted rate determined under this clause for such an item or service furnished in the previous year, increased by the percentage increase in the consumer price index for all urban consumers (United States city average) over such previous year.

(ii) NEW PLANS AND COVERAGE.—The term "median contracted rate" means, with respect to a sponsor of a group health plan or health

insurance issuer offering health insurance coverage in the group market in a geographic region in which such sponsor or issuer, respectively, did not offer any group health plan or health insurance coverage during 2019—

(I) for the first year in which such group health plan or health insurance coverage, respectively, is offered in such region, a rate (determined in accordance with a methodology established by the Secretary) for items and services that are covered by such plan and furnished during such first year; and

(II) for each subsequent year such group health plan or health insurance coverage, respectively, is offered in such region, the median contracted rate determined under this clause for such items and services furnished in the previous year, increased by the percentage increase in the consumer price index for all urban consumers (United States city average) over such previous year.

(iii) INSUFFICIENT INFORMATION; NEWLY COVERED ITEMS AND SERVICES.—In the case of a sponsor of a group health plan or health insurance issuer offering health insurance coverage in the group market that does not have sufficient information to calculate the median of the contracted rates described in clause (i)(I) in 2019 (or, in the case of a newly covered item or service (as defined in clause (iv)(III)), in the first coverage year (as defined in clause (iv)(I)) for such item or service with respect to such plan or coverage) for an item or service (including with respect to provider type, or amount, of claims for items or services (as determined by the Secretary) provided in a particular geographic region (other than in a case with respect to which clause (ii) applies)) the term "median contracted rate"—

(I) for an item or service furnished during 2022 (or, in the case of a newly covered item or service, during the first coverage year for such item or service with respect to such plan or coverage), means such rate for such item or service determined by the sponsor or issuer, respectively, through use of any database that is determined, in accordance with rulemaking described in paragraph (2)(B), to not have any conflicts of interest and to have sufficient information reflecting allowed amounts paid to a health care provider or facility for relevant services furnished in the applicable geographic region (such as a State all-payer claims database);

(II) for an item or service furnished in a subsequent year (before the first sufficient information year (as defined in clause (iv)(II)) for such item or service with respect to such plan or coverage), means the rate determined under subclause (I) or this subclause, as applicable, for such item or service for the year previous to such subsequent year, increased by the percentage increase in the consumer price index for all urban consumers (United States city average) over such previous year;

(III) for an item or service furnished in the first sufficient information year for such item or service with respect to such plan or coverage, has the meaning given the term median contracted rate in clause (i)(I), except that in applying such clause to such item or service, the reference to "furnished during 2022" shall be treated as a reference to furnished during such first sufficient information year, the reference to "in 2019" shall be treated as a reference to such sufficient information year, and the increase described in such clause shall not be applied; and

(IV) for an item or service furnished in any year subsequent to the first sufficient information year for such item or service with respect to such plan or coverage, has the meaning given such term in clause (i)(II), except that in applying such clause to such item or service, the reference to "furnished during 2023 or a subsequent year" shall be treated as a reference to furnished during the year after such first sufficient information year or a subsequent year.

(iv) DEFINITIONS.—For purposes of this subparagraph:

(I) FIRST COVERAGE YEAR.—The term "first coverage year" means, with respect to a group health plan or health insurance coverage offered by a health insurance issuer in the group market and an item or service for which coverage is not offered in 2019 under such plan or coverage, the first year after 2019 for which coverage for such item or service is offered under such plan or health insurance coverage.

(II) FIRST SUFFICIENT INFORMATION YEAR.—The term "first sufficient information year" means, with respect to a group health plan or health insurance coverage offered by a health insurance issuer in the group market—

(aa) in the case of an item or service for which the plan or coverage does not have sufficient information to calculate the median of the contracted rates described in clause (i)(I) in 2019, the first year subsequent to 2022 for which such sponsor or issuer has such sufficient information to calculate the median of such contracted rates in the year previous to such first subsequent year; and

(bb) in the case of a newly covered item or service, the first year subsequent to the first coverage year for such item or service with respect to such plan or coverage for which the sponsor or issuer has sufficient information to calculate the median of the contracted rates described in clause (i)(I) in the year previous to such first subsequent year.

(III) NEWLY COVERED ITEM OR SERVICE.—The term "newly covered item or service" means, with respect to a group health plan or health insurance issuer offering health insurance coverage in the group market, an item or service for which coverage was not offered in 2019

under such plan or coverage, but is offered under such plan or coverage in a year after 2019.

(F) NONPARTICIPATING EMERGENCY FACILITY; PARTICIPATING EMERGENCY FACILITY.—

(i) NONPARTICIPATING EMERGENCY FACILITY.—The term "nonparticipating emergency facility" means, with respect to an item or service and a group health plan or health insurance coverage offered by a health insurance issuer in the group market, an emergency department of a hospital, or an independent freestanding emergency department, that does not have a contractual relationship directly or indirectly with the plan or issuer, respectively, for furnishing such item or service under the plan or coverage, respectively.

(ii) PARTICIPATING EMERGENCY FACILITY.—The term "participating emergency facility" means, with respect to an item or service and a group health plan or health insurance coverage offered by a health insurance issuer in the group market, an emergency department of a hospital, or an independent freestanding emergency department, that has a contractual relationship directly or indirectly with the plan or issuer, respectively, with respect to the furnishing of such an item or service at such facility.

(G) NONPARTICIPATING PROVIDERS; PARTICIPATING PROVIDERS.—

(i) NONPARTICIPATING PROVIDER.—The term "nonparticipating provider" means, with respect to an item or service and a group health plan or health insurance coverage offered by a health insurance issuer in the group market, a physician or other health care provider who is acting within the scope of practice of that provider's license or certification under applicable State law and who does not have a contractual relationship with the plan or issuer, respectively, for furnishing such item or service under the plan or coverage, respectively.

(ii) PARTICIPATING PROVIDER.—The term "participating provider" means, with respect to an item or service and a group health plan or health insurance coverage offered by a health insurance issuer in the group market, a physician or other health care provider who is acting within the scope of practice of that provider's license or certification under applicable State law and who has a contractual relationship with the plan or issuer, respectively, for furnishing such item or service under the plan or coverage, respectively.

(H) RECOGNIZED AMOUNT.—The term "recognized amount" means, with respect to an item or service furnished by a nonparticipating provider or emergency facility during a year and a group health plan or health insurance coverage offered by a health insurance issuer in the group market—

(i) subject to clause (iii), in the case of such item or service furnished in a State that has in effect a specified State law with respect to such plan, coverage, or issuer, respectively, such a nonparticipating provider or emergency facility, and such an item or service, the amount determined in accordance with such law;

(ii) subject to clause (iii), in the case of such item or service furnished in a State that does not have in effect a specified State law, with respect to such plan, coverage, or issuer, respectively, such a nonparticipating provider or emergency facility, and such an item or service, an amount that is the median contracted rate (as defined in subparagraph (E)) for such year and determined in accordance with rulemaking described in paragraph (2)(B)) for such item or service; or

(iii) in the case of such item or service furnished in a State with an All-Payer Model Agreement under section 1115A of the Social Security Act, the amount that the State approves under such system for such item or service so furnished.

(I) SPECIFIED STATE LAW.—The term "specified State law" means, with respect to a State, an item or service furnished by a nonparticipating provider or emergency facility during a year and a group health plan or health insurance coverage offered by a health insurance issuer in the group market, a State law that provides for a method for determining the amount of payment that is required to be covered by such a plan, coverage, or issuer, respectively (to the extent such State law applies to such plan, coverage, or issuer, subject to section 514) in the case of a participant or beneficiary covered under such plan or coverage and receiving such item or service from such a nonparticipating provider or emergency facility.

(J) STABILIZE.—The term "to stabilize," with respect to an emergency medical condition (as defined in subparagraph (B)), has the meaning give in section 1867(e)(3) of the Social Security Act (42 U.S.C. 1395dd(e)(3)).

(c) ACCESS TO PEDIATRIC CARE.—

(1) PEDIATRIC CARE.—In the case of a person who has a child who is a participant or beneficiary under a group health plan, or health insurance coverage offered by a health insurance issuer in the group market, if the plan or issuer requires or provides for the designation of a participating primary care provider for the child, the plan or issuer shall permit such person to designate a physician (allopathic or osteopathic) who specializes in pediatrics as the child's primary care provider if such provider participates in the network of the plan or issuer.

(2) CONSTRUCTION.—Nothing in paragraph (1) shall be construed to waive any exclusions of coverage under the terms and conditions of the plan or health insurance coverage with respect to coverage of pediatric care.

(d) PATIENT ACCESS TO OBSTETRICAL AND GYNECOLOGICAL CARE.—

(1) GENERAL RIGHTS.—

(A) DIRECT ACCESS.—A group health plan, or health insurance issuer offering group health insurance coverage, described in paragraph (2) may not require authorization or referral by the plan, issuer, or any person (including a primary care provider described in paragraph (2)(B)) in the case of a female participant or beneficiary who seeks coverage for obstetrical or gynecological care provided by a participating health care professional who specializes in obstetrics or gynecology. Such professional shall agree to otherwise adhere to such plan's or issuer's policies and procedures, including procedures regarding referrals and obtaining prior authorization and

providing services pursuant to a treatment plan (if any) approved by the plan or issuer.

(B) OBSTETRICAL AND GYNECOLOGICAL CARE.—A group health plan or health insurance issuer described in paragraph (2) shall treat the provision of obstetrical and gynecological care, and the ordering of related obstetrical and gynecological items and services, pursuant to the direct access described under subparagraph (A), by a participating health care professional who specializes in obstetrics or gynecology as the authorization of the primary care provider.

(2) APPLICATION OF PARAGRAPH.—A group health plan, or health insurance issuer offering group health insurance coverage, described in this paragraph is a group health plan or coverage that—

(A) provides coverage for obstetric or gynecologic care; and

(B) requires the designation by a participant or beneficiary of a participating primary care provider.

(3) CONSTRUCTION.—Nothing in paragraph (1) shall be construed to—

(A) waive any exclusions of coverage under the terms and conditions of the plan or health insurance coverage with respect to coverage of obstetrical or gynecological care; or

(B) preclude the group health plan or health insurance issuer involved from requiring that the obstetrical or gynecological provider notify the primary care health care professional or the plan or issuer of treatment decisions.

(e) COVERAGE OF NON-EMERGENCY SERVICES PERFORMED BY NONPARTICIPATING PROVIDERS AT CERTAIN PARTICIPATING FACILITIES.—

(1) IN GENERAL.—In the case of items or services (other than emergency services to which subsection (b) applies) for which any benefits are provided or covered by a group health plan or health insurance issuer offering health insurance coverage in the group market furnished to a participant or beneficiary of such plan or coverage by a nonparticipating provider (as defined in subsection (b)(3)(G)(i)) (and who, with respect to such items and services, has not satisfied the notice and consent criteria of section 2799A–2(d) of the Public Health Service Act) with respect to a visit (as defined by the Secretary in accordance with paragraph (2)(B)) at a participating health care facility (as defined in paragraph (2)(A)), with respect to such plan or coverage, respectively, the plan or coverage, respectively—

(A) shall not impose on such participant or beneficiary a cost-sharing amount (expressed as a copayment amount or coinsurance rate) for such items and services so furnished that is greater than the cost-sharing amount that would apply under such plan or coverage, respectively, had such items or services been furnished by a participating provider (as defined in subsection (b)(3)(G)(ii));

(B) shall calculate such cost-sharing amount as if the total amount that would have been charged for such items and services by such participating provider were equal to the recognized amount (as defined in subsection (b)(3)(H)) for such items and services, plan or coverage, and year;

(C) shall pay to such provider furnishing such items and services to such participant or beneficiary the amount by which the recognized amount (as defined in subsection (b)(3)(H)) for such items and services and year involved exceeds the cost-sharing amount imposed under the plan or coverage, respectively, for such items and services (as determined in accordance with subparagraphs (A) and (B)); and

(D) shall count toward any in-network deductible and in-network out-of-pocket maximums (as applicable) applied under the plan or coverage, respectively, any cost-sharing payments made by the participant or beneficiary (and such in-network deductible and out-of-pocket maximums shall be applied) with respect to such items and services so furnished in the same manner as if such cost-sharing payments were with respect to items and services furnished by a participating provider.

(2) DEFINITIONS.—In this section:

(A) PARTICIPATING HEALTH CARE FACILITY.—

(i) IN GENERAL.—The term "participating health care facility" means, with respect to an item or service and a group health plan or health insurance issuer offering health insurance coverage in the group market, a health care facility described in clause (ii) that has a contractual relationship with the plan or issuer, respectively, with respect to the furnishing of such an item or service at the facility.

(ii) HEALTH CARE FACILITY DESCRIBED.—A health care facility described in this clause, with respect to a group health plan or health insurance coverage offered in the group market, is each of the following:

(I) A hospital (as defined in 1861(e) of the Social Security Act).

(II) A hospital outpatient department.

(III) A critical access hospital (as defined in section 1861(mm) of such Act).

(IV) An ambulatory surgical center (as defined in section 1833(i)(1)(A) of such Act).

(V) Any other facility that provides items or services for which coverage is provided under the plan or coverage, respectively.

(B) VISIT.—The term "visit" shall, with respect to items and services furnished to an individual at a participating health care facility, include equipment and devices, telemedicine services, imaging services, laboratory services, and such other items and services as the Secretary may specify, regardless of whether or not the provider furnishing such items or services is at the facility.

(f) AIR AMBULANCE SERVICES.—

(1) IN GENERAL.—In the case of a participant or beneficiary in a group health plan or health insurance coverage offered in the group market who receives air ambulance services from a nonparticipating provider (as defined in subsection (b)(3)(G)) with respect to such plan or coverage, if such services would be covered if provided by a participating provider (as defined in such subsection) with respect to such plan or coverage—

(A) the cost-sharing requirement (expressed as a copayment amount, coinsurance rate, or deductible) with respect to such services shall be the same

requirement that would apply if such services were provided by such a participating provider, and any coinsurance or deductible shall be based on rates that would apply for such services if they were furnished by such a participating provider;

(B) such cost-sharing amounts shall be counted toward the in-network deductible and in-network out-of-pocket maximum amount under the plan or coverage for the plan year (and such in-network deductible shall be applied) with respect to such items and services so furnished in the same manner as if such cost-sharing payments were with respect to items and services furnished by a participating provider; and

(C) the plan or coverage shall pay to such provider furnishing such services to such participant or beneficiary the amount by which the recognized amount (as defined in and determined pursuant to subsection (b)(3)(H)(ii)) for such services and year involved exceeds the cost-sharing amount imposed under the plan or coverage, respectively, for such services (as determined in accordance with subparagraphs (A) and (B)).

(2) AIR AMBULANCE SERVICE DEFINED.—For purposes of this section, the term "air ambulance service" means medical transport by helicopter or airplane for patients.

(g) CERTAIN ACCESS FEES TO CERTAIN DATABASES.—In the case of a sponsor of a group health plan or health insurance issuer offering health insurance coverage in the group market that, pursuant to subsection (b)(3)(E)(iii), uses a database described in such subsection to determine a rate to apply under such subsection for an item or service by reason of having insufficient information described in such subsection with respect to such item or service, such sponsor or issuer shall cover the cost for access to such database.

(h) DISCLOSURE OF CERTAIN PROTECTIONS AGAINST BALANCE BILLING.—Each group health plan and health insurance issuer offering group health insurance coverage shall make publicly available, and (if applicable) post on a public website of such plan or issuer—

(1) information in plain language on—

(A) the requirements and prohibitions applied under sections 2799A–1, 2799A–2 and 2799A–4 of the Public Health Service Act (relating to prohibitions on balance billing in certain circumstances);

(B) if provided for under applicable State law, any other requirements on providers and facilities regarding the amounts such providers and facilities may, with respect to an item or service, charge a participant, beneficiary, or enrollee of such plan or coverage with respect to which such a provider or facility does not have a contractual relationship for furnishing such item or service under the plan or coverage after receiving payment from the plan or coverage for such item or service and any applicable cost-sharing payment from such participant, beneficiary, or enrollee; and

(C) the requirements applied under subsections (b), (e), and (f); and

(2) information on contacting appropriate State and Federal agencies in the case that an individual believes that such a provider or facility has violated any requirement described in paragraph (1) with respect to such individual.

(i) STANDARDIZED REPORTING FORMAT.—

(1) IN GENERAL.—Not later than 1 year after the date of enactment of this subsection, the Secretary shall establish a standardized reporting format for the reporting, by group health plans (or health insurance coverage offered in connection with such a plan) to State All Payer Claims Databases, of medical claims, pharmacy claims, dental claims, and eligibility and provider files that are collected from private and public payers, and shall provide guidance to States on the process by which States may collect such data from such plans or coverage in the standardized reporting format.

(2) DEFINITION.—In this subsection, the term "State All Payer Claims Database" means, with respect to a State, a database that may include medical claims, pharmacy claims, dental claims, and eligibility and provider files, which are collected from private and public payers.

(j) TRANSPARENCY REGARDING IN-NETWORK AND OUT-OF-NETWORK DEDUCTIBLES AND OUT-OF-POCKET LIMITATIONS.—

(1) IN GENERAL.—A group health plan or a health insurance issuer offering group health insurance coverage and providing or covering any benefit with respect to items or services shall include, in clear writing, on any plan or insurance identification card issued to participants or beneficiaries in the plan or coverage the amount of the in-network and out-of-network deductibles and the in-network and out-of-network out-of-pocket maximum limitation that apply to such plan or coverage.

(2) GUIDANCE.—The Secretary, in consultation with the Secretary of Health and Human Services and Secretary of the Treasury, shall issue guidance to implement paragraph (1).

SEC. 717. PROTECTING PATIENTS AND IMPROVING THE ACCURACY OF PROVIDER DIRECTORY INFORMATION.

(a) NETWORK STATUS OF PROVIDERS.—

(1) IN GENERAL.—Beginning on the date that is one year after the date of enactment of this section, a group health plan (or health insurance coverage offered in connection with such a plan) shall—

(A) establish business processes to ensure that all participants and beneficiaries in such plan or coverage receive proof of a health care provider's network status, based on what a plan or issuer of such coverage knows or should know—

(i) upon a telephone inquiry by a participant or beneficiary—

(I) through a written electronic communication from the plan or issuer to the participant or beneficiary, as soon as practicable and not later than 1 business day after such inquiry is made by such participant or beneficiary for such information;

(II) through an oral communication from the plan or issuer to the participant or beneficiary, as soon as practicable and not later than

1 business day after such inquiry is made by such participant or beneficiary for such information, which communication shall be documented by such plan or issuer, and such documentation shall be kept in the participant's or beneficiary's file for a minimum of 5 years; and

(ii) in real-time through an online health care provider directory search tool maintained by the plan or issuer; and

(B) include in any print directory—

(i) a disclosure that the information included in the directory is accurate as of the date of the last data update and that participants or beneficiaries or prospective participants or beneficiaries should consult the group health plan's or issuer's electronic provider directory on its website or call a specified customer service telephone number to obtain the most current provider directory information; and

(ii) a list of the categories of providers of ancillary services for which the plan or coverage has no in-network providers.

(2) GROUP HEALTH PLAN AND HEALTH INSURANCE ISSUER BUSINESS PROCESSES.—Beginning on the date that is one year after the date of enactment of this section, a group health plan (or health insurance coverage offered in connection with such a plan) shall establish business processes to—

(A) verify and update, at least once every 90 days, the provider directory information for all providers included in the online health care provider directory search tool described in paragraph (1)(A)(ii); and

(B) remove any provider from such online directory search tool if such provider has not verified the directory information within the previous 6 months or the plan or issuer has been unable to verify the provider's network participation.

(b) COST-SHARING LIMITATIONS.—A group health plan (or health insurance coverage offered in connection with such a plan) shall not apply, and shall ensure that no provider applies, cost-sharing to a participant or beneficiary for treatment or services provided by a health care provider in excess of the normal cost-sharing applied for such treatment or services provided in-network (including any balance bill issued by the health care provider involved), if such participant or beneficiary, or health care provider referring such participant or beneficiary, demonstrates (based on the electronic, written information described in subsection (a)(1)(A)(i)(I), the oral confirmation described in subsection (a)(1)(A)(i)(II) received by the participant or beneficiary not more than 30 days before the date the treatment or services were received, or a copy of the online provider directory described in subsection (a)(1)(A)(ii) on a date not more than 30 days before the date the treatment or services were received), that the participant or beneficiary relied on the information described in subsection (a)(1) for which such participant or beneficiary provides such documentation, that indicated that the provider is an in-network provider, if the provider was out-of-network at the time the treatment or service involved was received.

(c) DEFINITION.—For purposes of this section, the term "provider directory information" includes the names, addresses, specialty, and telephone numbers of individual health care providers, and the names, addresses, and telephone numbers of

each medical group, clinic, or facility contracted to participate in any of the networks of the group health plan or health insurance coverage involved.

SEC. 718. PROVISION OF COST-SHARING INFORMATION.

A group health plan (or health insurance coverage offered in connection with such a plan) shall provide a participant or beneficiary in the plan or coverage with a good faith estimate of the participant's or beneficiary's cost-sharing (including deductibles, copayments, and coinsurance) for which the participant or beneficiary may be responsible for paying with respect to a specific health care service (including any service that is reasonably expected to be provided in conjunction with such specific service), as soon as practicable and not later than 2 business days after a request for such information by a participant or beneficiary. For purposes of the previous sentence, the Secretary shall develop and make available in multiple languages (as specified by the Secretary) a model form that is in easily understandable language and format.

SEC. 719. CONTINUITY OF CARE.

(a) ENSURING CONTINUITY OF CARE WITH RESPECT TO TERMINATIONS OF CERTAIN CONTRACTUAL RELATIONSHIPS RESULTING IN CHANGES IN PROVIDER NETWORK STATUS.—

(1) IN GENERAL.—In the case of an individual with benefits under a group health plan or health insurance coverage offered by a health insurance issuer in connection with a group health plan and with respect to a health care provider or facility that has a contractual relationship with such plan or such issuer (as applicable) for furnishing items and services under such plan or such coverage, if, while such individual is a continuing care patient (as defined in subsection (b)) with respect to such provider or facility—

(A) such contractual relationship is terminated (as defined in paragraph (b));

(B) benefits provided under such plan or such health insurance coverage with respect to such provider or facility are terminated because of a change in the terms of the participation of the provider or facility in such plan or coverage; or

(C) a contract between such group health plan and a health insurance issuer offering health insurance coverage in connection with such plan is terminated, resulting in a loss of benefits provided under such plan with respect to such provider or facility; the plan or issuer, respectively, shall meet the requirements of paragraph (2) with respect to such individual.

(2) REQUIREMENTS.—The requirements of this paragraph are that the plan or issuer—

(A) notify each individual enrolled under such plan or coverage who is a continuing care patient with respect to a provider or facility at the time of a termination described in paragraph (1) affecting such provider or facility on

a timely basis of such termination and such individual's right to elect continued transitional care from such provider or facility under this section;

(B) provide such individual with an opportunity to notify the plan or issuer of the individual's need for transitional care; and

(C) permit the patient to elect to continue to have benefits provided under such plan or such coverage, under the same terms and conditions as would have applied and with respect to such items and services as would have been covered under such plan or coverage had such termination not occurred, with respect to the course of treatment furnished by such provider or facility relating to such individual's status as a continuing care patient during the period beginning on the date on which the notice under subparagraph (A) is provided and ending on the earlier of—

(i) the 90-day period beginning on such date; or

(ii) the date on which such individual is no longer a continuing care patient with respect to such provider or facility.

(b) DEFINITIONS.—In this section:

(1) CONTINUING CARE PATIENT.—The term "continuing care patient" means an individual who, with respect to a provider or facility—

(A) is undergoing a course of treatment for a serious and complex condition from the provider or facility;

(B) is undergoing a course of institutional or inpatient care from the provider or facility;

(C) is scheduled to undergo nonelective surgery from the provide or facility, including receipt of postoperative care from such provider or facility with respect to such a surgery;

(D) is pregnant and undergoing a course of treatment for the pregnancy from the provider or facility; or

(E) is or was determined to be terminally ill (as determined under section 1861(dd)(3)(A) of the Social Security Act) and is receiving treatment for such illness from such provider or facility.

(2) SERIOUS AND COMPLEX CONDITION.—The term "serious and complex condition" means, with respect to a participant, beneficiary, or enrollee under a group health plan or health insurance coverage—

(A) in the case of an acute illness, a condition that is serious enough to require specialized medical treatment to avoid the reasonable possibility of death or permanent harm; or

(B) in the case of a chronic illness or condition, a condition that—

(i) is life-threatening, degenerative, potentially disabling, or congenital; and

(ii) requires specialized medical care over a prolonged period of time.

(3) TERMINATED.—The term "terminated" includes, with respect to a contract, the expiration or nonrenewal of the contract, but does not include a termination of the contract for failure to meet applicable quality standards or for fraud.

Internal Revenue Code of 1986

Subtitle K—Group Health Plan Requirements

Chapter 100—Group Health Plan Requirements

Subchapter B—Other Requirements

Sec. 9811. Standards relating to benefits for mothers and newborns.

Sec. 9815. Additional market reforms. Sec. 9816. Consumer protections.

Sec.9817. Protecting patients and improving the accuracy of provider directory information.

Sec. 9818. Provision of cost-sharing information.

SEC. 9816. CONSUMER PROTECTIONS.

(a) CHOICE OF HEALTH CARE PROFESSIONAL.—If a group health plan requires or provides for designation by a participant or beneficiary of a participating primary care provider, then the plan shall permit each participant or beneficiary to designate any participating primary care provider who is available to accept such individual.

(b) COVERAGE OF EMERGENCY SERVICES.—

(1) IN GENERAL.—If a group health plan provides or covers any benefits with respect to services in an emergency department of a hospital or with respect to emergency services in an independent freestanding emergency department (as defined in paragraph (3)(D)), the plan shall cover emergency services (as defined in paragraph (3)(C))—

(A) without the need for any prior authorization determination;

(B) whether the health care provider furnishing such services is a participating provider or a participating emergency facility, as applicable, with respect to such services;

(C) in a manner so that, if such services are provided to a participant or beneficiary by a nonparticipating provider or a nonparticipating emergency facility—

(i) such services will be provided without imposing any requirement under the plan for prior authorization of services or any limitation on coverage that is more restrictive than the requirements or limitations that apply to emergency services received from participating providers and participating emergency facilities with respect to such plan;

(ii) the cost-sharing requirement (expressed as a copayment amount or coinsurance rate) is not greater than the requirement that would apply if such services were provided by a participating provider or a participating emergency facility;

(iii) such cost-sharing requirement is calculated as if the total amount that would have been charged for such services by such participating provider or participating emergency facility were equal to the recognized amount (as defined in paragraph (3)(H)) for such services, plan, and year;

(iv) *the group health plan pays to such provider or facility, respectively, the amount by which the recognized amount for such services and year involved exceeds the cost-sharing amount for such services (as determined in accordance with clauses (ii) and (iii)) and year; and*

(v) *any cost-sharing payments made by the participant or beneficiary with respect to such emergency services so furnished shall be counted toward any in-network deductible or out-of-pocket maximums applied under the plan (and such in-network deductible and out-of-pocket maximums shall be applied) in the same manner as if such cost-sharing payments were made with respect to emergency services furnished by a participating provider or a participating emergency facility; and*

(D) *without regard to any other term or condition of such coverage (other than exclusion or coordination of benefits, or an affiliation or waiting period, permitted under section 2704 of this Act, including as incorporated pursuant to section 715 of the Employee Retirement Income Security Act of 1974 and section 9815 of this Act, and other than applicable cost-sharing).*

(2) *AUDIT PROCESS AND REGULATIONS FOR MEDIAN CONTRACTED RATES.—*

(A) *AUDIT PROCESS.—*

(i) *IN GENERAL.—Not later than July 1, 2021, the Secretary, in consultation with appropriate State agencies and the Secretary of Health and Human Services and the Secretary of Labor, shall establish through rulemaking a process, in accordance with clause (ii), under which group health plans are audited by the Secretary or applicable State authority to ensure that—*

(I) *such plans are in compliance with the requirement of applying a median contracted rate under this section; and*

(II) *such median contracted rate so applied satisfies the definition under paragraph (3)(E) with respect to the year involved, including with respect to a group health plan described in clause (ii) of such paragraph (3)(E).*

(ii) *AUDIT SAMPLES.—Under the process established pursuant to clause (i), the Secretary—*

(I) *shall conduct audits described in such clause, with respect to a year (beginning with 2022), of a sample with respect to such year of claims data from not more than 25 group health plans; and*

(II) *may audit any group health plan if the Secretary has received any complaint about such plan or coverage, respectively, that involves the compliance of the plan with either of the requirements described in subclauses (I) and (II) of such clause.*

(iii) *REPORTS.—Beginning for 2022, the Secretary shall annually submit to Congress a report on the number of plans and issuers with respect to which audits were conducted during such year pursuant to this subparagraph.*

(B) RULEMAKING.—Not later than July 1, 2021, the Secretary, in consultation with the Secretary of Labor and the Secretary of Health and Human Services, shall establish through rulemaking—

(i) the methodology the group health plan shall use to determine the median contracted rate, differentiating by line of business;

(ii) the information such plan or issuer, respectively, shall share with the nonparticipating provider or nonparticipating facility, as applicable, when making such a determination;

(iii) the geographic regions applied for purposes of this subparagraph, taking into account access to items and services in rural and underserved areas, including health professional shortage areas, as defined in section 332 of the Public Health Service Act; and

(iv) a process to receive complaints of violations of the requirements described in subclauses (I) and (II) of paragraph (2)(A)(i) by group health plans.

Such rulemaking shall take into account payments that are made by such plan that are not on a fee-for-service basis. Such methodology may account for relevant payment adjustments that take into account quality or facility type (including higher acuity settings and the case-mix of various facility types) that are otherwise taken into account for purposes of determining payment amounts with respect to participating facilities. In carrying out clause (iii), the Secretary shall consult with the National Association of Insurance Commissioners to establish the geographic regions under such clause and shall periodically update such regions, as appropriate.

(3) DEFINITIONS.—In this section:

(A) EMERGENCY DEPARTMENT OF A HOSPITAL.—The term "emergency department of a hospital" includes a hospital outpatient department that provides emergency services.

(B) EMERGENCY MEDICAL CONDITION.—The term "emergency medical condition" means a medical condition manifesting itself by acute symptoms of sufficient severity (including severe pain) such that a prudent layperson, who possesses an average knowledge of health and medicine, could reasonably expect the absence of immediate medical attention to result in a condition described in clause (i), (ii), or (iii) of section 1867(e)(1)(A) of the Social Security Act.

(C) EMERGENCY SERVICES.—

(i) IN GENERAL.—The term "emergency services," with respect to an emergency medical condition, means—

(I) a medical screening examination (as required under section 1867 of the Social Security Act, or as would be required under such section if such section applied to an independent freestanding emergency department) that is within the capability of the emergency department of a hospital or of an independent freestanding emergency department, as applicable, including ancillary services routinely

available to the emergency department to evaluate such emergency medical condition; and

(II) within the capabilities of the staff and facilities available at the hospital or the independent freestanding emergency department, as applicable, such further medical examination and treatment as are required under section 1867 of such Act, or as would be required under such section if such section applied to an independent freestanding emergency department, to stabilize the patient.

(ii) INCLUSION OF CERTAIN SERVICES OUTSIDE OF EMERGENCY DEPARTMENT.—

(I) IN GENERAL.—For purposes of this subsection and section 2799A–1, in the case of an individual enrolled in a group health plan or health insurance coverage offered by a health insurance issuer in the group or individual market who is furnished services described in clause (i) by a participating or nonparticipating provider or a participating or nonparticipating emergency facility to stabilize such individual with respect to an emergency medical condition, the term "emergency services" shall include, unless each of the conditions described in subclause (II) are met, in addition to the items and services described in clause (i), items and services for which benefits are provided or covered under the plan or coverage, respectively, furnished by a nonparticipating provider or nonparticipating facility, regardless of the department of the hospital in which such individual is furnished such items or services, if, after such stabilization but during such visit in which such individual is so stabilized, the provider or facility determines that such items or services are needed.

(II) CONDITIONS.—For purposes of subclause (I), the conditions described in this subclause, with respect to an individual who is stabilized and furnished additional items and services described in subclause (I) after such stabilization by a provider or facility described in subclause (I), are the following:

(aa) Such a provider or facility determines such individual is able to travel using nonmedical transportation or nonemergency medical transportation.

(bb) Such provider furnishing such additional items and services satisfies the notice and consent criteria of section 2799A–2(d) of the Public Health Service Act with respect to such items and services.

(cc) Such an individual is in a condition to receive (as determined in accordance with guidance issued by the Secretary) the information described in section 2799A–2 of the Public Health Service Act and to provide informed consent under such section, in accordance with applicable State law.

(D) INDEPENDENT FREESTANDING EMERGENCY DEPARTMENT.—The term "independent freestanding emergency department" means a facility that—

(i) *is geographically separate and distinct and licensed separately from a hospital under applicable State law; and*

(ii) *provides any emergency services (as defined in subparagraph (C)).*

(E) *MEDIAN CONTRACTED RATE.—*

(i) *IN GENERAL.—The term "median contracted rate" means, subject to clauses (ii) and (iii), with respect to a sponsor of a group health plan—*

(I) *for an item or service furnished during 2022, the median of the contracted rates recognized by the plan (determined with respect to all such plans of such sponsor that are offered within the same line of business as the total maximum payment (including the cost-sharing amount imposed for such item or service and the amount to be paid by the plan) under such plans on January 31, 2019 for the same or a similar item or service that is provided by a provider in the same or similar specialty and provided in the geographic region in which the item or service is furnished, consistent with the methodology established by the Secretary under paragraph (2)(B), increased by the percentage increase in the consumer price index for all urban consumers (United States city average) over 2019, such percentage increase over 2020, and such percentage increase over 2021; and*

(II) *for an item or service furnished during 2023 or a subsequent year, the median contracted rate determined under this clause for such an item or service furnished in the previous year, increased by the percentage increase in the consumer price index for all urban consumers (United States city average) over such previous year.*

(ii) *NEW PLANS AND COVERAGE.—The term "median contracted rate" means, with respect to a sponsor of a group health plan in a geographic region in which such sponsor, respectively, did not offer any group health plan or health insurance coverage during 2019—*

(I) *for the first year in which such group health plan is offered in such region, a rate (determined in accordance with a methodology established by the Secretary) for items and services that are covered by such plan and furnished during such first year; and*

(II) *for each subsequent year such group health plan is offered in such region, the median contracted rate determined under this clause for such items and services furnished in the previous year, increased by the percentage increase in the consumer price index for all urban consumers (United States city average) over such previous year.*

(iii) *INSUFFICIENT INFORMATION; NEWLY COVERED ITEMS AND SERVICES.—In the case of a sponsor of a group health plan that does not have sufficient information to calculate the median of the contracted rates described in clause (i)(I) in 2019 (or, in the case of a newly covered item or service (as defined in clause (iv)(III)), in the first coverage year (as defined in clause (iv)(I)) for such item or service with respect to such plan) for an item or service (including with respect to provider type, or amount, of claims for items or services (as determined by the Secretary) provided in a particular geographic region (other than in a case with respect to which clause (ii) applies)) the term "median contracted rate"—*

(I) for an item or service furnished during 2022 (or, in the case of a newly covered item or service, during the first coverage year for such item or service with respect to such plan), means such rate for such item or service determined by the sponsor through use of any database that is determined, in accordance with rulemaking described in paragraph (2)(B), to not have any conflicts of interest and to have sufficient information reflecting allowed amounts paid to a health care provider or facility for relevant services furnished in the applicable geographic region (such as a State all-payer claims database);

(II) for an item or service furnished in a subsequent year (before the first sufficient information year (as defined in clause (iv)(II)) for such item or service with respect to such plan), means the rate determined under subclause (I) or this subclause, as applicable, for such item or service for the year previous to such subsequent year, increased by the percentage increase in the consumer price index for all urban consumers (United States city average) over such previous year;

(III) for an item or service furnished in the first sufficient information year for such item or service with respect to such plan, has the meaning given the term median contracted rate in clause (i)(I), except that in applying such clause to such item or service, the reference to "furnished during 2022" shall be treated as a reference to furnished during such first sufficient information year, the reference to "on January 31, 2019" shall be treated as a reference to in such sufficient information year, and the increase described in such clause shall not be applied; and

(IV) for an item or service furnished in any year subsequent to the first sufficient information year for such item or service with respect to such plan, has the meaning given such term in clause (i)(II), except that in applying such clause to such item or service, the reference to "furnished during 2023 or a subsequent year" shall be treated as a reference to furnished during the year after such first sufficient information year or a subsequent year.

(iv) DEFINITIONS.—For purposes of this subparagraph:

(I) FIRST COVERAGE YEAR.—The term "first coverage year" means, with respect to a group health plan and an item or service for which coverage is not offered in 2019 under such plan or coverage, the first year after 2019 for which coverage for such item or service is offered under such plan.

(II) FIRST SUFFICIENT INFORMATION YEAR.—The term "first sufficient information year" means, with respect to a group health plan—

(aa) in the case of an item or service for which the plan does not have sufficient information to calculate the median of the contracted

rates described in clause (i)(I) in 2019, the first year subsequent to 2022 for which such sponsor has such sufficient information to calculate the median of such contracted rates in the year previous to such first subsequent year; and

(bb) in the case of a newly covered item or service, the first year subsequent to the first coverage year for such item or service with respect to such plan for which the sponsor has sufficient information to calculate the median of the contracted rates described in clause (i)(I) in the year previous to such first subsequent year.

(III) NEWLY COVERED ITEM OR SERVICE.—The term "newly covered item or service" means, with respect to a group health plan, an item or service for which coverage was not offered in 2019 under such plan or coverage, but is offered under such plan or coverage in a year after 2019.

(F) NONPARTICIPATING EMERGENCY FACILITY; PARTICIPATING EMERGENCY FACILITY.—

(i) NONPARTICIPATING EMERGENCY FACILITY.—The term "nonparticipating emergency facility" means, with respect to an item or service and a group health plan, an emergency department of a hospital, or an independent freestanding emergency department, that does not have a contractual relationship directly or indirectly with the plan for furnishing such item or service under the plan.

(ii) PARTICIPATING EMERGENCY FACILITY.—The term "participating emergency facility" means, with respect to an item or service and a group health plan, an emergency department of a hospital, or an independent free-standing emergency department, that has a contractual relationship directly or indirectly with the plan, with respect to the furnishing of such an item or service at such facility.

(G) NONPARTICIPATING PROVIDERS; PARTICIPATING PROVIDERS.—

(i) NONPARTICIPATING PROVIDER.—The term "nonparticipating provider" means, with respect to an item or service and a group health plan, a physician or other health care provider who is acting within the scope of practice of that provider's license or certification under applicable State law and who does not have a contractual relationship with the plan or issuer, respectively, for furnishing such item or service under the plan.

(ii) PARTICIPATING PROVIDER.—The term "participating provider" means, with respect to an item or service and a group health plan, a physician or other health care provider who is acting within the scope of practice of that provider's license or certification under applicable State law and who has a contractual relationship with the plan for furnishing such item or service under the plan.

(H) RECOGNIZED AMOUNT.—The term "recognized amount" means, with respect to an item or service furnished by a nonparticipating provider or emergency facility during a year and a group health plan—

(i) subject to clause (iii), in the case of such item or service furnished in a State that has in effect a specified State law with respect to such plan; such a nonparticipating provider or emergency facility; and such an item or service, the amount determined in accordance with such law;

(ii) subject to clause (iii), in the case of such item or service furnished in a State that does not have in effect a specified State law, with respect to such plan; such a nonparticipating provider or emergency facility; and such an item or service, an amount that is the median contracted rate (as defined in subparagraph (E)) for such year and determined in accordance with rulemaking described in paragraph (2)(B)) for such item or service; or

(iii) in the case of such item or service furnished in a State with an All-Payer Model Agreement under section 1115A of the Social Security Act, the amount that the State approves under such system for such item or service so furnished.

(I) SPECIFIED STATE LAW.—The term "specified State law" means, with respect to a State, an item or service furnished by a nonparticipating provider or emergency facility during a year and a group health plan, a State law that provides for a method for determining the amount of payment that is required to be covered by such a plan (to the extent such State law applies to such plan, subject to section 514 of the Employee Retirement Income Security Act of 1974) in the case of a participant or beneficiary covered under such plan and receiving such item or service from such a nonparticipating provider or emergency facility.

(J) STABILIZE.—The term "to stabilize," with respect to an emergency medical condition (as defined in subparagraph (B)), has the meaning give in section 1867(e)(3) of the Social Security Act (42 U.S.C. 1395dd(e)(3)).

(c) ACCESS TO PEDIATRIC CARE.—

(1) PEDIATRIC CARE.—In the case of a person who has a child who is a participant or beneficiary under a group health plan, if the plan requires or provides for the designation of a participating primary care provider for the child, the plan shall permit such person to designate a physician (allopathic or osteopathic) who specializes in pediatrics as the child's primary care provider if such provider participates in the network of the plan or issuer.

(2) CONSTRUCTION.—Nothing in paragraph (1) shall be construed to waive any exclusions of coverage under the terms and conditions of the plan with respect to coverage of pediatric care.

(d) PATIENT ACCESS TO OBSTETRICAL AND GYNECOLOGICAL CARE.—

(1) GENERAL RIGHTS.—

(A) DIRECT ACCESS.—A group health plan described in paragraph (2) may not require authorization or referral by the plan or any person (including a primary care provider described in paragraph (2)(B)) in the case of a female participant or beneficiary who seeks coverage for obstetrical or gynecological care provided by a participating health care professional who specializes in obstetrics or gynecology. Such professional shall agree to otherwise adhere to such plan's policies and procedures, including

procedures regarding referrals and obtaining prior authorization and providing services pursuant to a treatment plan (if any) approved by the plan.

(B) OBSTETRICAL AND GYNECOLOGICAL CARE.—A group health plan described in paragraph (2) shall treat the provision of obstetrical and gynecological care, and the ordering of related obstetrical and gynecological items and services, pursuant to the direct access described under subparagraph (A), by a participating health care professional who specializes in obstetrics or gynecology as the authorization of the primary care provider.

(2) APPLICATION OF PARAGRAPH.—A group health plan described in this paragraph is a group health plan that—

(A) provides coverage for obstetric or gynecologic care; and

(B) requires the designation by a participant or beneficiary of a participating primary care provider.

(3) CONSTRUCTION.—Nothing in paragraph (1) shall be construed to—

(A) waive any exclusions of coverage under the terms and conditions of the plan with respect to coverage of obstetrical or gynecological care; or

(B) preclude the group health plan involved from requiring that the obstetrical or gynecological provider notify the primary care health care professional or the plan of treatment decisions.

(e) COVERAGE OF NON-EMERGENCY SERVICES PERFORMED BY NON-PARTICIPATING PROVIDERS AT CERTAIN PARTICIPATING FACILITIES.—

(1) IN GENERAL.—In the case of items or services (other than emergency services to which subsection (b) applies) for which any benefits are provided or covered by a group health plan furnished to a participant or beneficiary of such plan by a nonparticipating provider (as defined in subsection (b)(3)(G)(i)) (and who, with respect to such items and services, has not satisfied the notice and consent criteria of section 2799A–2(d) of the Public Health Service Act) with respect to a visit (as defined by the Secretary in accordance with paragraph (2)(B)) at a participating health care facility (as defined in paragraph (2)(A)), with respect to such plan, the plan—

(A) shall not impose on such participant or beneficiary a cost-sharing amount (expressed as a copayment amount or coinsurance rate) for such items and services so furnished that is greater than the cost-sharing amount that would apply under such plan had such items or services been furnished by a participating provider (as defined in subsection (b)(3)(G)(ii));

(B) shall calculate such cost-sharing amount as if the total amount that would have been charged for such items and services by such participating provider were equal to the recognized amount (as defined in subsection (b)(3)(H)) for such items and services, plan, and year;

(C) shall pay to such provider furnishing such items and services to such participant or beneficiary the amount by which the recognized amount (as defined in subsection (b)(3)(H)) for such items and services and year involved exceeds the cost-sharing amount imposed under the plan for such items and services (as determined in accordance with subparagraphs (A) and (B)); and

(D) shall count toward any in-network deductible and in-network out-of-pocket maximums (as applicable) applied under the plan, any cost-sharing payments

made by the participant or beneficiary (and such in-network deductible shall be applied) with respect to such items and services so furnished in the same manner as if such cost-sharing payments were with respect to items and services furnished by a participating provider.

(2) *DEFINITIONS.—In this section:*

(A) *PARTICIPATING HEALTH CARE FACILITY.—*

(i) *IN GENERAL.—The term "participating health care facility" means, with respect to an item or service and a group health plan, a health care facility described in clause (ii) that has a contractual relationship with the plan, with respect to the furnishing of such an item or service at the facility.*

(ii) *HEALTH CARE FACILITY DESCRIBED.—A health care facility described in this clause, with respect to a group health plan, is each of the following:*

(I) *A hospital (as defined in 1861(e) of the Social Security Act).*

(II) *A hospital outpatient department.*

(III) *A critical access hospital (as defined in section 1861(mm) of such Act).*

(IV) *An ambulatory surgical center (as defined in section 1833(i)(1)(A) of such Act).*

(V) *Any other facility that provides items or services for which coverage is provided under the plan or coverage, respectively.*

(B) *VISIT.—The term "visit" shall, with respect to items and services furnished to an individual at a participating health care facility, include equipment and devices, telemedicine services, imaging services, laboratory services, and such other items and services as the Secretary may specify, regardless of whether or not the provider furnishing such items or services is at the facility.*

(f) *AIR AMBULANCE SERVICES.—*

(1) *IN GENERAL.—In the case of a participant or beneficiary in a group health plan who receives air ambulance services from a nonparticipating provider (as defined in subsection (b)(3)(G)) with respect to such plan or coverage, if such services would be covered if provided by a participating provider (as defined in such subsection) with respect to such plan—*

(A) *the cost-sharing requirement (expressed as a copayment amount, coinsurance rate, or deductible) with respect to such services shall be the same requirement that would apply if such services were provided by such a participating provider, and any coinsurance or deductible shall be based on rates that would apply for such services if they were furnished by such a participating provider;*

(B) *such cost-sharing amounts shall be counted toward the in-network deductible and in-network out-of-pocket maximum amount under the plan for the plan year (and such in-network deductible shall be applied) with respect to such items and services so furnished in the same manner as if such cost-sharing payments were with respect to items and services furnished by a participating provider; and*

(C) the plan or coverage shall pay to such provider furnishing such services to such participant or beneficiary the amount by which the recognized amount (as defined in and determined pursuant to subsection (b)(3)(H)(ii)) for such services and year involved exceeds the cost-sharing amount imposed under the plan for such services (as determined in accordance with subparagraphs (A) and (B)).

(2) AIR AMBULANCE SERVICE DEFINED.—For purposes of this section, the term "air ambulance service" means medical transport by helicopter or airplane for patients.

(g) CERTAIN ACCESS FEES TO CERTAIN DATABASES.—In the case of a sponsor of a group health plan that, pursuant to subsection (b)(3)(E)(iii), uses a database described in such subsection to determine a rate to apply under such subsection for an item or service by reason of having insufficient information described in such subsection with respect to such item or service, such sponsor shall cover the cost for access to such database.

(h) TRANSPARENCY REGARDING IN-NETWORK AND OUT-OF-NETWORK DEDUCTIBLES AND OUT-OF-POCKET LIMITATIONS.—

(1) IN GENERAL.—A group health plan providing or covering any benefit with respect to items or services shall include, in clear writing, on any plan or insurance identification card issued to participants or beneficiaries in the plan the amount of the in-network and out-of-network deductibles and the in-network and out-of-network out-of-pocket maximum limitation that apply to such plan.

(2) GUIDANCE.—The Secretary, in consultation with the Secretary of Health and Human Services and Secretary of Labor, shall issue guidance to implement paragraph (1).

SEC. 9817. PROTECTING PATIENTS AND IMPROVING THE ACCURACY OF PROVIDER DIRECTORY INFORMATION.

(a) NETWORK STATUS OF PROVIDERS.—

(1) IN GENERAL.—Beginning on the date that is one year after the date of enactment of this section, a group health plan shall—

(A) establish business processes to ensure that all participants or beneficiaries in such plan receive proof of a health care provider's network status, based on what a plan or issuer knows or should know—

(i) upon a telephone inquiry by a participant or beneficiary—

(I) through a written electronic communication from the plan to the participant or beneficiary, as soon as practicable and not later than 1 business day after such inquiry is made by such participant or beneficiary for such information;

(II) through an oral communication from the plan to the participant or beneficiary, as soon as practicable and not later than 1 business day after such inquiry is made by such participant or beneficiary for such information, which communication shall be documented by such plan, and such documentation shall be kept in the participant's or beneficiary's file for a minimum of 2 years; and

(ii) in real-time through an online health care provider directory search tool maintained by the plan; and

(B) include in any print directory—

(i) a disclosure that the information included in the directory is accurate as of the date of the last data update and that participants or beneficiaries or prospective participants or beneficiaries should consult the group health plan's electronic provider directory on its website or call a specified customer service telephone number to obtain the most current provider directory information; and

(ii) a list of the categories of providers of ancillary services for which the plan or coverage has no in-network providers.

(2) GROUP HEALTH PLAN BUSINESS PROCESSES.—Beginning on the date that is one year after the date of enactment of this section, a group health plan shall establish business processes to—

(A) verify and update, at least once every 90 days, the provider directory information for all providers included in the online health care provider directory search tool described in paragraph (1)(A)(ii); and

(B) remove any provider from such online directory search tool if such provider has not verified the directory information within the previous 6 months or the plan or issuer has been unable to verify the provider's network participation.

(b) COST-SHARING LIMITATIONS.—A group health plan shall not apply, and shall ensure that no provider applies, cost-sharing to a participant or beneficiary for treatment or services provided by a health care provider in excess of the normal cost-sharing applied for such treatment or services provided in-network (including any balance bill issued by the health care provider involved), if such participant or beneficiary, or health care provider referring such participant or beneficiary, demonstrates (based on the electronic, written information described in subsection (a)(1)(A)(i)(I), the oral confirmation described in subsection (a)(1)(A)(i)(II) received by the participant or beneficiary not more than 30 days before the date the treatment or services were received, or a copy of the online provider directory described in subsection (a)(1)(A)(ii) on a date not more than 30 days before the date the treatment or services were received), that the participant or beneficiary relied on the information described in subsection (a)(1) for which such participant or beneficiary provides such documentation, that indicated that the provider is an in-network provider, if the provider was out-of-network at the time the treatment or service involved was received.

(c) DEFINITION.—For purposes of this section, the term "provider directory information" includes the names, addresses, specialty, and telephone numbers of individual health care providers, and the names, addresses, and telephone numbers of each medical group, clinic, or facility contracted to participate in any of the networks of the group health plan involved.

(d) RULE OF CONSTRUCTION.—Nothing in this section shall be construed to preempt any provision of State law relating to health care provider directories.

SEC. 9818. PROVISION OF COST-SHARING INFORMATION.

A group health plan shall provide a participant or beneficiary in the plan with a good faith estimate of the participant's or beneficiary's cost-sharing (including deductibles, copayments, and coinsurance) for which the participant or beneficiary may be responsible for paying with respect to a specific health care service (including any service that is reasonably expected to be provided in conjunction with such specific service), as soon as practicable and not later than 2 business days after a request for such information by a participant or beneficiary.

Title 5, United States Code

Part III—Employees

Subpart G—Insurance and Annuities

Chapter 89—Health Insurance

§ 8902. Contracting Authority

(a) The Office of Personnel Management may contract with qualified carriers offering plans described by section 8903 or 8903a of this title, without regard to section 6101(b) to (d) of title 41 or other statute requiring competitive bidding. Each contract shall be for a uniform term of at least 1 year, but may be made automatically renewable from term to term in the absence of notice of termination by either party.

(b) To be eligible as a carrier for the plan described by section 8903(2) of this title, a company must be licensed to issue group health insurance in all the States and the District of Columbia.

(c) A contract for a plan described by section 8903(1) or (2) of this title shall require the carrier—

  (1) to reinsure with other companies which elect to participate, under an equitable formula based on the total amount of their group health insurance benefit payments in the United States during the latest year for which the information is available, to be determined by the carrier and approved by the Office; or

  (2) to allocate its rights and obligations under the contract among its affiliates which elect to participate, under an equitable formula to be determined by the carrier and the affiliates and approved by the Office.

(d) Each contract under this chapter shall contain a detailed statement of benefits offered and shall include such maximums, limitations, exclusions, and other definitions of benefits as the Office considers necessary or desirable.

(e) The Office may prescribe reasonable minimum standards for health benefits plans described by section 8903 or 8903a of this title and for carriers offering the plans. Approval of a plan may be withdrawn only after notice and opportunity for hearing to the carrier concerned without regard to subchapter II of chapter 5 and chapter 7 of this title. The Office may terminate the contract of a carrier effective at the end of the contract term, if the Office finds that at no time during the preceding two contract terms did the carrier have 300 or more employees and annuitants, exclusive of family members, enrolled in the plan.

(f) A contract may not be made or a plan approved which excludes an individual because of race, sex, health status, or, at the time of the first opportunity to enroll, because of age.

(g) A contract may not be made or a plan approved which does not offer to each employee, annuitant, family member, former spouse, or person having continued coverage under section 8905a of this title whose enrollment in the plan is ended, except by a cancellation of enrollment, a temporary extension of coverage during which he may exercise the option to convert, without evidence of good health, to a nongroup contract providing health benefits. An employee, annuitant, family member, former spouse, or person having continued coverage under section 8905a of this title who exercises this option shall pay the full periodic charges of the nongroup contract.

(h) The benefits and coverage made available under subsection of this section are noncancelable by the carrier except for fraud, over-insurance, or nonpayment of periodic charges.

(i) Rates charged under health benefits plans described by section 8903 or 8903a of this title shall reasonably and equitably reflect the cost of the benefits provided. Rates under health benefits plans described by section 8903(1) and (2) of this title shall be determined on a basis which, in the judgment of the Office, is consistent with the lowest schedule of basic rates generally charged for new group health benefit plans issued to large employers. The rates determined for the first contract term shall be continued for later contract terms, except that they may be readjusted for any later term, based on past experience and benefit adjustments under the later contract. Any readjustment in rates shall be made in advance of the contract term in which they will apply and on a basis which, in the judgment of the Office, is consistent with the general practice of carriers which issue group health benefit plans to large employers.

(j) Each contract under this chapter shall require the carrier to agree to pay for or provide a health service or supply in an individual case if the Office finds that the employee, annuitant, family member, former spouse, or person having continued coverage under section 8905a of this title is entitled thereto under the terms of the contract.

(k)(1) When a contract under this chapter requires payment or reimbursement for services which may be performed by a clinical psychologist, optometrist, nurse midwife, nursing school administered clinic, or nurse practitioner/clinical specialist, licensed or certified as such under Federal or State law, as applicable, or by a qualified clinical social worker as defined in section 8901(11), an employee, annuitant, family member, former spouse, or person having continued coverage under section 8905a of this title covered by the contract shall be free to select, and shall have direct access to, such a clinical psychologist, qualified clinical social worker, optometrist, nurse midwife, nursing school administered clinic, or nurse practitioner/nurse clinical specialist without supervision or referral by another health practitioner and shall be entitled under the contract to have payment or reimbursement made to him or on his behalf for the services performed.

(2) Nothing in this subsection shall be considered to preclude a health benefits plan from providing direct access or direct payment or reimbursement to a provider in a health care practice or profession other than a practice or profession listed in

paragraph (1), if such provider is licensed or certified as such under Federal or State law.

(3) The provisions of this subsection shall not apply to comprehensive medical plans as described in section 8903(4) of this title.

(l) The Office shall contract under this chapter for a plan described in section 8903(4) of this title with any qualified health maintenance carrier which offers such a plan. For the purpose of this subsection, "qualified health maintenance carrier" means any qualified carrier which is a qualified health maintenance organization within the meaning of section 1310(d)(1) of title XIII of the Public Health Service Act (42 U.S.C. 300c–9(d)).

(m)(1) The terms of any contract under this chapter which relate to the nature, provision, or extent of coverage or benefits (including payments with respect to benefits) shall supersede and preempt any State or local law, or any regulation issued thereunder, which relates to health insurance or plans.

(2)(A) Notwithstanding the provisions of paragraph (1) of this subsection, if a contract under this chapter provides for the provision of, the payment for, or the reimbursement of the cost of health services for the care and treatment of any particular health condition, the carrier shall provide, pay, or reimburse up to the limits of its contract for any such health service properly provided by any person licensed under State law to provide such service if such service is provided to an individual covered by such contract in a State where 25 percent or more of the population is located in primary medical care manpower shortage areas designated pursuant to section 332 of the Public Health Service Act (42 U.S.C. 254e).

(B) The provisions of subparagraph (A) shall not apply to contracts entered into providing prepayment plans described in section 8903(4) of this title.

(n) A contract for a plan described by section 8903(1), (2), or (3), or section 8903a, shall require the carrier—

(1) to implement hospitalization-cost-containment measures, such as measures—

(A) for verifying the medical necessity of any proposed treatment or surgery;

(B) for determining the feasibility or appropriateness of providing services on an outpatient rather than on an inpatient basis;

(C) for determining the appropriate length of stay (through concurrent review or otherwise) in cases involving inpatient care; and

(D) involving case management, if the circumstances so warrant; and

(2) to establish incentives to encourage compliance with measures under paragraph (1).

(o) A contract may not be made or a plan approved which includes coverage for any benefit, item, or service for which funds may not be used under the Assisted Suicide Funding Restriction Act of 1997.

(p) Each contract under this chapter shall require the carrier to comply with requirements described in the provisions of section 2719A of the Public Health Service Act and sections 2730 and 2731 of such Act, sections 716, 717, and 718 of the Employee Retirement Income Security Act of 1974, sections 9816, 9817, and 9818 of the Internal Revenue Code of 1986 (as applicable), and section 2(d) of the Ban Surprise Billing Act in the same manner as such provisions apply to a group health plan or health insurance issuer offering health insurance coverage, as described in such sections.

The provisions of sections 2799A–1, 2799A–2, 2799A–3, and 2799A–4 of the Public Health Service Act shall apply to a health care provider and facility and an air ambulance provider described in such respective sections with respect to a participant, beneficiary, or enrollee in a health benefits plan under this chapter in the same manner as such provisions apply to such a provider and facility with respect to an enrollee in a group health plan or health insurance coverage offered by a health insurance issuer in the group or individual market, as described in such sections.

Patient Protection and Affordable Care Act

Title I—Quality, Affordable Health Care for All Americans

Subtitle C—Quality Health Insurance Coverage for All Americans

Part 2—Other Provisions

SEC. 1251. PRESERVATION OF RIGHT TO MAINTAIN EXISTING COVERAGE.

(a) NO CHANGES TO EXISTING COVERAGE.—
- (1) IN GENERAL.—Nothing in this Act (or an amendment made by this Act) shall be construed to require that an individual terminate coverage under a group health plan or health insurance coverage in which such individual was enrolled on the date of enactment of this Act.
- (2) CONTINUATION OF COVERAGE.—Except as provided in paragraph (3), with respect to a group health plan or health insurance coverage in which an individual was enrolled on the date of enactment of this Act, this subtitle and subtitle A (and the amendments made by such subtitles) shall not apply to such plan or coverage, regardless of whether the individual renews such coverage after such date of enactment.
- (3) APPLICATION OF CERTAIN PROVISIONS.—The provisions of sections 2715 and 2718 of the Public Health Service Act (as added by subtitle A) shall apply to grandfathered health plans for plan years beginning on or after the date of enactment of this Act.
- (4) APPLICATION OF CERTAIN PROVISIONS.—
  - (A) IN GENERAL.—The following provisions of the Public Health Service Act (as added by this title) shall apply to grandfathered health plans for plan years beginning with the first plan year to which such provisions would otherwise apply:
    - (i) Section 2708 (relating to excessive waiting periods).
    - (ii) Those provisions of section 2711 relating to lifetime limits.
    - (iii) Section 2712 (relating to rescissions).
    - (iv) Section 2714 (relating to extension of dependent coverage).
  - (B) PROVISIONS APPLICABLE ONLY TO GROUP HEALTH PLANS.—

(i) PROVISIONS DESCRIBED.—Those provisions of section 2711 relating to annual limits and the provisions of section 2704 (relating to pre-existing condition exclusions) of the Public Health Service Act (as added by this subtitle) shall apply to grandfathered health plans that are group health plans for plan years beginning with the first plan year to which such provisions otherwise apply.

(ii) ADULT CHILD COVERAGE.—For plan years beginning before January 1, 2014, the provisions of section 2714 of the Public Health Service Act (as added by this subtitle) shall apply in the case of an adult child with respect to a grandfathered health plan that is a group health plan only if such adult child is not eligible to enroll in an eligible employer-sponsored health plan (as defined in section 5000A(f)(2) of the Internal Revenue Code of 1986) other than such grandfathered health plan.

(5) *APPLICATION OF ADDITIONAL PROVISIONS.—Subsections (b), (e), (f), (g), and (h) of section 2719A of the Public Health Service Act shall apply to grandfathered health plans for plan years beginning on or after January 1, 2022.*

(b) ALLOWANCE FOR FAMILY MEMBERS TO JOIN CURRENT COVERAGE.—With respect to a group health plan or health insurance coverage in which an individual was enrolled on the date of enactment of this Act and which is renewed after such date, family members of such individual shall be permitted to enroll in such plan or coverage if such enrollment is permitted under the terms of the plan in effect as of such date of enactment.

(c) ALLOWANCE FOR NEW EMPLOYEES TO JOIN CURRENT PLAN.— A group health plan that provides coverage on the date of enactment of this Act may provide for the enrolling of new employees (and their families) in such plan, and this subtitle and subtitle A (and the amendments made by such subtitles) shall not apply with respect to such plan and such new employees (and their families).

(d) EFFECT ON COLLECTIVE BARGAINING AGREEMENTS.—In the case of health insurance coverage maintained pursuant to one or more collective bargaining agreements between employee representatives and one or more employers that was ratified before the date of enactment of this Act, the provisions of this subtitle and subtitle A (and the amendments made by such subtitles) shall not apply until the date on which the last of the collective bargaining agreements relating to the coverage terminates. Any coverage amendment made pursuant to a collective bargaining agreement relating to the coverage which amends the coverage solely to conform to any requirement added by this subtitle or subtitle A (or amendments) shall not be treated as a termination of such collective bargaining agreement.

(e) DEFINITION.—In this title, the term “grandfathered health plan” means any group health plan or health insurance coverage to which this section applies.

Index

D

E

F

Index

D

E

F

M

N

O

P

R